The SAGES Manual of Surgical Referral for Primary and Emergency Care

Geoffrey P. Kohn • Bethany J. Slater
Diane Alligood • Danielle S. Walsh
Editors

The SAGES Manual of Surgical Referral for Primary and Emergency Care

Springer

Editors
Geoffrey P. Kohn
Department of Surgery
Monash University
Melbourne, VIC, Australia

Bethany J. Slater
Surgery
University of Chicago
Chicago, IL, USA

Diane Alligood
Alligood Medical Acupuncture, PLLC
Greenville, NC, USA

Danielle S. Walsh
Surgery
University of Kentucky
Lexington, KY, USA

ISBN 978-3-031-92677-8 ISBN 978-3-031-92678-5 (eBook)
https://doi.org/10.1007/978-3-031-92678-5

This Springer imprint is published by the registered company Springer Nature Switzerland AG
The registered company address is: Gewerbestrasse 11, 6330 Cham, Switzerland

Foreword

In an era where efficient and accurate decision-making is paramount, determining when a patient requires surgical consultation can profoundly impact patient outcomes. This comprehensive guide serves as a unique and important companion for primary care physicians, emergency room clinicians, advanced practitioners, and all healthcare providers tasked with making crucial referral decisions. While there are plenty of resources that outline management of the topics covered in this volume, none are written from the surgeon's perspective. Here is an opportunity to have a trusted surgical colleague by your side, explaining not only how to identify the need for surgical evaluation but also providing guidance on selecting appropriate diagnostic tests and studies, ensuring that referrals can be both timely and justified.

These authors are your trusted colleagues, recognized globally for their expertise and commitment to surgical guidelines and education. They have compiled evidence-based criteria that delineate between emergent situations requiring immediate surgical intervention and elective cases that can be managed conservatively or scheduled appropriately. Most importantly, this text helps the non-surgeon to think like a surgeon, bridging the gap between primary care, emergency care, and surgical specialties, enhancing interdisciplinary collaboration and streamlining patient care.

As a practicing primary care physician and an educator deeply invested in training medical students and residents, I recognize the value a "when to refer" guide can offer. This is the book we have been missing. It empowers healthcare professionals at every level to make informed, confident decisions regarding the consultation of surgical colleagues, ultimately leading to improved patient care, optimized resource utilization, and stronger professional collaboration. Don't just add this book to your library—read it, share it, teach it, and use it.

Jonathon M. Firnhaber
Max R. & Catherine S. Joyner
Distinguished Professor in Primary
Care Medicine, Professor and Vice Chair
for Academic Affairs, Family Medicine
Residency Program Director
Brody School of Medicine
East Carolina University
Greenville, NC, USA

Preface

Primary care and emergency room clinicians manage a complex array of disorders and are commonly the first to encounter a surgical or potentially surgical disorder. The purpose of this text is to assist non-surgeons in determining when a patient should, or need not, be referred for surgical assessment of disorders in the thoracoabdominal domain. Additionally, it provides guidance on diagnostic evaluation through provision of relevant history and clinical examination findings, recommended laboratory and radiographic assessment, and timing of referral, if indicated.

We provided chapters divided into four parts. In the first part, we have endeavored to provide chapters with guidance for the management of symptoms described by a patient to their treating clinician where the true diagnosis has yet to be established. The second part advises on treatment options for findings elicited on examination of the patient. Part three directs the assessment of findings notified to the treating clinician in the report of an investigation such as radiology or endoscopy. The fourth and final part details management sometimes required of non-surgeons in the postoperative care of the placement of certain surgical devices. All parts are arranged in an approximation of anatomical location from superior to inferior.

Readers are provided high-impact tables and summative flowcharts for rapid decision-making and text chapters for more in-depth consideration.

This text grew out of the Society of American Gastrointestinal and Endoscopic Surgeons (SAGES) Guidelines Committee, which is dedicated to the development of evidence-based guidelines for safe and effective surgical care. While our society has a growing body of resources to guide the surgeon, we recognized the need to supplement these with guidance for the many clinicians who encounter the patient before the surgeon has been invited to assess and provide care. In editing these chapters, we took care to consider adult and pediatric patients, rural and urban settings, and countries beyond the "America" in our organization's title.

This editorial team greatly appreciates the support we have received from SAGES and Springer in completing this project. We would especially like to thank the SAGES Guidelines Committee and all the authors who provided their time, effort, patience, and expertise to build the content and information within this book. An appendix to the text is included wherein details are provided of the significant and important output of this Committee to direct readers to further information.

It is our goal to help trainees, primary care physicians, pediatricians, surgeons, and others to obtain practical knowledge for improving the care of pediatric and adult surgical patients.

From Dr. Geoffrey P. Kohn

I have been fortunate to have been involved for many years with the Guidelines Committee of SAGES. Our committee has aimed to position ourselves at the forefront of societies producing clinical practice guidelines. We have adapted as the field itself as evolved, moving from the production of expert opinion reviews to our current processes of producing high-quality systematic reviews and development of evidence-based guidelines. While we hope that our guidelines are readily available and implemented by our target group of member surgeons, we have noted that much of the collated knowledge was not being disseminated effectively among our referrer base. It was in acknowledging this that our idea for this Manual was formed. Working closely with my coeditor surgeons, Dr. Slater and Dr. Walsh, we developed a plan for this Manual with the enthusiastic support of the Guidelines Committee and the wider SAGES community. Dr. Alligood soon joined our team from a Family Medicine background, and her advice was invaluable for tailoring this publication to be appropriate to, and accepted by, our target readership of primary care physicians, pediatricians and emergency physicians. This group of co-editors has my deep appreciation for the hard work and significant time commitment which they have contributed to make what we hope is a valuable addition to the literature. We hope that our patients will benefit by experiencing best-practice evidence-based care, provided in a streamlined manner no matter their geographical location, with great efficiency and optimal outcomes.

I also am deeply appreciative and humbled by the support of my wife Michelle and our beautiful children Justin and Amelie. They tolerated all the time I was unavailable to them while I sat in my office by my computer and committed to this endeavor. They accepted this because they understood this project always held the aim to help others, a value that I am proud to say is always at the front of their minds. Thank you.

From Dr. Bethany J. Slater

I really enjoyed being an editor on this book. It was very fun and educational to work on all aspects of the process, to be able to review all of the chapters, and especially to focus on the aspects of when and what to refer to the surgeon.

From Dr. Diane Alligood

As a family practice physician, I was drawn to this project as a way to address the progressive challenges to communication and collegiality I had observed over my three plus decades in practice. The days of being able to pick up the phone and speak to a specialist about a clinic patient have been overtaken by phone trees with voicemail boxes that may not reach the clinician for days. Meanwhile, the science of medicine has continued to rapidly evolve, insurance companies requiring increasing pre-authorization for testing, and electronic record "inboxes" are filled with hundreds of messages from patients, pharmacies, and clinical colleagues of all types. It's no wonder that clinicians struggle at times to keep up with the "right" work up and timing for referral to a surgeon for a variety of disorders. It is my sincere hope that you find this book to be a valuable tool toward overcoming these challenges in your clinical work.

The diagnosis-based organization of this book with the flow diagrams and summary charts allows rapid access to the critical information to streamline your patient's assessment and treatment. But beyond facilitating timely evaluations and referrals, several other benefits became apparent.

The diagrams and charts are fleshed out with more in-depth material including details of the other conditions in the differential and of the surgical approach to the diagnosis—a quick educational refresher and a reference to help field your patient's questions. Serendipitously, reacquainting yourself with medical knowledge in the evaluation of one case often serves to bring into focus your approach to subsequent cases.

Also, in today's practice environment, multiple providers working as a team may interact with the patient over time. The guidelines on future follow-up and surveillance testing can be incorporated into the patient's medical record at the time of initial contact—serving as a reminder to the primary provider, as well as allowing other collaborating caregivers to help ensure the plan is followed through to completion. While many texts offer a comprehensive review of a particular diagnosis, few bridge the gap between primary care and the specialist. It is my hope that this resource can do so for you.

On a personal note, I'd like to thank the bright minds of the early 1990s Internal Medicine department at David Grant USAF Medical Center. In an era that predated the on-line "peripheral brain," you inspired me with your encyclopedic knowledge and never-ending quest to understand and serve our patients.

From Dr. Danielle S. Walsh

Lao Tsu once said that if you give a hungry man a fish, you feed him for a day. But if you teach him how to fish, you feed him for a lifetime. It is my hope that the efforts of this book will "feed" the many physicians and other clinicians who earnestly want to provide outstanding care of their patients using dependable clinical algorithms in a cost conscious manner. A special thank you to my husband, Stephen, and children, Kamryn and Christian, who put up with my hours on the couch at night in support of this handbook. Thanks for forgiving me for taking on another book after my promise to not do so again in the past. Know that your understanding is supporting the health of others.

Melbourne, VIC, Australia — Geoffrey P. Kohn
Chicago, IL, USA — Bethany J. Slater
Greenville, NC, USA — Diane Alligood
Lexington, KY, USA — Danielle S. Walsh

Disclaimer for Society of American Gastrointestinal and Endoscopic Surgeons (SAGES) Manual

The contents of this manual are intended exclusively for educational and informational purposes only, and nothing contained within constitutes medical advice. Neither this manual nor its contents have been subject to formal peer-review. The information provided herein does not represent, nor should it be interpreted as, the official position, view, or endorsement of the Society of American Gastrointestinal and Endoscopic Surgeons (SAGES) or its governing body. This manual is not intended for use in diagnosing or treating any health problem, condition, or disease. Individuals seeking personal medical advice should consult an appropriate licensed professional.

Neither SAGES, nor its officers, directors, employees, members, nor any of the contributors to this manual, make any representation or warranty, express or implied, regarding the accuracy, completeness, fitness for any intended purpose, or suitability of the information contained herein for any specific use or function. Neither access to, nor use of, this manual creates or implies any physician-patient relationship, and reliance on any information provided, contained, or implied herein is solely at the user's own risk.

Contents

Contributors

Qais AbuHasan Department of Surgery, Indiana University School of Medicine, Indianapolis, IN, USA

John Agzarian McMaster University, Hamilton, ON, Canada

Vamsi V. Alli Penn State Milton S. Hershey Medical Center, Hershey, PA, USA

Mazen R. Al-Mansour University of Florida, Gainesville, FL, USA

Ziad T. Awad Department of Surgery, University of Florida College of Medicine-Jacksonville, Jacksonville, FL, USA

Joy Ayemoba University of Chicago, Comer Children's Hospital, Chicago, IL, USA

Emily J. Baker Eastern Health, Melbourne, VIC, Australia

Nicholas Bartschat Department of Surgery, University of Iowa, Iowa City, IA, USA

Joe Bean Department of Surgery, University of Pittsburgh, Pittsburgh, PA, USA

Colin Bohannan University of Kentucky, Lexington, KY, USA

Lindsay T. Bryant University of Kentucky, Lexington, KY, USA

Elisa C. Calabrese Department of Surgery, University of California San Francisco-East Bay, Oakland, CA, USA

Department of Surgery, University of Adelaide, The Queen Elizabeth Hospital, Adelaide, SA, Australia

Kylie M. Callier University of Chicago, Comer Children's Hospital, Chicago, IL, USA

Robert A. Catania Southern New Hampshire Medical Center, Nashua, NH, USA

Lawrence Cetrulo University of Washington – Northwest Hospital, Seattle, WA, USA

Daniel Chase Carle Illinois College of Medicine, Urbana, IL, USA

Carle Hoopeston Regional Medical Center, Hoopeston, IL, USA

Marina Robson Chase Division of General, Endocrine, and Metabolic Surgery, Department of Surgery, University of Kentucky, Lexington, KY, USA

Hamza Nasir Chatha University Hospitals, Cleveland, OH, USA

Clark H. Cunningham Department of Surgery, Division of Gastrointestinal Surgery, The University of North Carolina at Chapel Hill, Chapel Hill, NC, USA

Nicholas Dalkie Department of Surgery, University of Melbourne, Austin Health, Heidelberg, VIC, Australia

Shaun Daly Department of Surgery, University of California Irvine Medical Center, Orange, CA, USA

Brynley Dean Inova Fairfax Medical Campus, Falls Church, VA, USA

Sergio Mazzola Poli de Figueiredo University of North Carolina, Chapel Hill, NC, USA

Lindel Dewberry University of Kentucky, Lexington, KY, USA

Mackenzie Donoho University of Kentucky, Lexington, KY, USA

Jonathan Dort Inova Fairfax Medical Campus, Falls Church, VA, USA

Colston A. Edgerton New Hanover Regional Medical Center/ Novant Health, Wilmington, NC, USA

Aldo Fafaj The University of Tennessee Health Sciences Center, Knoxville, TN, USA

Timothy M. Farrell Department of Surgery, Division of Gastrointestinal Surgery, The University of North Carolina at Chapel Hill, Chapel Hill, NC, USA

Jenny M. Guido Department of Surgery, University of South Dakota Sanford School of Medicine, Sioux Falls, SD, USA

Stephen P. Haggerty Department of Surgery, Division of Gastrointestinal and General Surgery, Endeavor Health, Evanston, IL, USA

Abdelazeem Hamed Department of Surgery, University of Florida College of Medicine-Jacksonville, Jacksonville, FL, USA

Nader Hanna McMaster University, Hamilton, ON, Canada

Ivy N. Haskins Department of Surgery, University of Nebraska Medical Center, Omaha, NE, USA

Imran Hassan Department of Surgery, University of Iowa, Iowa City, IA, USA

Chrys Hensman Monash University, University of Adelaide, Swinburne University, LapSurgery Australia, Dandenong North, VIC, Australia

Madeleine S. Higgins Department of Surgery, Division of Gastrointestinal Surgery, The University of North Carolina at Chapel Hill, Chapel Hill, NC, USA

Celeste Hollands Texas Tech University Health Sciences Center, Amarillo, USA

William W. Hope New Hanover Regional Medical Center/ Novant Health, Wilmington, NC, USA

Charlotte Horne Mayo Clinic, Rochester, MN, USA

Travis Hughes University of Kentucky, Lexington, KY, USA

Bright Huo McMaster University, Hamilton, ON, Canada

Alexandra Ibewuike, MD Department of Surgery, University of Kentucky, Lexington, KY, USA

Romeo C. Ignacio Jr Department of Surgery, University of California San Diego School of Medicine, La Jolla, CA, USA

William B. Inabnet III Division of General, Endocrine, and Metabolic Surgery, Department of Surgery, University of Kentucky, Lexington, KY, USA

Aayma Irfan University of California Riverside School of Medicine, Riverside, CA, USA

D. Rohan Jeyarajah Methodist Richardson Medical Center, Richardson, TX, USA

TCU Burnett School of Medicine, Fort Worth, TX, USA

Noah Jordan University of Kentucky, Lexington, KY, USA

Andreas M. Kaiser City of Hope National Medical Center, Duarte, CA, USA

Anna Katz Advocate Medical Group, Park Ridge, IL, USA

Julie E. Kim Department of Surgery, University of Nebraska Medical Center, Omaha, NE, USA

Geoffrey P. Kohn Monash University, Melbourne, VIC, Australia

Melbourne Upper GI Surgical Group, Melbourne, VIC, Australia

Monash University, Eastern Health Clinical School, Melbourne, VIC, Australia

Justin D. Leavitt New Hanover Regional Medical Center/ Novant Health, Wilmington, NC, USA

Joseph Lee Department of Surgery, Naval Medical Center San Diego, San Diego, CA, USA

Yung Lee Department of Surgery, Division of General Surgery, McMaster University, Hamilton, ON, Canada

Brittany E. Levy University of Kentucky, Lexington, KY, USA

Paige E. Likes John Peter Smith Hospital, Fort Worth, TX, USA

Joshua L. Lyons University Hospitals, Cleveland, OH, USA

Juan S. Malo Methodist Richardson Medical Center, Richardson, TX, USA

Katie Marrero Carle Health, Urbana, IL, USA

Carle Illinois College of Medicine, Urbana, IL, USA

Pennsylvania State University Milton S. Hershey Medical Center, Hershey, PA, USA

Kareem Marwan Colorectal & Robotic Surgeon, Melbourne, VIC, Australia

Michelle McCarthy Lahey Hospital and Medical Center, Department of General Surgery, Burlington, MA, USA

Sophia K. McKinley Department of Surgery, Harvard Medical School, Massachusetts General Hospital, Boston, MA, USA

Emily Miraflor UCSF East Bay, San Francisco, CA, USA

Aditi Mishra Department of Surgery, University of Iowa, Iowa City, IA, USA

Nisha Narula Department of Surgery, Rutgers New Jersey Medical School, Newark, NJ, USA

Pramod Nepal Beth Israel Deaconess Medical Center, Harvard Medical School, Boston, MA, USA

Paul J. Nguyen-Lee Department of Surgery, University of Nebraska Medical Center, Omaha, NE, USA

Mehrdad Nikfarjam Department of Surgery, University of Melbourne, Austin Health, Heidelberg, VIC, Australia

Vahagn C. Nikolian Oregon Health & Science University, Portland, OR, USA

Uretz Oliphant Carle Health, Urbana, IL, USA

University of Illinois College of Medicine at Chicago, Chicago, IL, USA

George Orthopoulos Winchester Hospital, Tufts University School of Medicine, Winchester, MA, USA

Rodolfo J. Oviedo Department of Surgery, Nacogdoches Medical Center, Nacogdoches, TX, USA

University of Houston Tilman J. Fertitta Family College of Medicine, Houston, TX, USA

Sam Houston State University College of Osteopathic Medicine, Conroe, TX, USA

Francesco Palazzo Thomas Jefferson University Hospital, Philadelphia, PA, USA

Jalpa Patel Department of Surgery, Rutgers New Jersey Medical School, Newark, NJ, USA

Neil Patel Creighton University Medical Center, Omaha, NE, USA

Sydney Pekarek Advocate Medical Group, Park Ridge, IL, USA

Amanda C. Purdy Department of Surgery, University of California Irvine Medical Center, Orange, CA, USA

Nicholas A. Rawson Carle Health, Urbana, IL, USA

Eric J. Rellinger University of Kentucky, Lexington, KY, USA

William S. Richardson Oschner Medical Center, New Orleans, LA, USA

Yashasvini Sampathkumar Department of Surgery, Rutgers New Jersey Medical School, Newark, NJ, USA

Sophia M. V. Schermerhorn Department of Surgery, Naval Medical Center San Diego, San Diego, CA, USA

Stefan Scholz Department of Surgery, University of Pittsburgh, Piitsburgh, PA, USA

Division of General and Thoracic Pediatric Surgery, UPMC Children's Hospital of Pittsburgh, Piitsburgh, PA, USA

Saamia Shaikh St. Joseph's University Medical Center, Paterson, NJ, USA

Bethany J. Slater University of Chicago, Chicago, IL, USA

Dean C. Spilias Monash Medical Centre, Clayton, VIC, Australia

Melbourne Upper GI Surgical Group, Melbourne, VIC, Australia

Dimitrios Stefanidis Department of Surgery, Indiana University School of Medicine, Indianapolis, IN, USA

Andrew T. Strong Digestive Disease Institute, Cleveland Clinic, Cleveland, OH, USA

Cleveland Clinic Lerner College of Medicine of Case Western Reserve University, Cleveland, OH, USA

Tanvi Subramanian Department of Surgery, University of Chicago, Chicago, IL, USA

Léa Tessier Department of Surgery, Division of General Surgery, McMaster University, Hamilton, ON, Canada

Oscar Paredes Torres Department of Abdominal Surgery, National Institute of Neoplastic Diseases, Lima, Peru

Crystal Totten Department of Surgery, University of Kentucky, Lexington, KY, USA

Sage A. Vincent Thomas Jefferson University Hospital, Philadelphia, PA, USA

R. Wesley Vosburg HCA Grand Strand Medical Center, Myrtle Beach, SC, USA

Danielle S. Walsh Department of Surgery, University of Kentucky, Lexington, KY, USA

Martin Walsh Department of Surgery, Advocate Lutheran General Hospital, Park Ridge, IL, USA

Brittany Wheelock University of Kentucky, Lexington, KY, USA

Andrew Whipkey Department of Surgery, University of Kentucky, Lexington, KY, USA

Markey Cancer Center, University of Kentucky, Lexington, KY, USA

Elizabeth D. Winter Oschner Medical Center, New Orleans, LA, USA

Part I

Symptoms

Dysphagia

1

Geoffrey P. Kohn

Dysphagia describes a difficulty in swallowing or a subjective sensation of food getting stuck. It can arise from oropharyngeal or esophageal causes, with the level of delineation being the upper esophageal sphincter. Dysphagia can arise from multiple pathologies, including inflammatory, mechanical, functional, and esophageal motility problems.

Mainstays of investigation include a detailed history and examination, endoscopy, contrast esophagram, and esophageal manometry. This chapter will describe some of the underlying conditions and their diagnostic features, but does not aim to be an exhaustive textbook chapter on the topic. Rather, guidance is provided to the primary care physician and the Emergency Room physician regarding relevant initial workup, urgency of investigation and criteria for referral. With the overlap of responsibilities between foregut surgeons and gastroenterologists in the field of esophagology, referral to either is appropriate for the conditions detailed below, dependent on local expertise and practice pattern.

G. P. Kohn (✉)
Monash University, Melbourne, VIC, Australia

Melbourne Upper GI Surgical Group, Melbourne, VIC, Australia

Monash University, Eastern Health Clinical School, Melbourne, VIC, Australia
e-mail: gkohn@uppergi.net

G. P. Kohn et al. (eds.), *The SAGES Manual of Surgical Referral for Primary and Emergency Care*,
https://doi.org/10.1007/978-3-031-92678-5_1

1.1 Location of Dysphagia

A thorough history and examination should be able to define the location of the dysphagia. Symptoms commencing immediately upon consuming food or liquid may indicate an oropharyngeal cause. Immediate symptoms of cough, regurgitation, dysphonia, or a perception of incoordination of swallowing will have occurred before the bolus has entered the esophagus and therefore must arise from above the upper esophageal sphincter. Neurological examination, particularly of the cranial nerves, can be very helpful, as is simply watching the patient consume food or liquid and noting what occurs, and the timeframe thereof. If oropharyngeal dysphagia is suspected based on history, involvement of a speech pathologist and investigation by video fluoroscopy will assist. Frequently such problems are seen in the elderly and in patients having suffered strokes, though many neurological conditions can be the origin.

It is noteworthy that the subjective location of the food getting stuck in the throat is not a useful indicator as to the true location of the pathology. Subjective holdup at the level of the sternal notch or in the retrosternal area is more likely to suggest an esophageal problem than an oropharyngeal cause, though again the actual location of the problem is not reliably indicated. Occasionally, local neck issues such as a very large thyroid goiter may cause the sensation of dysphagia at the level of the sternal notch.

The single most important investigation of esophageal causes of dysphagia is upper gastrointestinal endoscopy with biopsy. This will confirm any mechanical obstruction, particularly the presence of malignancy, but may also diagnose inflammation, stricture, hiatal hernia, or suggest the presence of a motility disorder.

1.2 Acuity of Presentation

Once a physician determines that it is probable that the symptom of dysphagia is related to the esophagus, information regarding the acuity of onset is very helpful (Table 1.1).

Table 1.1 When to refer to a surgeon for the symptoms of dysphagia

Emergent, refer to the emergency room	Acute-onset dysphagia, especially with pain Inability to tolerate oral secretions Dysphagia with a history of ingesting a sharp foreign object or button battery
Urgent	Onset over weeks or months, particularly with solid dysphagia worse than liquid dysphagia Greater than 10% unintentional weight loss
Non-urgent	Onset over weeks or months, particularly if solid dysphagia has always been equal to liquid dysphagia

Sudden-onset dysphagia is likely from food bolus obstruction. Often presenting with complete obstruction and inability to tolerate secretions, saliva, or oral fluids, this is very distressing to the patient and often painful. Food bolus obstruction is often the first presentation of an underlying and more chronic problem, such as a cancer or a motility disorder.

Rapid progression over weeks to months, with greater difficulty of tolerating solids rather than liquids, suggests a mechanical problem such as an esophageal malignancy. Occasionally acute volvulus of a hiatal hernia may present similarly.

In cases of gradual onset, with difficulty to both solids and liquids, consideration should be given to motility disorders. However, advanced mechanical problems can also result in this presentation. Certain medications, particularly opiates, can have negative effects of esophageal motility, causing dysphagia.

1.3 Investigation of Dysphagia

Again, the most important investigation is upper GI endoscopy (Table 1.2). Only once this has been performed, and should the symptoms and patient's comorbidities warrant, then further investigation is required. An exception to this rule may be a history of foreign body ingestion, particularly relevant to the pediatric population; where radio-opaque foreign body ingestion is suspected,

Table 1.2 Investigations to order so as to be available for surgeon's review

Upper GI endoscopy. Please attach the histology results of any biopsies
Contrast esophagram may be helpful, though obtaining this study should not delay the referral
Chest radiograph is useful if foreign body ingestion is suspected but should not delay the referral

initial plain chest radiograph and possible contrast esophagram may aid in planning for subsequent endoscopy.

Esophageal manometry: Esophageal manometry is the gold-standard evaluation of esophageal motor function by measuring pressure changes within the esophagus with swallowing. Manometry has supplanted contrast esophagram as the investigation of choice for these conditions. Specific manometric criteria have been defined for various esophageal motility disorders and follow a classification system based on evaluation of the lower esophageal sphincter pressure, amplitude of esophageal body contractions, duration between the initiation of the swallow and esophageal contraction, and bolus emptying of the esophagus. A number of disorders are diagnosed by manometry and most cannot be reliably diagnosed without.

Contrast esophagram: This is a fluoroscopic study performed after ingestion by the patient of a contrast medium, usually barium. Caution must be employed when using alternative media that may cause pneumonitis if aspirated into the airways. Esophagram is a dynamic evaluation of the anatomy and function of the esophagus. It is useful to evaluate the anatomy of the esophagus, highlighting pouches, laryngeal penetration or aspiration, diverticula, and bolus transit. Mucosal pathology may be identified, but with lesser sensitivity and specificity than endoscopy. Motility disorders may be identified but with lesser sensitivity and specificity than manometry. Contrast esophagram supplements manometry by evaluating different aspects of the esophagus.

1.4 Functional Luminal Impedance Planimetry (FLIP)

This is a newer technology evaluating the distensibility of the esophagus, particularly the lower esophageal sphincter. It is useful in diagnosing many of the same motility conditions as esophageal manometry by use of different metrics. It may be seen as complementary to manometry. It is less accessible than manometry but is becoming more widely available.

1.5 Specific Conditions Resulting in Dysphagia

1. Esophageal tumors: The incidence of esophageal cancer is increasing in the Western world, while the cell type of origin is rapidly changing from proximal esophageal squamous cell cancer to distal esophageal adenocarcinoma. The major risk factor for the now much more common adenocarcinoma is gastroesophageal reflux disease, often secondary to obesity. The frequent presenting complaint of esophageal cancer is dysphagia. Diagnosis is by endoscopy with biopsy. Depending on the cell type and the location of the cancer, different management strategies can be employed. Staging usually requires CT scan, PET scan, often endoscopic ultrasound, and sometimes staging laparoscopy. Treatment often involves neoadjuvant therapy (either chemotherapy alone or combined chemoradiation). Resection is often recommended for appropriate patients, particularly for adenocarcinoma, with definitive chemoradiation more frequently being used for proximal squamous cell cancers.

   Benign tumors of the esophagus do exist, including stromal tumors and leiomyomas, and some of these can cause dysphagia from mechanical obstruction and effects on motility. Esophageal duplication cysts may similarly cause obstructive symptoms.

2. Hiatal Hernia: Another mechanical cause for dysphagia is a large hiatal hernia. Simple sliding hiatal hernias, in which the gastroesophageal junction alone has migrated into the chest, are unlikely to cause distortion to prevent the passage of a food bolus. Larger hiatal hernias may do so with volvulus of the stomach, a possibility in larger paraoesophageal hernias. Acute strangulation of the intrathoracic stomach is a surgical emergency, manifest by pain, obstruction, and regurgitation.

   Matters are more complex with dysphagia arising in a patient who has previously undergone foregut surgery, such as previous antireflux surgery, bariatric surgery, hiatal hernia repair, gastroesophageal resection, and others. In these specific cases, where possible the original operating surgeon should be contacted for advice, with the urgency of referral based on the severity and acuity of the symptoms.
3. Inflammatory Conditions

   Eosinophilic esophagitis is a cause of dysphagia, caused by the immune-mediated infiltration of the esophageal wall with eosinophils, with subsequent fibrosis. While there are pathognomic features seen at endoscopy, these are sometimes subtle and overlooked. This author suggests therefore that esophageal biopsies should be performed at every upper endoscopy to avoid missing this diagnosis. Exact recommendations vary by jurisdiction, but it is reasonable to take multiple biopsies from both the mid- and distal esophagus. It is important to note that inflammation secondary to gastroesophageal reflux disease must be treated before a conclusive diagnosis of eosinophilic esophagitis can be made.
4. Strictures

   These may be caused by malignancy, gastroesophageal reflux, or caustic ingestion. These can be diagnosed by endoscopy and biopsy. Treatment is often by dilatation, though results are not always satisfactory.
5. Diverticula

   These include Zenker's pharyngeal diverticulum, mid-esophageal diverticulum (often caused by traction from extrinsic pathology such as mediastinal inflammation), and epiphrenic diverticulum. Depending on the size and orientation of such diverticula, compression of the adjacent esophagus may occur. Though theoretically visible at endoscopy, they are frequently overlooked, particularly if the neck of the diverticulum is very small. Contrast esophagram is usually diagnostic.

6. Motility Disorders

These are most commonly classified by the Chicago Classification of Esophageal Motility Disorders. This hierarchical system defines the type of motility defect, and is reproducible and clinically useful. It is required reading for those with an interest in dysphagia management and esophagology in general.[1]

The classical motility disorder causing dysphagia is achalasia. Manometry will reveal a high-pressure, nonrelaxing lower esophageal sphincter and an absence of effective esophageal peristalsis. It can frequently be relieved by targetting the lower esophageal sphincter either by division or by injected pharmacologic means. Other causes of dysphagia include hypercontractile esophagus and gastroesophageal junction outflow obstruction.

It is important to note that gastroesophageal reflux disease can cause secondary esophageal dysmotility that can resolve after acid suppression or antireflux surgery. There is frequently supportive endoscopic evidence for reflux, and the esophageal specialist will often institute investigation for reflux as part of dysphagia assessment.

---

[1]Yadlapati, Rena et al. "Esophageal motility disorders on high-resolution manometry: Chicago classification version 4.0©." *Neurogastroenterology and motility* vol. 33(1) (2021): e14058. https://doi.org/10.1111/nmo.14058

Impactions of the Esophagus and Upper Gastrointestinal Tract

2

Bright Huo, Nader Hanna,
and John Agzarian

2.1 Background

Most impactions (80%) pass without the need for treatment, but <20% of patients require endoscopic intervention and 1% will need surgery [1].

In adults, most esophageal impactions are due to food and can occur if patients have a preexisting condition, including an esophageal stricture, gastroesophageal reflux disease, hiatal hernia, eosinophilic esophagitis, or Schatzki's ring, or underlying motility disorder. Fish bones and other bony fragments are the most commonly ingested foreign bodies in adults and carry an elevated risk of perforation.

The esophagus demonstrates physiologic narrowing at the upper esophageal sphincter (cricopharyngeus muscle), the level of the aortic arch, and the diaphragmatic hiatus.

Most food impactions occur at the level of the cricopharyngeus muscle. Structural or functional abnormalities increase the risk of

---

The original version of the chapter has been revised. A correction to this chapter can be found at https://doi.org/10.1007/978-3-031-92678-5_52

B. Huo (✉) · N. Hanna · J. Agzarian
McMaster University, Hamilton, ON, Canada
e-mail: brighthuo@dal.ca

G. P. Kohn et al. (eds.), *The SAGES Manual of Surgical Referral for Primary and Emergency Care*,
https://doi.org/10.1007/978-3-031-92678-5_2

Table 2.1 Location of esophageal foreign body impactions by conditions

Location	Frequency	Predisposition
Proximal one-third	Rare	Central nervous system lesions
		Zenker's diverticulum
		Cervical web
Middle one-third	Frequent	Cancer (primary or extrinsic)
		Eosinophilic esophagitis
		Radiation stricture
		Traction esophageal diverticula
		Spastic dysmotility
Distal one-third	Common	Peptic stricture
		Eosinophilic esophagitis
		Esophageal mucosal ring
		Cancer
		Achalasia
		Pulsion esophageal diverticula
		Spastic dysmotility

Adapted from *UpToDate*

impactions, including tumors, strictures, diverticula, postsurgical anatomy, and achalasia (Table 2.1).

A focused history should include the type of foreign body, the timing of ingestion with respect to presentation, and the nature, persistence, and severity of their symptoms. Symptoms may include choking, low appetite, retrosternal fullness, regurgitation, wheezing, blood-stained saliva, and odynophagia. Respiratory symptoms may develop such as choking, stridor, or dyspnea due to aspiration of saliva or tracheal compression.

Assess for the risk of esophageal perforation by remaining attentive to signs, including fever, tachycardia, peritonitis, subcutaneous emphysema, and/or swelling around the neck and chest. The physical examination must include an inspection of the neck, chest, abdomen, oropharynx, and hypopharynx. Though patients may point to an area of discomfort, this does not correlate well anatomically to the location of the impaction.[2]

If untreated, complications include perforation of the gastrointestinal tract, ulceration, lacerations, erosions, and fistulae formation.

2.2 Diagnosis and Management

In patients with non-bony food bolus impactions without complications, radiologic evaluation is not necessary. In all other patients, including those who have swallowed a radiopaque blunt foreign body or if the type of object is unknown, plain radiographs aid in characterizing the presence, location, size, configuration, and number of ingested objects. Food boluses, fish or chicken bones, wood, plastic, glass, and thin metal objects are not reliably observed on x-ray. Failure to locate an object on radiographic examination does not exclude foreign body ingestion. For patients with persistent esophageal symptoms, endoscopy must be performed even if the radiographic examination is negative.

Computed tomography (CT) without contrast enables the characterization of the shape, size, location, and depth of the foreign body with respect to surrounding tissues. Note that the use of contrast may increase the risk of aspiration and can impact proper visualization on endoscopy (though this is of more importance with barium esophagrams rather than the oral contrast used with CT scans). However, in the case of suspected perforation, oral contrast is needed. Additionally, information with respect to staging is provided in the context of food bolus impaction secondary to malignancy. This anatomical information, in addition to the presence or absence of complications, guides management and facilitates the evaluation of the risks of endoscopic management. CT is indicated for patients with

- Suspected perforation based on either clinical or radiographic findings
- Sharp or pointed foreign body ingestion
- Narcotic ingestion
- Ingestion of other drugs with an unclear history

Generally, investigations will be completed in the emergency department setting for new patients presenting with esophageal impactions. For patients presenting to their family physician with impactions in the esophagus and gastrointestinal tract, all patients should be referred to the emergency department. Table 2.2 outlines the timing of referral based on patient presentation and foreign body ingestion.

Once imaging is obtained in the emergency department, for patients who are asymptomatic following the ingestion of blunt and small objects <2 cm in diameter and < 5 cm in length in the stomach, clinical observation is appropriate. These patients should be instructed to return emergently if they develop symptoms or

Table 2.2 Timing of referral based on presentation and foreign body

Presentation	Foreign body	Initial investigations	Timing of referral to ED
Concern for perforation (febrile, peritonitis, hemoptysis, hematemesis)	N/A	CT with oral contrast if stable, then OR	Emergent (<2 h, maximum 6 h)
Patient presenting with complete obstruction (drooling and/or hypersalivation with inability to tolerate liquids)	Sharp objects Button battery Disk battery Food bolus	Straight to endoscopy	Emergent (<2 h, maximum 6 h)
Patients NOT presenting with complete obstruction (drooling and/or hypersalivation with inability to tolerate liquids)	Blunt object <5 cm Large foreign body >5 cm Magnets	Plain radiograph	Urgent (<24 h)
Asymptomatic patients and those NOT presenting with complete obstruction (drooling and/or hypersalivation with inability to tolerate liquids)	Blunt and small objects <2–2.5 cm in diameter and 5-6 cm in length	Plain radiograph	Urgent (<24 h)

signs of perforation such as sudden and/or severe abdominal pain and fever/chills, or small bowel obstruction including signs of obstipation. They can also be instructed to monitor their stools continuously for the passage of the object. These patients may receive outpatient management, but weekly radiographs are recommended to monitor the progression of the foreign body. Endoscopic intervention is needed if the foreign body does not pass beyond the stomach by 3–4 weeks.

The exception to this is in the setting of acute ingestion of batteries and/or magnets. Ingestion of button (or disk) batteries (these are small, round lithium batteries most commonly ingested by children) is a surgical emergency as batteries erode through tissue, leading to perforation.

Once foreign bodies pass the esophagus, most pass out of the body within 4–6 days. Objects >2 cm in diameter will frequently be blocked at the pylorus or ileocecal valve, and objects >5 cm may not pass the convexity of the duodenum (also termed the duodenal sweep). Patients with these impactions will need endoscopic intervention.

For patients with suspected non-bony food impaction without evidence of complications, endoscopy without radiographic imaging is a reasonable option. Urgent (<24 h) endoscopy is indicated for esophageal foreign body impactions without complete obstruction. Delay beyond this timeframe increases the risk for complications such as perforation, abscess, and fistula formation.

Emergent (<2 h, maximum 6 h) esophagogastroduodenoscopy, preferably in the operating room setting for appropriate patient sedation and monitoring, is warranted for patients presenting with complete obstruction (drooling and/or hypersalivation with an inability to tolerate fluids) as well as those who have swallowed sharp objects. Patients with button/disk batteries in the esophagus must also undergo emergent endoscopic retrieval as these patients are at high risk for perforation, necrosis, or fistulization due to pressure necrosis, electrical discharge, or chemical injury. Table 2.3 summarizes the timing of referral for endoscopic retrieval of foreign body.

Table 2.3 Timing of endoscopic intervention based on foreign body and presentation in the esophagus

Timing	Foreign body/presentation
Emergent (<2 h, maximum 6 h)	Concern for perforation (febrile, peritonitis, hemoptysis, hematemesis)
Emergent (<2 h, maximum 6 h)	Patient presenting with complete obstruction (drooling and/or hypersalivation with inability to tolerate liquids
	Sharp objects
	Button battery in the esophagus
	Disk battery in the esophagus
	Food bolus
Urgent (<24 h)	Blunt object <5 cm
	Large foreign body >5 cm
	Magnets
Observation with weekly radiographs, self-monitoring until 3–4 weeks	Blunt and small objects <2–2.5 cm in diameter and 5-6 cm in length that have passed beyond the esophagus

ED emergency department

For sharp-pointed objects, magnets, blunt objects >5 cm in length or > 2 cm in diameter, and disk batteries in the stomach >24 h, endoscopic intervention is indicated.

For foreign bodies in the stomach, urgent (<24 h) endoscopic removal is indicated for sharp objects, magnets, batteries, and large/long objects. Nonurgent (<72 h) endoscopic is appropriate for medium-sized blunt foreign bodies in the stomach (Table 2.4).

Following endoscopy, outpatient follow-up is appropriate unless the following indications are present:

- Ingestion of multiple objects
- Ingestion of foreign bodies with a high risk for complications (sharp-pointed objects, batteries, magnets, objects >5 cm in length)
- Extensive mucosal injury

Table 2.4 Timing of endoscopic intervention based on foreign body and presentation in the stomach

Timing	Foreign body/presentation
Urgent (<24 h)	Large/long objects >5 cm
	Sharp objects
	Magnets
	Disk batteries
Nonurgent (<72 h)	Blunt objects <5 cm
Observation with weekly radiographs, self-monitoring until 3–4 weeks	Blunt and small objects <2–2.5 cm in diameter and 5-6 cm in length

Biopsies are typically taken to rule out eosinophilic esophagitis. In patients with foreign bodies that cannot be removed endoscopically, daily radiographs should be performed to assess the object's passage through the gastrointestinal tract.

Surgery is indicated for patients who develop complications such as obstruction, perforation, or non-progression of blunt objects (e.g., object remaining in the same location distal to duodenum for >1 week or sharp foreign body in the same location for 3 consecutive days).

2.2.1 Recurrent Esophageal Foreign Body Impactions

Upper endoscopy is indicated in all patients with recurrence and extensive mucosal injury on initial endoscopy to evaluate mucosal healing. Endoscopy is also needed to biopsy the esophagus to rule out eosinophilic esophagitis and manage underlying structural defects (e.g., Schatzki's ring) if not completed on initial endoscopy. Those without structural abnormalities should be referred for the evaluation of an esophageal motility disorder.

2.1.1 Special Populations

Some patients may be involved with packing drugs in the gastrointestinal tract, typically using latex condoms or balloons in parcels. These can typically be identified radiographically. As rupture and leakage of contents may result in fatal intoxication, conservative management has a success rate of up to 98% and is favored over endoscopic removal. This consists of clinical observation as an inpatient, whole bowel irrigation, and serial radiographic examinations to monitor the passage of the parcels.

For symptomatic patients with intoxication or bowel obstruction, surgical intervention is needed.

Overall, esophageal impactions in adults can be time-sensitive, life-threatening emergencies. Expeditious assessment in the form of investigative workup is needed. Table 2.5 lists the investigations needed prior to surgical referral.

Table 2.5 Investigations required prior to surgical referral

Presentation	Initial investigations	Timing of referral to surgery
Concern for perforation (febrile, peritonitis, hemoptysis, hematemesis)	CT with oral contrast if stable	Emergent (<2 h, maximum 6 h)
Patient presenting with complete obstruction (drooling and/or hypersalivation with inability to tolerate liquids)	Nil, straight to endoscopy	Emergent (<2 h, maximum 6 h)
Patients NOT presenting with complete obstruction (drooling and/or hypersalivation with inability to tolerate liquids)	Plain radiograph	Urgent (<24 h)
Asymptomatic patients and those NOT presenting with complete obstruction (drooling and/or hypersalivation with inability to tolerate liquids)	Plain radiograph	Urgent (<24 h)

Resources for Readers:

1. Ingested foreign bodies and food impactions in adults https://www.uptodate.com/contents/ingested-foreign-bodies-and-food-impactions-in-adults?search=esophageal%20impaction&source=search_result&selectedTitle=1~150&usage_type=default&display_rank=1#H3
2. Birk M, Bauerfeind P, Deprez PH, et al. Removal of foreign bodies in the upper gastrointestinal tract in adults: European Society of Gastrointestinal Endoscopy (ESGE) Clinical Guideline. Endoscopy. 2016;48(5):489–496. https://doi.org/10.1055/s-0042-100456

Reference

Birk M, Bauerfeind P, Deprez PH, et al. Removal of foreign bodies in the upper gastrointestinal tract in adults: European Society of Gastrointestinal Endoscopy (ESGE) Clinical Guideline. Endoscopy. 2016;48(5):489–496. https://doi.org/10.1055/s-0042-100456.

2. A P CA, P W waring G. Ingested Foreign Bodies: Patient-Guided Localization Is a Useful Clinical Tool. Vol 17.; 1992.

Hematemesis

3

Rodolfo J. Oviedo

3.1 Background

The word hematemesis comes from the Greek *hemato*, for blood, and *emesis*, for vomiting. It represents the evident and external manifestation of acute upper gastrointestinal bleeding (UGIB) from a variety of possible etiologies that ultimately express themselves with bleeding per mouth and that may be accompanied by hemodynamic compromise and cardiovascular collapse. Hematemesis has long been regarded as a medical and potential surgical emergency that requires close attention to detail in the implementation of life-saving algorithms in compliance with some basic tenets of resuscitation, including an ABC approach. Such methodology is well known in medicine for its emphasis on protecting the *airway*, ensuring that *breathing* is taking place, and securing access to the *circulatory* system via intravenous cannula-

R. J. Oviedo (✉)
Department of Surgery, Nacogdoches Medical Center,
Nacogdoches, TX, USA

University of Houston Tilman J. Fertitta Family College of Medicine,
Houston, TX, USA

Sam Houston State University College of Osteopathic Medicine,
Conroe, TX, USA

G. P. Kohn et al. (eds.), *The SAGES Manual of Surgical Referral for Primary and Emergency Care*,
https://doi.org/10.1007/978-3-031-92678-5_3

tion and fluid resuscitation, which usually begins with crystalloid and which may require blood products. The most important aspect when treating a patient who is experiencing hematemesis is to follow these basic resuscitation tenets and to eventually reach a phase in the treatment algorithm that will require gastric decompression and lavage via insertion of a nasogastric tube (NGT) or an equivalent device to diagnose and treat the acute process of UGIB.

3.2 Rationale for Surgeon Referral

Referral to a surgeon will depend on the availability of resources and the context of the environment in which the patient is being seen. For example, the workplace could be an academic or urban center where gastroenterologists may be available versus a rural or community practice where surgeons typically perform endoscopy for diagnostic and therapeutic purposes given the lack of availability of gastroenterologists, or simply due to the philosophy of care that has become the norm within that environment [1]. In either case, referral to a surgeon must be ensured if the process of acute UGIB cannot be stopped by conventional measures and if endoscopy must be performed due to lack of stabilization of the hemoglobin and hematocrit (H/H) with or without hemodynamic compromise. It is important to understand that before thinking of obtaining advanced radiographic studies such as a nuclear tagged red blood cell scan or a computerized tomography (CT) angiogram, or even a visceral angiogram, all of which have powerful diagnostic and/or therapeutic potential, the gold standard continues to be an upper gastrointestinal endoscopy or esophagogastroduodenoscopy (EGD). Such endoscopic procedure is typically performed by a gastroenterologist or a surgeon, but can also be done by primary care professionals (PCPs) in many communities where specialist referral may be logistically challenging. The most important aspect of understanding when to refer a patient to a surgical specialist is the fact that the resuscitation efforts are not productive and the patient continues to bleed at a rate that, if not properly addressed and treated, will lead to cardiovascular collapse due to hemorrhagic shock and hypovolemia despite blood product resuscitation and indicated pharmacotherapy [2]. If the hematemesis persists and the gastric aspirate via NGT reveals fresh blood from the lumen, referral to a surgeon must take place as soon as possible to perform an EGD under an airway protection protocol and treat the source of bleeding, ideally with endoscopic techniques and, less frequently, with a surgical approach.

3.3 Types of Hematemesis

There are typically two recognized types of hematemesis that manifest themselves on a clinical basis as soon as the patient is evaluated and the color and quality of the effluent is analyzed. The types are coffee-grounds emesis and bloody hematemesis. The first type represents the fact that the patient may have bled at a slow rate and eventually vomited this processed blood, which appears to have a coffee grounds consistency. However, the second type represents high-volume or ongoing acute UGIB that is clearly distinguished from coffee-grounds emesis and that represents a medical and potential surgical emergency in comparison to the first type. Although both are considered an emergency, the latter carries a sense of urgency and requires a quicker response and a focused multidisciplinary approach. Although bloody emesis has not been shown to be associated with more severe bleeding in comparison to coffee-grounds emesis, it has been proven to be associated with higher rates of endoscopic bleeding control and re-bleeding episodes. If, on the other hand, melena (dark blood per rectum) occurs with hematemesis, the clinical outcomes are worse compared to hematemesis without melena. If bloody emesis is seen with melena at the same time, usually the decision to intervene with upper GI endoscopy takes precedence and must be made sooner rather than later [3].

3.4 Potential Sources of Hematemesis

The potential causes of hematemesis can be regarded in terms of their organ of origin. If the oral cavity is the beginning and the ligament of Treitz is considered the end of the upper GI tract, the organs of interest are the esophagus, the stomach, and the duodenum. On the other hand, there are other less frequent sources of acute UGIB that may not have their origin in the lumen of these organs but that eventually enter their lumen from a different organ or structure. The esophagus has possible etiologies such as esophageal varices, erosive esophagitis, malignancy, infectious esophagitis, Mallory–Weiss tear, or black esophagus (due to ischemia). The stomach may be the source of acute UGIB due to peptic ulcer disease (PUD), gastric varices, malignancy, or a Dieulafoy lesion. The duodenum may be the source due to PUD or malignancy. Examples of these less frequent causes are an aortoenteric fistula, hemosuccus pancreaticus, and hemobilia [4, 5].

3.5 Patient Evaluation Prior to Surgeon Referral

Whether a decision has been made to refer the patient to a surgeon or not yet, along with the resuscitation efforts described above, equally important is the evaluation of the patient's laboratory studies that are relevant to the episode of acute UGIB, including the complete blood count (CBC), and basic metabolic profile (BMP), along with coagulation studies such as prothrombin time (PT), partial thromboplastin time (PTT), and international normalized ratio (INR). On the other hand, a type and screen (T&S) and a type and cross (T&C) are mandatory in the context of acute UGIB to guide the resuscitation efforts with appropriate blood products depending on the acuity of the situation. Other laboratory studies that may prove useful include the hepatic function panel as well as the arterial blood gas (ABG), especially if the patient is experiencing hemorrhagic shock and if tissue perfusion is a concern due to massive intraluminal hemorrhage. However, what should not delay a prompt endoscopic intervention is a nuclear-tagged red blood cell scan, a CT abdomen/pelvis angiogram, or a visceral angiogram. These advanced radiologic studies should not be performed before the gold standard, that is, upper GI endoscopy, takes place. The reason is the important diagnostic and therapeutic potential that upper GI endoscopy carries and the fact that it can offer a solution to the diagnostic dilemma and the bleeding etiology in a shorter amount of time and more efficiently compared to advanced radiologic studies that are typically available at larger centers with more resources. Hematemesis also requires resuscitation with IV fluids, blood product transfusion, as well as a surgical evaluation after clinical surveillance demonstrates ongoing bleeding, an unfavorable response to blood product transfusion, and labile hemodynamics with development of an acute abdomen/peritonitis. Such findings from clinical surveillance would require a surgical consultation on an emergency basis. Serial physical exams are indicated, too, since peritonitis will usually become evident if hematemesis is associated with a hollow viscus perforation such as the stomach, the duodenum, or the distal esophagus in some cases. Attention to detail and clinical surveillance in an ICU setting or a closely monitored ward setting take precedence as part of the algorithm for the treatment of hematemesis, including surgical consultation and evaluation. Table 3.1 describes the key steps in the clinical decision-making process when evaluating and treating a patient with hematemesis. Table 3.2 introduces the most important evaluation maneuvers that are necessary prior to consulting a surgical specialist.

Table 3.1 Key features of the clinical decision-making process when evaluating and treating patients with hematemesis

Features of emergency presentation	Criteria for urgent surgical review/ consultation	Criteria for nonurgent surgical review-consultation	Conditions for management by PCP versus referral to GI medicine
Hemodynamic instability	Hemodynamic instability	Hemodynamic stability	Hemodynamic stability
Need for significant blood product transfusion without improvement (> 4 units of PRBC) over the first 24 h	Inability to respond to massive transfusion protocol	Appropriate response to blood transfusion	Appropriate response to blood transfusion
Acute/surgical abdomen	Acute/surgical abdomen	Abdominal pain (without peritonitis)	No abdominal pain and resolution of hematemesis

Table 3.2 Diagnostic testing maneuvers prior to consultation with a surgical specialist

Physical exam and clinical maneuvers	Laboratory studies	Radiographic studies
Thorough or focused abdominal physical exam (depending on patient's instability)	CBC	Chest X-ray
Nasogastric tube decompression and lavage	BMP	Abdominal X-ray
Large bore peripheral IV lines with isotonic crystalloid fluids	PT, PTT, INR	CT abdomen/pelvis (unless an acute/surgical abdomen prohibits it)
Blood product transfusion (possible need for massive transfusion protocol)	Hepatic function panel, amylase, lipase	CT abdomen/pelvis angiogram (in cases when surgical consultation cannot be obtained immediately, and only if the patient's hemodynamics allow it)

3.6 Summary and Treatment Algorithm

After initial assessment and resuscitation with the ABC approach, IVF and blood product resuscitation along with laboratory studies evaluation will be followed by referral to a surgical specialist when these efforts do not lead to resolution of the hemorrhagic process and if the H/H and cardiovascular status of the patient continue to decompensate. Surgical judgment regarding the need for an operation after UGI endoscopy is not the subject of this chapter, but the decision to operate (if indicated) should be discussed by the surgeon with the referring physician depending on the endoscopic findings and the rate of success of intraluminal therapeutic intervention at controlling the source of bleeding with a nonsurgical approach.

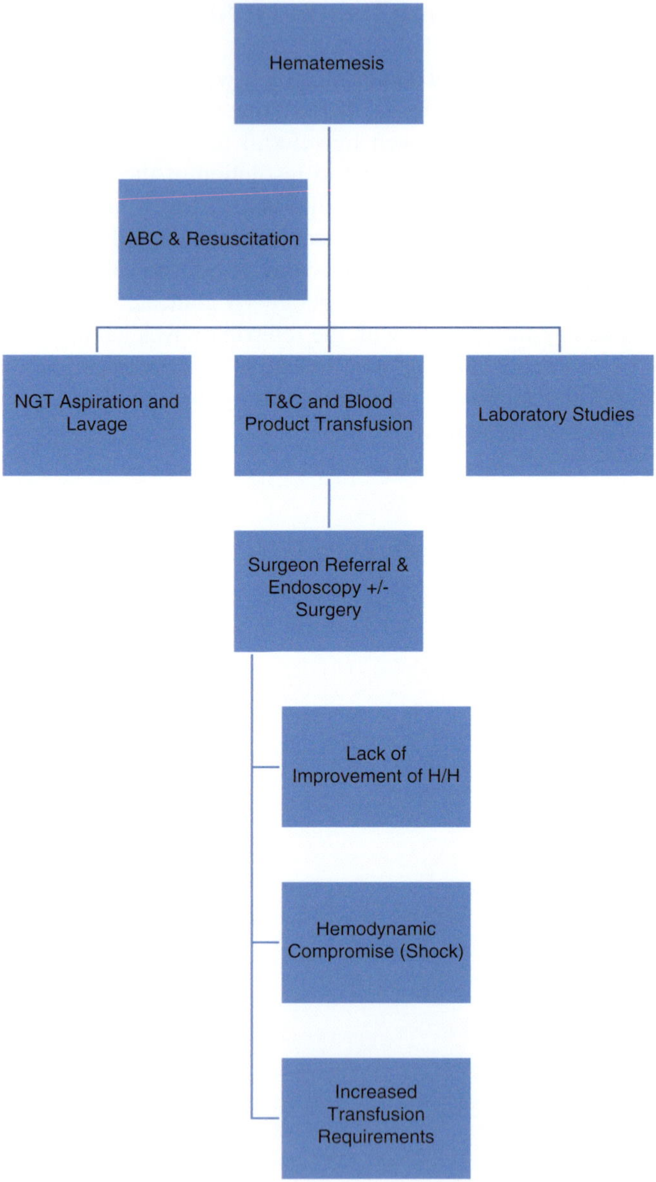
Hematemesis
ABC & Resuscitation
NGT Aspiration and Lavage
T&C and Blood Product Transfusion
Laboratory Studies
Surgeon Referral & Endoscopy +/- Surgery
Lack of Improvement of H/H
Hemodynamic Compromise (Shock)
Increased Transfusion Requirements

Selected Readings

1. Morgenthal CB, Richards WO, Dunkin BJ, Forde KA, Vitale G, Lin E. SAGES Flexible Endoscopy Committee. The role of the surgeon in the evolution of flexible endoscopy. Surg Endosc. 2007;21(6):838–53. https://doi.org/10.1007/s00464-006-9109-4. Epub 2006 Dec 16. PMID: 17180263
2. Barkun AN, Almadi M, Kuipers EJ, Laine L, Sung J, Tse F, Leontiadis GI, Abraham NS, Calvet X, Chan FKL, Douketis J, Enns R, Gralnek IM, Jairath V, Jensen D, Lau J, Lip GYH, Loffroy R, Maluf-Filho F, Meltzer AC, Reddy N, Saltzman JR, Marshall JK, Bardou M. Management of nonvariceal upper gastrointestinal bleeding: guideline recommendations from the International Consensus Group. Ann Intern Med. 2019;171(11):805–22. https://doi.org/10.7326/M19-1795. Epub 2019 Oct 22. PMID: 31634917; PMCID: PMC7233308
3. Laine L, Laursen SB, Zakko L, Dalton HR, Ngu JH, Schultz M, Stanley AJ. Severity and outcomes of upper gastrointestinal bleeding with bloody vs coffee-grounds hematemesis. Am J Gastroenterol. 2018;113(3):358–66. https://doi.org/10.1038/ajg.2018.5. Epub 2018 Jan 30. PMID: 29380820
4. Kamboj AK, Hoversten P, Leggett CL. Upper gastrointestinal bleeding: etiologies and management. Mayo Clin Proc. 2019;94(4):697–703. https://doi.org/10.1016/j.mayocp.2019.01.022. PMID: 30947833
5. Martino A, Di Serafino M, Orsini L, Giurazza F, Fiorentino R, Crolla E, Campione S, Molino C, Romano L, Lombardi G. Rare causes of acute non-variceal upper gastrointestinal bleeding: a comprehensive review. World J Gastroenterol. 2023;29(27):4222–35. https://doi.org/10.3748/wjg.v29.i27.4222. PMID: 37545636; PMCID: PMC10401659

4 Substernal Chest Pain

Madeleine S. Higgins,
Clark H. Cunningham,
and Timothy M. Farrell

4.1 Inflammatory and Anatomic Pathologies

Gastroesophageal reflux disease (GERD) involves the retrograde flow of acidic gastric contents into the lower esophagus, most often due to an incompetent lower esophageal sphincter. Over time the chronic presence of acidic contents can lead to esophagitis, ulceration, or intestinal metaplasia (Barrett's esophagus) with or without dysplasia.

The classic symptom of GERD is heartburn (pyrosis), which is felt as a burning pain in the substernal area that worsens with high-acidity or spicy foods, or when supine. Regurgitation is another common complaint where the patient experiences retrograde movement of gastric fluid or undigested food. Other well-known, but atypical, symptoms of GERD include substernal chest pain, globus sensation, chronic cough, nausea, hoarseness, and wheezing.

The initial approach to the management of GERD should include lifestyle modification and avoidance of trigger foods.

M. S. Higgins (✉) · C. H. Cunningham · T. M. Farrell
Department of Surgery, Division of Gastrointestinal Surgery, The University of North Carolina at Chapel Hill, Chapel Hill, NC, USA

G. P. Kohn et al. (eds.), *The SAGES Manual of Surgical Referral for Primary and Emergency Care*,
https://doi.org/10.1007/978-3-031-92678-5_4

Data have shown that weight loss and head-of-bed elevation are most efficacious. Medical treatment of mild GERD should begin with antacid medications, such as H2 blockers. If patients have severe or refractory symptoms, escalation to proton pump inhibitors (PPIs) is appropriate. Most patients will have at least some response to these medications, and in fact a positive response to medical therapy is a positive predictor of response to antireflux surgery.

Upper endoscopy is not always necessary in patients with typical GERD symptoms who respond to medical treatment. It should be pursued in cases of severe or alarm symptoms (dysphagia, odynophagia, anemia, weight loss) to evaluate for erosive esophagitis, stricture, Barrett's esophagus, or malignancy.

Factors that should prompt consideration of surgical management of GERD include suboptimal response, intolerance or contraindication to chronic antireflux medications, esophageal mucosal damage on upper endoscopy, or the presence of a large hiatal hernia. A diagnosis of a hiatal hernia is best established with an upper gastrointestinal contrast study such as a barium swallow. An abdominal computed tomography (CT) scan is a secondary option; however, unlike barium swallow, this does not evaluate esophageal swallowing function in real time. Additional studies required in the preoperative workup of GERD include an upper endoscopy, and in some cases 24-hour pH monitoring, esophageal manometry, and gastric emptying assessment.

Surgical management of reflux disease involves reducing any hiatal hernia, closing the diaphragmatic hiatus, and performing a fundoplication, which involves wrapping the upper part of the stomach around the lower esophagus to augment the lower esophageal sphincter for reflux control. A surgeon may tailor the degree of fundoplication based on the strength and function of the esophagus, which is established with esophageal manometry.

A related yet independent etiology of noncardiac substernal chest pain is a large *hiatal hernia,* with or without the presence of reflux. Hiatal hernias can be classified into five types:

I. *Type I or sliding hiatal hernia* involves intermittent upward movement of the esophagogastric junction (EGJ)

II. Types II–IV are *paraesophageal hernias*
   (a) *Type II* occurs when the EGJ remains in the correct anatomic location, but the fundus rolls into the chest along the esophagus through a localized defect in the phreno-esophageal membrane
   (b) *Type III* involves the herniation of both the EGJ and the fundus. They are considered mixed type, with components of both types I and II
   (c) *Type IV* involves herniation of the EGJ, stomach, and other organ(s)
   (d) *Type V* is a recurrence after previous repair

Chest pain related to a paraesophageal hernia is a diagnosis made after exclusion of cardiac causes. Presentation varies; however, it is often described as a substernal and related to oral intake, especially consumption of more solid/tough foods like meats and improved with a liquid/pureed diet. Dysphagia and regurgitation are often present. Patients whose primary complaint is pain are more likely to have a gastric volvulus, where the stomach twists or folds, putting the patient at risk for gastric ischemia and perforation (1% per year).

A patient with an acute gastric volvulus often presents with profound intolerance of oral intake and dehydration in the setting of upper abdominal/chest pain. Initial workup and management of suspected acute gastric volvulus should entail prompt intravenous fluid resuscitation, full labs including complete blood count (CBC) and lactate, a CT of the chest/abdomen/pelvis, administration of IV PPI and broad spectrum antibiotics, and placement of a nasogastric tube for decompression to help prevent the risk of perforation and/or ischemia. The latter is particularly important if a patient is to be transferred to a tertiary facility for a higher level of care.

The workup of a hiatal/paraesophageal hernia in the outpatient setting is similar to that of GERD. The initial imaging test of choice is a barium swallow or upper GI series (Fig. 4.1), followed by an upper endoscopy. We recommend that all patients with a true symptomatic paraesophageal hernia be referred for surgical evaluation.

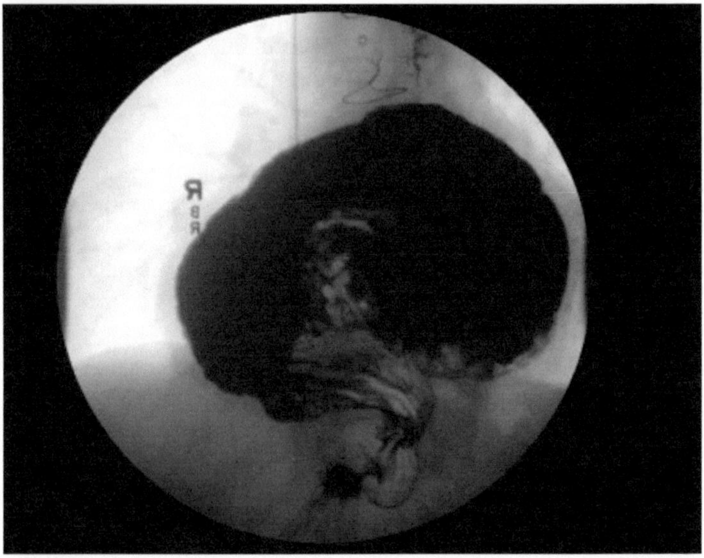

Fig. 4.1 Upper GI contrast study of a patient who presented with substernal postprandial chest pain, showing a large type III paraesophageal hernia with organo-axial volvulus

Peptic ulcer disease (PUD) is marked by erosion of the mucosa and muscularis mucosa with extension into the submucosa or muscular layers of the stomach or duodenum. The most common etiology of PUD is infection with *Helicobacter pylori*, which is present in most cases. Use of nonsteroidal anti-inflammatory drugs (NSAIDs), corticosteroids, and salicylates such as aspirin are also risk factors for PUD due to inhibition of cyclooxygenase 1 (cox-1). Cox-1 inhibition disrupts prostaglandin synthesis, which decreases local blood flow, mucus production, and bicarbonate secretion that protect gastrointestinal mucosa from gastric acid and pepsin. Tobacco use is an additional risk factor for PUD. While alcohol is known to promote gastric acid secretion, its role in ulcerogenesis remains uncertain.

PUD can be asymptomatic but often presents with epigastric or substernal chest pain, bloating, nausea, vomiting, and lack of appetite. Classically, pain associated with gastric ulcers is worse with eating and is associated with lack of appetite, while the pain associated with duodenal ulcers is relieved with food and worsens several hours after eating. PUD can also be a source of occult GI bleeding, presenting with melena and anemia. Acute presentations of PUD that require emergent surgical consultation include hematemesis or "coffee-ground" emesis, and acute abdominal pain with focal or generalized peritonitis concerning for perforation.

Diagnosis of PUD should begin with complete history and physical examination, with particular attention to noted risk factors. The gold standard for diagnosis of PUD is upper endoscopy with biopsy to evaluate for malignancy and active *H. pylori* infection. Other studies that are useful in diagnosing suspected PUD include testing for *H. pylori* infection with a stool antigen assay or urea breath test. Serological testing for *H. pylori* antibodies can also be used; however, titers will remain elevated in patients who have previously been treated for *H. pylori* infection even if acute infection is not present. Blood hemoglobin and iron studies and fecal occult blood testing can provide evidence of anemia and occult gastrointestinal bleeding from PUD. CT scan evidence of PUD includes mural thickening of the stomach or duodenum with mucosal hyperenhancement and inflammatory stranding. Pneumoperitoneum on CT or upright abdominal X-ray can also be observed in the setting of perforated PUD.

Medical management of PUD should begin by addressing the underlying etiology, namely, risk factor avoidance, and eradication of active *H. pylori* infection, if present. Gastric acid suppression therapy with PPIs is the first-line medical management of uncomplicated PUD. Additional adjunctive therapies including sucralfate and misoprostol may be used to facilitate mucosal healing.

Active upper gastrointestinal bleeding from PUD warrants upper endoscopy with endoscopic control of hemorrhage using combination of sclerotherapy, hemostatic clips, thermal coagulation, and intralesional epinephrine. Perforated PUD requires emergent surgical consultation. Perforated pyloric channel ulcers <1 cm may be repaired primarily followed by coverage with an omental flap. For perforated pyloric ulcers with friable edges and those not amenable to a tension-free primary repair, omental (Graham) patching may be employed. Large (>3 cm) perforated duodenal ulcers are managed differently through a combination of omental patching, duodenostomy tube drainage, temporary pyloric exclusion with absorbable suture or noncutting staples, and gastrojejunostomy to reestablish gastrointestinal continuity. Adjunctive medical management, treatment of any infection, and avoidance of NSAIDs must be part of the overall treatment of these acute presentations, or recurrence is possible.

Surgical management of chronic PUD is reserved for patients who fail to respond to medical management or present with gastric outlet obstruction. Obstructing or refractory ulcers should be completely excised and sent for pathological evaluation to assess for underlying malignancy. Antrectomy is performed for ulcers on the distal lesser curve, combined distal lesser curve and duodenum, and prepyloric antrum. Transection of the vagus nerves at the gastroesophageal junction (truncal vagotomy) may be performed in addition to antrectomy to further decrease gastric acid production in severe cases, although this is much less commonly applied than in prior years due to improved understanding of the role of *H. pylori* and NSAIDs in ulcer etiology. To restore gastrointestinal continuity, either gastroduodenostomy (Billroth I) or gastrojejunostomy (Billroth II) reconstruction may be performed. Ulcers on the proximal lesser curve or gastric cardia are managed differently, with options including local excision or near-total gastrectomy with Roux-en-Y reconstruction. After surgical therapy, chronic PUD patients must avoid NSAID use, or recurrence is possible.

4.2 Disorders of Esophageal Motility

Esophageal dysmotility can also cause noncardiac, substernal chest pain. Additional common symptoms are dysphagia, heartburn, regurgitation, odynophagia, and weight loss.

Achalasia is a rare esophageal motility disorder that results from the degeneration/dysfunction of the ganglion cells in the myenteric plexus of the esophageal wall. The etiology of primary achalasia is unknown; secondary achalasia is the result of another condition such as a tumor or other cause of esophageal outflow obstruction that presents with similar manometric and imaging findings.

The most common presenting complaint of achalasia is progressive dysphagia with regurgitation. Additionally, many patients will complain of short bursts of chest/epigastric pain, occasionally with radiation. The pain is typically post-prandial in nature but can be spontaneous. Heartburn that persists despite antacid therapy is another common finding. Of note, many patients are treated for GERD prior to ultimately receiving a diagnosis of achalasia. Proper diagnosis can take years due to the common misattribution of the symptoms to another clinical entity.

The workup of suspected achalasia can begin with a barium swallow, which may show the classic bird's-beak finding (Fig. 4.2). Esophageal manometry is required to diagnose achalasia and will show aperistalsis of the esophageal body with incomplete relaxation of the lower esophageal sphincter (LES). Upper endoscopy should be performed in all patients with suspected or newly diagnosed achalasia to exclude malignancy or another cause of esophageal junction outflow obstruction.

The goal for the treatment of achalasia is to decrease the tone of the lower esophagus to allow for improved esophagogastric transit. Medical therapy can include nitrates or calcium channel blockers; however, their use is limited by their side effect profile and the loss of response with time. Endoscopic botulinum toxin injection into the distal esophagus is efficacious at controlling symptoms, but effects fade as the toxin is metabolized over months. More invasive endoscopic therapeutic options include pneumatic dilation, which involves disruption of the muscular fibers in the LES with forceful endoscopic balloon dilation, or a per-oral endoscopic myotomy (POEM), where a mucosotomy is performed and the circular muscular layer of the esophagus is divided down onto the upper stomach. This is compared with a minimally invasive Heller myotomy, which is a surgical method to divide the LES muscle that is typically combined with a loose fundoplication, to help mitigate the risk of postprocedural reflux.

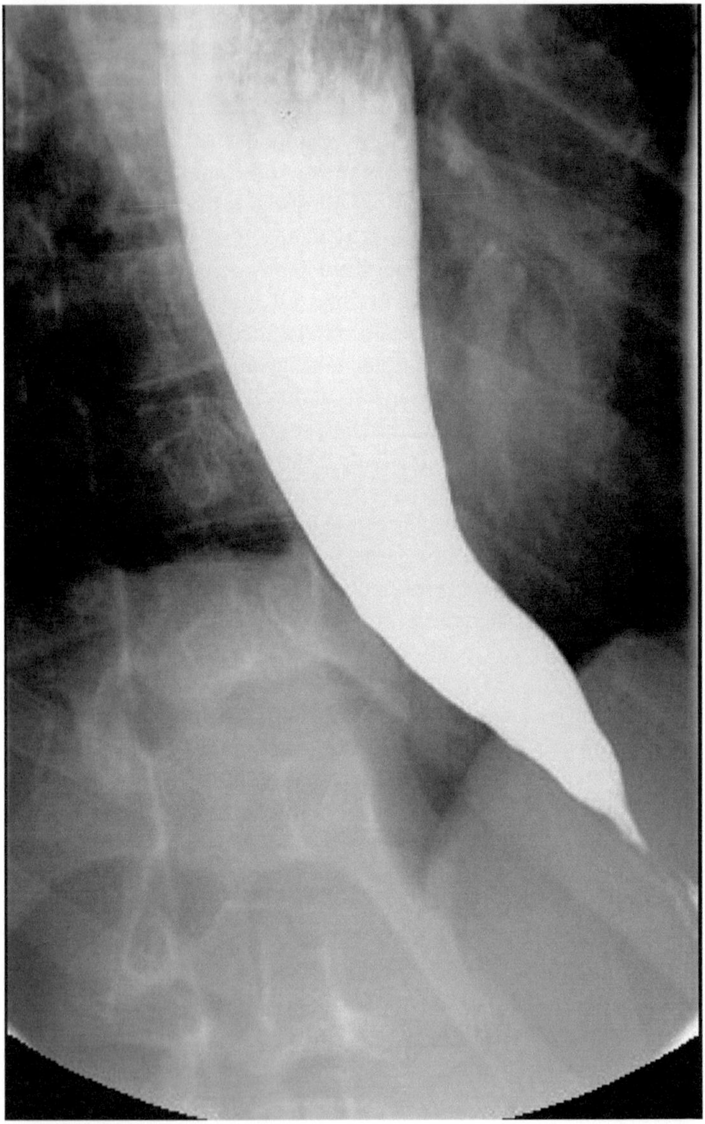

Fig. 4.2 Upper GI contrast study of a patient with achalasia showing classic birds beak finding

A particular limitation of POEM is the potential for uncontrolled reflux and reflux esophagitis on EGD due to the complete disruption of the natural antireflux valve. Of note, the 2021 SAGES guidelines for the use of POEM for achalasia cite a moderate risk for the most mild form of reflux esophagitis (grade A esophagitis), but a small risk for grade B-D reflux esophagitis, which are more clinically significant. Subsequent data seems to support the higher rate of GERD symptoms after POEM compared to Heller, though the judicious use of acid suppressant medications can result in comparable, or even improved, quality of life scores after the endoscopic myotomy.

It is therefore prudent to consider a patient's reflux history prior to specialty referral.

We recommend that all patients with suspected or confirmed achalasia be referred to either a gastroenterologist or a general surgeon with a focus on esophageal disease.

Distal esophageal spasm (DES) is a rare clinical entity where there are premature and rapidly propagated contractions in the distal esophagus, thought secondary to impaired inhibitory innervation. Typical symptoms are dysphagia, substernal chest pain with oral intake, +/− heartburn. Diagnosis is via esophageal manometry and requires >20% premature contractions with normal relaxation of the distal esophagus (normal IRP) *in addition to* the presence of dysphagia and/or noncardiac chest pain (as per the Chicago classification version 4).

Another esophageal motor condition associated with chest pain is *hypercontractile esophagus (HE)*, where there are coordinated but high-pressure esophageal body contractions. Patients will present with dysphagia, substernal chest pain, and sometimes heartburn. Manometric diagnosis requires >20% hypercontractile swallows, with normal LES relaxation, *in addition to* the presence of dysphagia and/or noncardiac chest pain. HE is further broken down into three subsets, including *jackhammer esophagus* where there are repetitive and prolonged contractions.

Management of both DES and HE is aimed at control of symptoms rather than normalization of manometric readings. If GERD-like symptoms are present, PPI therapy should be initiated. Additional treatments to be considered include peppermint oil, antispasmodic agents, nitrates, calcium channel blockers, tricyclic antidepressants, botulinum toxin injections, or rarely myotomy. We recommend all patients with suspected DES or HE be referred to a gastroenterologist with a focus on esophageal disease.

4.3 Functional Esophageal Disorders

Functional esophageal disorders are marked by typical and atypical foregut symptoms (heartburn, dysphagia, regurgitation, substernal chest pain, globus) that cannot be explained by inflammatory or anatomic etiologies, nor disordered motility. These are rare and are diagnoses of exclusion.

Functional chest pain presents with recurrent substernal chest pain that is assumed esophageal in origin with a negative workup for foregut pathology. The pain is different from heartburn and occurs at least once a week.

Functional heartburn is retrosternal burning that is refractory to maximal antireflux medications, not associated with pathologic GERD or other structural/motility diagnoses. Symptoms occur at least 2x per week.

Reflux hypersensitivity (esophageal hypersensitivity) presents with classic esophageal symptoms (heartburn, chest pain, dysphagia/regurgitation) without esophagitis on endoscopy or pathologic reflux on pH testing, *but with a symptomatic correlation with physiologic reflux.* Symptoms occur 2x per week.

Diagnosis of the above functional esophageal disorders requires criteria be met for at least 3 months, with a historical symptom onset of at least 6 months prior to diagnosis. The workup involves upper endoscopy to rule out mucosal/anatomic pathology, 24-hour pH monitoring to show absence of pathologic reflux, and esophageal manometry to rule out dysmotility. Suspicion or diagnosis of any of the above requires referral to a gastroenterologist with a focus on esophageal disease.

4.4 Conclusion

A patient with substernal chest pain should promptly be evaluated for cardiopulmonary causes. If none are found, the possible diagnoses are typically gastroesophageal in nature and can include inflammatory disorders, anatomic derangements, esophageal dysmotility, and functional disorders. Upper endoscopy, barium swallow, pH testing, and manometry are fundamental in refining the diagnosis. Referral to a specialist in foregut disease is indicated when a provider has confirmed a relevant diagnosis, or if uncertainty remains and further workup is indicated.

Pathology	Findings requiring ER presentation	Findings requiring surgical referral	Appropriate for GI referral	Appropriate for PCP management
GERD	Severe chest pain	Refractory symptoms with objective evidence for GERD	Complications of GERD including Barrett's esophagus, grade C or D esophagitis, peptic stricture, or if refractory symptoms	Without complication
Paraesophageal hernia				
With gastric obstruction (acute)	Severe chest/abdominal pain, refractory nausea/ vomiting, hematemesis, food impaction, aspiration	Symptomatic with obstruction, hemorrhage, concern for necrosis, radiographic evidence of volvulus	Need for luminal evaluation to evaluate for necrosis or to facilitate decompression, non- surgical candidate	Never
Without gastric obstruction (chronic)		Symptomatic or with paraesophageal component (type II-IV), Cameron's ulcers, iron deficiency anemia	Need for luminal evaluation or additional workup	Management of nutritional or hematologic sequela before or after specialist treatment
Peptic ulcer disease	Severe chest/abdominal pain, peritonitis, hematemesis	Concern for perforation or neoplasm, refractory ulcers, gastric outlet obstruction	Need for luminal evaluation or additional workup, bleeding	After GI evaluation, if within PCP scope of practice

Esophageal motility disorders				
Achalasia	Severe chest pain, food impaction, aspiration	Diagnosis on high resolution manometry	Diagnosis on high-resolution manometry	Never
Distal esophageal spasm		Rarely indicated, per GI discretion	With high degree of suspicion	After GI evaluation, if within PCP scope of practice
Hypercontractile esophagus				
Jackhammer esophagus				
Functional esophageal disorders				
Functional chest pain	Severe chest pain	Rarely indicated	With high degree of suspicion	After GI evaluation, if within PCP scope of practice
Functional heartburn				
Reflux hypersensitivity/ esophageal hypersensitivity				

Pathology	Initial management	Tests
GERD	Empiric medical management with antisecretory agent, consider EGD	EGD, barium swallow. If no grade C or D esophagitis, Barrett's esophagus, peptic stricture, large hiatal hernia, proceed with 24 h pH/impedence testing (preferred off PPI)[a]
Paraesophageal hernia		
With gastric obstruction (acute)	NGT placement, fluid resuscitation, IV PPI, broad-spectrum antibiotics, bloodwork including CBC, CMP, lactate	CT chest/abdomen. Consider EGD if concern for necrosis or unable to decompress stomach
Without gastric obstruction (chronic)	Empiric medical management with antisecretory agent, consider EGD	EGD, barium swallow, or CT chest/abdomen
Peptic ulcer disease	Empiric medical management with antisecretory agent	EGD with biopsy for *H. pylori*
Esophageal motility disorders		
Achalasia	Early high suspicion, nutritional support, acid suppression, symptom management, early referral to specialist	Barium swallow, EGD, high-resolution esophageal manometry
Distal esophageal spasm	Early referral to gastroenterology Symptom management	EGD, high-resolution esophageal manometry
Hypercontractile esophagus		
Jackhammer esophagus		

(continued)

Pathology	Initial management	Tests
Functional esophageal disorders		
Functional chest pain	Referral to gastroenterology after ruling out above diagnoses	
Functional heartburn		
Reflux hypersensitivity/ esophageal hypersensitivity		

[a]For all pathology, first objective is to rule out cardiopulmonary causes of chest pain with EKG, troponin, and any other indicated tests

Suggested Readings

1. Kohn GP, Dirks RC, Ansari MT, et al. SAGES guidelines for the use of peroral endoscopic myotomy (POEM) for the treatment of achalasia. Surg Endosc. 2021;35:1931–48. https://doi.org/10.1007/s00464-020-08282-0.
2. Daly S, Kumar SS, Collings AT, et al. SAGES guidelines for the surgical treatment of hiatal hernias. Surg Endosc. 2024;38:4765–75. https://doi.org/10.1007/s00464-024-11092-3.

Gastroesophageal Reflux Disease

5

Aayma Irfan, Amanda C. Purdy, and Shaun Daly

5.1 Presentation

5.1.1 Typical Symptoms

Typical esophageal symptoms of gastroesophageal reflux disease (GERD) include heartburn and regurgitation. Patients with heartburn may describe postprandial burning epigastric and/or chest pain. Those with regurgitation often describe a sensation of fluid or food regurgitating after eating, a sour taste in the back of their throat, and/or a globus sensation. Symptoms are often worse after eating or if the patient lies down or bends over too soon after eating. Symptoms may also be worsened after eating a large meal or after eating spicy or acidic foods.

A. Irfan
University of California Riverside School of Medicine, Riverside, CA, USA

A. C. Purdy · S. Daly (✉)
Department of Surgery, University of California Irvine Medical Center, Orange, CA, USA
e-mail: shaund@hs.uci.edu

G. P. Kohn et al. (eds.), *The SAGES Manual of Surgical Referral for Primary and Emergency Care*,
https://doi.org/10.1007/978-3-031-92678-5_5

5.1.2 Atypical Symptoms

Atypical, extraesophageal, symptoms of GERD occur due to irritation of structures other than the esophagus. The more common atypical symptoms include cough, wheezing, frequent throat clearing, belching, sore throat, hoarseness, and dental erosion. These cases pose a diagnostic challenge and may require further diagnostics to rule out alternative etiologies, particularly in the case of respiratory symptoms.

5.1.3 Alarm Symptoms

Alarm symptoms should clue practitioners into the possible development of GERD complications. These symptoms most commonly include dysphagia, early satiety, vomiting, unintentional weight loss, hematemesis, melena, and iron deficiency anemia. These may be signs of esophageal strictures, erosive esophagitis, or malignancy. In addition to initiating medical therapy for suspected GERD, these patients should undergo further workup with an upper gastrointestinal series and an esophagogastroduodenoscopy (EGD) and should prompt a surgical consultation.

5.2 Complications of GERD and Hiatal Hernias

5.2.1 Esophagitis

Untreated GERD commonly leads to esophagitis. Esophagitis varies in severity, from mild inflammation to more severe cases with large erosions. Over time, esophagitis can lead to occult gastrointestinal bleeding, Barrett's esophagus, strictures, and adenocarcinoma. Esophagitis is diagnosed with EGD, where the endoscopist will grade the esophagitis based on the Los Angeles (LA) classification. LA grade A is the least severe and LA grade D is the most severe. In cases of LA grade C and D esophagitis, gastroenterologists will often repeat an EGD after 8 weeks of medical therapy.

5.2.2 Esophageal Stricture

Esophageal strictures can be the result of long-standing GERD. Patients often present with dysphagia. The definitive diagnosis is made with EGD, which can be diagnostic and therapeutic. Initial management involves treating the patient's underlying GERD as well as endoscopic dilation to relieve the obstruction and ruling out malignancy. Many patients will require serial dilations. Patients with recurrent or nonhealing strictures despite appropriate medical management should be referred to a surgeon for consideration of an antireflux operation.

5.2.3 Barrett's Esophagus

Barrett's esophagus is a potential serious consequence of long-standing esophageal inflammation. Barrett's esophagus is defined as intestinal metaplasia of the esophagus, and it is associated with a higher risk of developing esophageal adenocarcinoma. Barrett's esophagus is diagnosed by EGD with biopsies. The endoscopist and pathologist will describe the length of the esophagus involved and if there is any dysplasia present (low- or high-grade). According to the American College of Gastroenterology (ACG) guidelines, patients with any evidence of dysplasia on pathology should undergo an endoscopic eradication procedure.

Regular endoscopic surveillance is required for those with Barrett's esophagus to screen for the advancement to adenocarcinoma. According to the ACG guidelines, the timing of repeat endoscopic surveillance depends on multiple factors, including the length of the Barrett's esophagus segment (short-segment is defined as <3 cm, long-segment is defined as ≥ 3 cm), whether or not dysplasia is present, the grade of dysplasia, and if an endoscopic eradication procedure was performed. Repeat surveillance EGD should be performed in 5 years for short-segment (<3 cm) Barrett's esophagus without dysplasia, and in 3 years for long-segment (≥ 3 cm) Barrett's esophagus without dysplasia. In Barrett's esophagus with low-grade dysplasia that did not undergo endoscopic eradication, surveillance EGD should be performed every 6 months for 1 year, then annually thereafter. In Barrett's esophagus with low-grade dysplasia that underwent endoscopic eradication, surveillance EGD should be performed after 1 year, then every 2 years thereafter. After endoscopic eradication of Barrett's esophagus with high-grade dysplasia, surveillance EGD should be performed at 3 months, 6 months, 12 months, then annually thereafter.

Patients with GERD and Barrett's esophagus should be managed initially with PPIs and lifestyle modifications. Barrett's esophagus alone is not an indication for an antireflux operation, and antireflux operations have not been definitively shown to decrease the risk of progression to cancer compared to medical management. However, many patients with Barrett's may require surgical management for refractory GERD. It is important to note that if a patient with Barrett's undergoes an antireflux operation they must continue endoscopic surveillance.

5.2.4 Esophageal Adenocarcinoma

Esophageal adenocarcinoma is a feared complication of long-standing GERD and can develop in the setting of Barrett's esophagus. It is essential to proceed with early endoscopic evaluation to evaluate for esophageal cancer in patients with alarm symptoms, including dysphagia, early satiety, iron deficiency anemia, or gastrointestinal bleeding.

5.2.5 Cameron's Ulcer

Cameron's ulcers are linear gastric mucosal erosions that occur in the setting of hiatal hernias, located at the diaphragm. This can cause upper gastrointestinal bleeding and iron deficiency anemia. If patients are diagnosed with a Cameron's ulcer and hiatal hernia on EGD, they should be referred to a surgeon in addition to initiating medical management for GERD.

5.2.6 Acute Gastric Volvulus

Gastric volvulus is an abnormal rotation of the stomach, which causes a closed-loop obstruction and may progress to gastric ischemia and perforation. This emergent complication can occur in patients with hiatal hernias. Patients often present with acute abdominal and/or chest pain, oral intolerance, nausea, and dry heaving. Patients with suspected gastric volvulus should be evaluated in the emergency department as prompt decompression and surgical management are essential to avoid gastric ischemia. Chest and abdominal X-ray can help clue clinicians into the diagnosis, which may show a large gastric bubble superior to the diaphragm. Upon the suspicion of gastric volvulus, a nasogastric tube should be inserted for decompression and urgent surgical consultation should be obtained.

5.3 Initial Management

The initial management for a patient with typical GERD symptoms and no alarm symptoms includes both lifestyle modifications and medical management.

5.3.1 Lifestyle Modification

Lifestyle modifications for the treatment of GERD include minimizing the modifiable GERD risk factors. This includes weight loss in patients with obesity, waiting 2–3 hours after eating prior to lying down, avoiding trigger foods, smoking cessation, and consuming smaller, more frequent meals.

5.3.2 Medical Management

Initial medical management for patients with GERD symptoms is an 8-week trial of daily proton pump inhibitor (PPI) therapy.

Patients should be counseled about the correct way to take a PPI: they should be taken in the morning, on an empty stomach, 30 min prior to eating or drinking. If patients have refractory GERD symptoms after an initial PPI trial, it is first important to ensure they are taking the PPI correctly. If patients are taking the PPI correctly, refractory GERD should prompt further diagnostic testing, including upper gastrointestinal series, EGD, and pH +/− impedance testing. If the diagnosis of GERD is confirmed, patients should be referred to a surgeon.

5.4 Diagnostic Testing

Three categories of diagnostic tests are available: those that help define anatomy, those that definitively diagnose GERD, and those that evaluate for esophageal dysmotility. Diagnostic testing available for GERD is summarized in Table 5.1. Most patients with typical GERD symptoms, without alarm symptoms, and without a contraindication to PPI therapy can be initially managed with lifestyle modifications and medications without the need for diagnostic testing.

There are cases where diagnostic testing is necessary. Patients with alarm symptoms that raise concern for malignancy should undergo upper gastrointestinal series (UGI) and EGD. Patients with atypical symptoms or those who do not respond to initial medical therapy should undergo confirmatory testing to evaluate for GERD. Patients who complain of dysphagia should undergo UGI and motility testing in addition to EGD to assess for partially obstructing lesions and/or motility disorders.

If referring a patient to a surgeon to be evaluated for an antireflux operation, basic diagnostic studies should be performed prior to surgical referral. All patients should have an upper gastrointestinal series (UGI) and esophagogastroduodenoscopy (EGD) completed prior to surgical referral. This may be sufficient in patients with large paraesophageal hernias where the primary goal of surgery is to address the hiatal hernia. However, the majority of patients being referred for an antireflux operation should have ambulatory pH +/− impedance testing to confirm the diagnosis of

Table 5.1 Summary of relevant diagnostic studies for patients with gastroesophageal reflux disease

Study	Description and logistics	Findings	Notes	Necessary to complete before surgical referral?
Studies that evaluate the anatomy and mucosa of the upper GI tract				
Upper gastrointestinal series (UGI)	In this study, performed by radiology, a patient drinks contrast while multiple X-rays are taken using fluoroscopy. The radiologist follows the contrast from the mouth, esophagus, stomach, and duodenum	UGI is most useful to see if a hiatal hernia is present It may also show reflux, abnormal esophageal motility, esophageal diverticuli, or filling defects that may indicate stricture or malignancy	In patients requiring further workup for GERD or requiring a surgical consultation, UGI and EGD are often the initial diagnostic studies UGI should be completed prior to surgical consultation	Yes, always
Upper endoscopy (EGD)	This study, performed by gastroenterologists (GI), involves the direct visual inspection of the esophageal, gastric, and proximal duodenal mucosa. Biopsies may be taken. Sedation or anesthesia is required.	EGD is useful to diagnose hiatal hernias, esophagitis, Barrett's esophagus, strictures, malignancy, and gastritis EGD may also be therapeutic, such as in the setting of strictures (that can be endoscopically dilated)	EGD should be completed prior to surgical consultation for an antireflux operation Also indicated in patients with alarm symptoms that raise concern for underlying malignancy, or in patients that don't respond appropriately to initial PPI therapy	Yes, always

(continued)

Table 5.1 (continued)

Study	Description and logistics	Findings	Notes	Necessary to complete before surgical referral?
Studies that confirm the diagnosis of GERD				
Ambulatory pH testing	This can use a catheter-based system or a wireless capsule. In the former, a catheter is placed through the nose into the stomach, and in the latter, a small wireless, pH-sensing capsule is clipped to the distal esophagus during endoscopy. This capsule will fall off and pass through the GI tract on its own For both techniques, patients have a receiver with a button that they press when they experience symptoms, as well as a symptom diary The data is reviewed and includes tracking symptoms, along with esophageal acid exposure, for 48 h For accurate results, PPIs must be held 7 days prior to the study, and H2 blockers must be held 48 h prior to the study	The report will have a "DeMeester score," which if greater than 14.72, is considered consistent with pathologic GERD. A second assessment is acid exposure time (AET) that should be less than 4%. It will also have a symptom association probability, which helps discern which specific symptoms are most likely due to the patient's reflux	This is a useful study to confirm (or rule out) the presence of GERD, especially in a patient with atypical symptoms Logistically, if you are referring a patient for an EGD for GERD evaluation, ambulatory pH wireless capsule testing might be requested at the same time so the patient doesn't have to undergo a repeat endoscopy In patients with severe symptoms when off medication, clinicians can consider switching from PPI to H2 blocker 7 days prior to the study, then holding the H2 blocker 48 h prior to the study	Yes, most of the time (when is it not needed: If the patient has known LA grade C or D esophagitis, or in the case of a large paraesophageal hernia, where the GERD is not the indication to repair)

Impedance testing	This procedure involves placing a small catheter through the nose into the esophagus, where it remains in place for 24 h. The study uses impedance measurements to see if reflux is present. The patient keeps a receiver with them and a diary to record symptoms Similar to pH testing, PPIs should be held for 7 days and H2 blockers for 48 h prior to testing.	The report will show if the patient has pathologic reflux, and how their symptoms correlate One benefit over testing for pH alone is that it can diagnose all reflux, even in the absence of acid reflux. This includes bile reflux.	Similar to pH testing, it is a useful study to confirm (or rule out) the presence of GERD, especially in a patient with atypical symptoms Impedance testing is often more uncomfortable for patients than pH monitoring Impedance testing is favored in patients with GERD that doesn't improve with PPI (indicating that they may have non-acid reflux), and in patients with altered gastric anatomy (such as a prior Whipple or partial gastrectomy, as they are predisposed to bile reflux).	No, usually not (it may be helpful in patients where bile reflux is suspected)

(continued)

Table 5.1 (continued)

Study	Description and logistics	Findings	Notes	Necessary to complete before surgical referral?
Studies to evaluate for motility disorders				
High-resolution manometry	In this procedure, a catheter with pressure sensors along its length is placed into the nose, through the esophagus, and into the stomach. After the catheter is placed, the patient performs a series of swallows, while the catheter measures the pressure along the esophagus. The catheter is then removed. This does not require sedation or anesthesia	This study will show if there is any evidence of esophageal dysmotility. It is also the gold standard in diagnosis of achalasia, which may mimic the symptoms of GERD	Ruling out esophageal motility disorders is important prior to surgical management of GERD. They are particularly important in patients who endorse dysphagia Many patients complain that this test is uncomfortable. This includes the placement itself, which is similar to nasogastric tube placement, as well as swallowing with the catheter in place	Yes, most of the time (especially important in patients who endorse dysphagia)

EndoFLIP	This procedure is performed at the same time as endoscopy. It uses a balloon attached to a catheter to measure the diameter and distensibility of the esophagus. The patient does not need to actively swallow as in manometry. This is performed when the patient is sedated during EGD	This study will show if there is any evidence of esophageal dysmotility. It may be helpful in diagnosing achalasia	EndoFLIP is better tolerated in patients than manometry as it can be done while the patient is sedated for EGD If referring a patient for surgical evaluation, it may be helpful to order EGD, pH monitoring, and EndoFLIP together as they can all be performed in the same procedure	No, usually not

pathologic GERD. The information from these studies can help set expectations for symptomatic improvement after an antireflux operation. Studies to confirm the diagnosis of GERD are typically not necessary prior to surgery in patients with LA grade C or D esophagitis or Barrett's esophagus since these are pathognomonic of GERD. In addition, many patients referred to surgery will undergo esophageal motility testing with either manometry or EndoFLIP. This is especially important for patients who endorse dysphagia. These studies are important to rule out achalasia, which can mimic the symptoms of GERD and requires a different operative approach. Motility testing also helps surgeons determine which surgical intervention to offer. Some surgeons will tailor the extent of the fundoplication (i.e., complete or partial fundoplication) to preoperative motility studies, and only patients with normal esophageal motility are candidates for magnetic lower esophageal augmentation.

5.5 When to Refer the Patient for Surgical Evaluation

A summary of when GERD can be managed by primary care, what requires surgical referral, what should be referred to gastroenterology (GI), and what constitutes an emergency is summarized below and in Table 5.2.

5.5.1 Failure of Medical Management

Failure of medical management is defined as no improvement, partial improvement, residual GERD complications (such as esophagitis), or recurrent/nonhealing stricture despite optimal medical therapy for 6–8 weeks. When failure of medical management is suspected, clinicians should first ensure patients are taking their PPI correctly.

It is important to note that patients with typical GERD symptoms that respond to PPI therapy significantly benefit from an antireflux operation as their symptoms are most likely a direct

Table 5.2 Summary of when GERD can be managed by primary care physician and when referrals should be made to a surgeon, gastroenterologist, or emergency department

Clinical scenario	PCP management	Should the patient be referred to GI?	Should the patient be referred to a surgeon?	Should the patient be sent to the emergency department?
GERD without alarm symptoms and without a hiatal hernia	Daily PPI Lifestyle modifications	No	No	No
GERD without alarm symptoms, with a sliding hiatal hernia	Daily PPI Lifestyle modifications Inform the patient that surgical options are available	Sometimes, for EGD and bravo—Only if the patient prefers surgical over medical management, or has a contraindication to long-term PPI use	Sometimes: If the patient prefers surgical over medical management, has a contraindication to long-term PPI use, or would like to discuss surgical options	No
GERD with alarm symptoms	Daily PPI Lifestyle modifications Order UGI	Yes, for endoscopic evaluation	Probably: Depending on findings on workup (UGI, endoscopy, and GI evaluation)	Only if hemodynamically unstable, acute gastrointestinal bleed, or inability to tolerate oral intake

(continued)

Table 5.2 (continued)

Clinical scenario	PCP management	Should the patient be referred to GI?	Should the patient be referred to a surgeon?	Should the patient be sent to the emergency department?
GERD that does not respond to 8 weeks of medical management	Ensure patients are taking the PPI correctly Order UGI Consider other diagnoses and initiate workup if applicable	Yes, for EGD and bravo	Yes, if the diagnosis of GERD is confirmed	No
Large hiatal hernia	Daily PPI Lifestyle modifications Order UGI	Yes, for EGD	Yes	No
Symptoms of acute gastric volvulus (nausea, retching)	Send patient to ER	No	Yes	Yes

result of GERD. Patients with no or minimal symptomatic improvement with optimal PPI therapy should have confirmatory diagnostic testing with ambulatory pH monitoring or impedance testing prior to surgical referral. If pathologic reflux is confirmed, patients should be referred to a surgeon to discuss an antireflux operation.

5.5.2 When Long-Term Medical Management Is Not Appropriate

There are two situations in which long-term medical management may not be appropriate. First, in patients with osteoporosis since long-term PPI therapy is associated with an increased risk of osteoporotic fracture. Clinicians should consider early surgical referral in these patients. In addition, many patients prefer to avoid long-term medical management with daily pills requiring a strict schedule to be effective. It is important for primary care providers to counsel patients and inform them that surgery is an alternative to long-term medical management.

5.5.3 When the Primary Symptom Is Regurgitation

Some patients' chief complaint is regurgitation. Those patients with both heartburn and regurgitation may see an improvement in their heartburn symptoms with PPI therapy, but still suffer from regurgitation. While PPIs ensure the gastric contents refluxing back into the esophagus is not acidic, they do not correct anatomic abnormalities (such as hiatal hernias) that result in the regurgitation itself. These patients, especially in the setting of a hiatal hernia, should be referred for surgical consultation.

5.5.4 Large, Symptomatic Hiatal Hernia

Medical management and lifestyle modifications alone are often sufficient to treat GERD in the setting of a small sliding hiatal hernia. Patients with larger paraesophageal hernias may have symptoms resulting from their altered anatomy and warrant surgical consultation. Symptoms of early satiety, oral intolerance, nausea, and vomiting can occur as a result of the mid-stomach being compressed by the diaphragm, causing slow passage of ingested contents through the hiatus. Another possible manifestation of a symptomatic hiatal hernia on EGD is Cameron's erosions, which is a source of upper gastrointestinal bleeding. The primary goal of surgery in these cases is to reduce the stomach (and other herniated abdominal structures) back into the abdomen to allow healing.

5.5.5 Acute Gastric Volvulus

Gastric volvulus is a complication of hiatal hernias that requires urgent management to avoid gastric ischemia and perforation. These patients should be sent to the emergency department for nasogastric decompression, resuscitation, and urgent surgical consultation.

Suggested Readings

1. Slater BJ, Collings A, Dirks R, et al. Multi-society consensus conference and guideline on the treatment of gastroesophageal reflux disease (GERD). Surg Endosc. 2023;37(2):781–806. https://doi.org/10.1007/s00464-022-09817-3.
2. Slater BJ, Dirks RC, McKinley SK, et al. SAGES guidelines for the surgical treatment of gastroesophageal reflux (GERD). Surg Endosc. 2021;35(9):4903–17. https://doi.org/10.1007/s00464-021-08625-5.

3. Katz PO, Dunbar KB, Schnoll-Sussman FH, Greer KB, Yadlapati R, Spechler SJ. ACG clinical guideline for the diagnosis and management of gastroesophageal reflux disease. Am J Gastroenterol. 2022;117(1):27–56. https://doi.org/10.14309/ajg.0000000000001538.
4. Shaheen NJ, Falk GW, Iyer PG, et al. Diagnosis and management of Barrett's esophagus: an updated ACG guideline. Am J Gastroenterol. 2022;117(4):559–87. https://doi.org/10.14309/ajg.0000000000001680.

6 Nonreflux Emesis: Bilious and Nonbilious in Adults

Alexandra Ibewuike, Jenny M. Guido, and Crystal Totten

6.1 Introduction

The etiology of emesis can be bundled into the four major biochemical pathways that lead to vomiting. These pathways include involvement of the cerebral cortex due to increased intracranial pressure, the vestibular apparatus via inner ear dysfunction, activation of chemoreceptor trigger zones from toxins or medications, and activation via the gastrointestinal tract. This chapter will primarily focus on the gastrointestinal pathways triggering emesis via endoluminal dilation of the gut from obstruction, ingested toxins, mucosal inflammation, or ulceration. However, the ability to rule out other pathways is important in the patient's evaluation and ultimately the correct diagnosis. Primary testing strategies and when to refer to a surgeon or endoscopist will be categorized using emergent, urgent and nonurgent descriptors, and probable diagnosis.

A. Ibewuike · C. Totten (✉)
Department of Surgery, University of Kentucky, Lexington, KY, USA
e-mail: crystal.totten@uky.edu

J. M. Guido
Department of Surgery, University of South Dakota Sanford School of Medicine, Sioux Falls, SD, USA

G. P. Kohn et al. (eds.), *The SAGES Manual of Surgical Referral for Primary and Emergency Care*,
https://doi.org/10.1007/978-3-031-92678-5_6

6.2 Defining Details

Obtaining a thorough history is required to it patient symptoms, to understand the timing and possible urgency of treatment, and to determine which of the above pathways causes emesis.

Clarity in the description of patient symptoms can act as a window into the cause of emesis.

Emesis, or vomiting, is the result of contents from the stomach traversing out the mouth due to gastric muscular contraction. The force can vary depending on the cause. Projectile vomiting describes quick, forceful episodes that travel a few feet from the body. Nonprojectile emesis refers to emptying of the stomach with less force, urgency, and distance. Regurgitation refers to passive, retrograde movement of esophageal or gastric contents up through the mouth without diaphragmatic or gastric muscular contraction. This can often be initiated by bending over promptly after a meal for those with a hiatal hernia or poor esophageal emptying. Retching is the result of repetitive spasmodic contraction of the abdomen; however, no contents pass a closed glottis leaving the body.

The quality of the emesis should be elucidated and can help narrow a differential diagnosis. Emesis may consist of whole food or partially digested food contents and may be nonbilious or bilious depending upon where along the proximal gastrointestinal (GI) tract the problem arises. Emesis of whole food is commonly seen with esophageal narrowing or a hiatal hernia. Whole food is promptly expelled from the GI tract and may occur immediately following consumption. Expulsion of partially digested food contents occurs with gastroparesis, proximal obstruction, reaction to a toxin, or bulimia. Nonbilious emesis from a source proximal to the Ampulla of Vater (second portion of the duodenum) can be caused by obstruction near the pylorus, gastritis, ulcers, motion sickness, food poisoning, or viral gastroenteritis. Alternatively, bilious emesis (output includes contents distal to the Ampulla of Vater containing bile) can be present due to a distal obstruction, biliary disease, repetitive emesis, or infection. If emesis is described as feculent, concern for more chronic or distal intestinal obstruction is raised.

The duration of symptoms is important for narrowing down the etiology. It may be easier to identify a cause when a patient experiences acute symptoms less than 24 hours or 1 week. However, as symptoms become more chronic, it is important to elucidate the frequency, severity of events, and associated symptoms.

Once you have a good understanding of the quality and quantity of the emesis, the following questions or relationships should be elucidated:

- Could the patient be pregnant?
- Have they experienced this before? If so, what was the cause?
- Is emesis preceded by nausea?
- Is there accompanying dysphagia or changes in voice?
- If emesis is related to food intake, assess the time relationship with intake and emesis.
- Is there associated abdominal pain? If yes, ask severity and location and if there is relief with emesis or not.
- Have they experienced unintended weight loss? If yes, quantify amount and duration.
- Are there changes in bowel function? Ask about melena, obstipation, diarrhea, and hematochezia.
- Have they had an endoscopy or colonoscopy?
- Is there a personal history of prior abdominal surgeries, inflammatory bowel disease, hernias, diabetes, liver, or kidney disease?
- Is there a family history of gastric, pancreatic, colon cancer, or neurologic disorders?
- Obtain a substance abuse history (alcohol, tobacco, marijuana/cannabinoids).
- Are there exposures to toxins (alcohol, iron, aspirin, lead, arsenic, insecticides), food sources, nonprescription supplements, sick contacts, recent radiation or chemotherapy?
- Have they started any new medications or undergone dose changes (consider medication side effects, i.e., metformin, GLP-1 agonist, digoxin, estrogen, antibiotics, opioids, antidepressants)?

- Are there urinary symptoms, such as polyuria or dysuria? If yes, rule out urinary tract infection.
- Is there concern for untreated anxiety/depression, vomiting related to stress, risk factors of self-induced vomiting? If yes, consider directed management of these disorders.
- Is there an associated migraine, headache, or change in mental status? If yes, rule out increases in intracranial pressure and cerebral cortex pathway dysfunction.
- Is there associated motion sickness, hearing loss/ringing, dizziness, or syncope? If yes, rule out vestibular apparatus pathway dysfunction.
- Is there association with acute chest or arm pain? If yes, rule out myocardial infarction.

6.3 Initial Triage and Identifying Alarm Signs

While a head-to-toe physical exam is ideal to complete for all patients, determining hydration status and obtaining vital signs is paramount to recognizing urgent scenarios. Assessment of hydration status should include evaluating for skin turgor, dry mucous membranes, increased respiratory rate, fruity odor to the breath, obtaining baseline vital signs, and calculating orthostatic blood pressure in the setting of persistent emesis or poor oral intake. A rectal exam should be performed, with consent, if a patient reports melena or hematochezia. Blood glucose levels are important to obtain in the office to rule out diabetic ketoacidosis or hypoglycemia. For those presenting with chest pain as an associated symptom, an electrocardiogram is a necessary time-sensitive step to rule out myocardial ischemia. Patients with neurologic or vestibular symptoms need a focused neurologic exam, Dix–Hallpike maneuver, Weber and Rinne hearing tests, and gait assessment for postural instability. The presence of lymphadenopathy, jaundice, and abdominal masses should be noted if concern for malignancy if present. Evaluation for obstruction should include visualizing prior surgical scars with inspection and palpation of the abdomen

Table 6.1 "Alarm signs"

Age older than 55 years	Evidence of gastrointestinal bleeding	Abdominal pain
Unintended weight loss	Family history of gastric cancer	Feculent vomiting
Progressive dysphagia	Altered mental status	Hematochezia, melena
Persistent vomiting	Severe headache	Focal neurologic defect

for distention or hernias. For any hernias identified on examination, bedside reduction efforts must be attempted if there are no overlying skin changes or associated fevers.

"Alarm Signs," coined by Anderson et al. in the American Academy of Family Physicians paper on Evaluating Nausea and Emesis, are factors that would increase your index of suspicion for an acute process requiring further imaging or biochemical evaluation. These are defined, but not limited to, in Table 6.1.

Alarm signs paired with abnormal vital signs, orthostatic hypotension, severe abdominal pain, uncontrollable projectile emesis, altered mental status, hyperglycemia with fruity breath suspiscious for ketoacidosis, or incarcerated or strangulated hernias are considered an emergent diagnosis and need to be referred to the closest emergency room for prompt biochemical testing and imaging assessment.

Urgent and nonurgent scenarios can have variable chronicity of symptoms. A focus on the patient's ability to remain hydrated and tolerance of accompanying pain permits outpatient evaluation to dictate treatment and guides specialty consultation.

6.4 Acute Nausea and Emesis, Duration Less Than 1 Week

The first step is to rule out and treat etiologies of emesis that are clear from the patient's history. Persons of childbearing potential must be tested for pregnancy prior to radiographic imaging. Acute 24–48-hour duration of projectile emesis will be more consistent with exposure to toxins, a food source, recent radiation, chemotherapy, or sick contacts. Acute nonprojectile emesis is more commonly associated with viral illnesses, urinary tract infection, or due to medication reactions and side effects. Patients with alarm signs should be sent to the emergency room for rapid further evaluation. Those without alarm signs can undergo urgent outpatient biochemical evaluation, including urinalysis, complete blood count (CBC), comprehensive metabolic panel (CMP), lipase, C-reactive protein (CRP), thyroid-stimulating hormone (TSH), and stool studies, if diarrhea is an associated symptom.

Laboratory abnormalities need to be treated accordingly along with source elimination and rehydration. Those able to tolerate oral intake without alarm signs initiate supportive care including antiemetics, oral hydration, and education on worsening symptoms. Those who fail supportive care and cannot tolerate oral intake require IV rehydration and should be referred for these resources.

6.5 Acute Symptoms with Abdominal Pain/Distension

Patients without etiologies described in the above section whose emesis is accompanied by abdominal pain or distension need further diagnostic laboratory and radiographic testing. Pathophysiology causing acute, severe abdominal pain includes perforated viscus, high-grade bowel obstructions, incarcerated hernias, pancreatitis, or acute cholecystitis/appendicitis. These commonly have associated alarm signs requiring emergent evaluation with surgical consultation as indicated.

Patients remaining hemodynamically stable with mild-to-moderate pain or abdominal distension and able to maintain oral hydration will need outpatient urgent CBC, CMP, C-reactive protein (CRP), lipase, and radiographic imaging (Table 6.2) to aid in diagnosis.

Abdominal radiographs can yield important information regarding ileus, obstruction, or kidney stones. The probability of correctly diagnosing a bowel obstruction on plain X-rays has been

Table 6.2 Pain and distension workup checklist

	Pain and distension workup list
☐	Hernias, if present, are reducible
☐	CBC
☐	CMP
☐	Lipase
☐	CRP
☐	Abdominal X-ray
☐	Focused US or CT abdomen/pelvis

studied. By combining any two of the six most common patient factors (distended abdomen, increased bowel sounds, history of constipation, previous abdominal surgery, age over 50, and vomiting), the probability of a correct diagnosis of bowel obstruction is threefold over a single patient factor. The combination of three of the above patient factors increases prognostic probability by at least fivefold.

Focused ultrasound (US), such as right upper quadrant (RUQ) ultrasound, is used when patients have RUQ pain or biliary colic is suspected. Focused US of hernias can be used if defect is reducible and less than 3 cm to determine the size and characteristics of the contents. Focused ultrasound also may have utility in diagnosing abdominal free fluid resulting from a perforated viscus.

Computed tomography (CT) of the abdomen and pelvis should be used in the urgent moderate pain scenario to rule out inflammatory bowel disease, diverticulitis, appendicitis, larger hernias with obstructions, etc. The use of intravenous (IV) contrast is dependent on the patient's renal function; however, it is generally preferred to evaluate perfusion, detect an abscess or mass, and allow for improved delineation of intraabdominal structures. Oral contrast is preferred in outpatient settings if oral intake can be tolerated to determine the location of obstruction or enteric association with a hernia when present.

Abnormal biochemical or radiographic results are to be treated accordingly. Patients diagnosed in the urgent outpatient setting with cholecystitis, appendicitis, perforated diverticulitis, or an acute bowel obstruction require urgent surgical referral with a direct provider-to-provider conversation. Most of these cases will result in hospital admission and prompt surgical intervention. If this cannot be achieved, the patient should be referred to emergency room for expedited care.

Diagnosis such as inflammatory bowel disease and nonperforated diverticulitis require medical management and referral to a gastroenterologist for endoscopy prior to consideration of surgical referral, as detailed later in the chapter.

6.6 Chronic Nausea and Emesis

Individuals with chronic nausea and emesis with symptoms lasting greater than one month are still assessed for alarm signs and, if present, referred for emergency department evaluation. Many patients, by nature of the chronicity of symptoms, can undergo elective, outpatient testing. Ruling out pregnancy, toxin ingestion, medication side effects, and obtaining a thorough neuropsychiatric history are important. Patients with neurologic changes or signs of vestibular dysfunction need inner ear evaluation as described in the initial triage and exam. If positive vestibular findings, this subset of patients warrants CT or magnetic resonance imaging (MRI) of the head to rule out vascular or inner ear pathology.

The initial workup for chronic nausea and emesis includes CBC, CMP, magnesium, phosphate, Hemoglobin A1C (HgbA1C), thyroid stimulating hormone, and abdominal radiograph (Table 6.3). Secondary testing is differentiated by nonbilious and bilious quality as well as associated symptoms to narrow the diagnosis.

Chronic nonbilious emesis suggests a source for the emesis proximal to Ampulla of Vater. Patients who report bloating but can remain hydrated and experience a large volume emesis of partially or undigested food consumed days prior should be evaluated for gastric outlet obstruction. A KUB may reveal significant gastric dilation, and this finding necessitates a CT Abdomen/Pelvis with oral as tolerated and IV contrast to diagnose dilation, mass, or significant food bezoar. Urgent surgical referral for management is required.

Table 6.3 Chronic nausea and emesis workup checklist

	Chronic nausea and emesis workup list
☐	CBC
☐	CMP
☐	Magnesium
☐	Phosphate
☐	HgbA1C
☐	Thyroid-stimulating hormone
☐	Abdominal X-ray

Patients with suspected gastroparesis will have nonbilious emesis of partially digested foods. They tolerate liquids more than solids, and can experience significant unintentional weight loss, recurrent episodes of dehydration, or electrolyte disturbances. Medications that can delay gastric emptying should be discontinued, including: opioids; calcium channel blockers; progesterone; anticholinergic; and GLP-1 agonists. Delayed gastric emptying can also occur with cannabis and nicotine use; poorly controlled diabetes mellitus; neuromuscular disorders including Parkinson's disease, multiple sclerosis, amyloidosis Ehlers–Danlos, and scleroderma; or from prior injury to the vagus nerve from hiatal surgery or cardiac ablation. Patients may have an elevated HgbA1c. A fluid-filled stomach may be noted on abdominal radiograph, increasing the probability of this diagnosis that is confirmed by a gastric emptying study and nonurgent referral for an upper endoscopy.

Patients with concern for a hiatal hernia, and likely associated with reflux, may vomit portions of their meal that are undigested or partially digested. They also may report regurgitation. Their initial labs are often within normal limits, but mild anemia may be present if the hernia is associated with Cameron's ulcerations. Patients may have an air bubble above the diaphragm on chest X-ray (CXR) or KUB. This diagnosis is best confirmed by a fluoroscopic upper GI study with subsequent referral to a gastroenterologist or surgical endoscopist for an upper endoscopy. If patient fails an antiacid medication trial and behavior modifications, refer in a nonurgent pathway to a surgeon.

Chronic bilious emesis is due to source distal to the Ampulla of Vater. Patients with a partial or low-grade bowel obstruction from a mass, adhesions in the setting of prior surgeries, or reducible hernias can present with chronic bilious and infrequently feculent emesis. Abdominal radiographs will demonstrate dilated loops of bowel and laboratory values can be normal in patients sustaining hydration. An outpatient CT Abdomen/Pelvis with oral and IV contrast should be obtained to aid in diagnosis prior to surgical referral.

Patients with recurrent bilious or nonbilious emesis associated with RUQ pain need a RUQ US to rule out symptomatic cholelithiasis or chronic cholecystitis. If RUQ US is negative, then a hepatobiliary iminodiacetic acid (HIDA) scan with calculated ejection fraction should be obtained prior to surgical referral.

In the setting of low-grade chronic abdominal pain, managed without narcotics, a CT Abdomen/Pelvis with oral and IV contrast should be obtained to evaluate vasculature, as well as bowel gas pattern to rule out diverticulitis, inflammatory bowel disease, or vascular calcifications causing inflow reduction prior to general surgery referral. Direct referral to vascular surgery is recommended if mesenteric calcifications or chronic mesenteric ischemia are diagnosed. If diverticulitis or inflammatory bowel disease is diagnosed, the patient will need a colonoscopy by a surgeon or gastroenterologist.

6.7 Referral Destinations

The supportive testing and timeline for surgical referral have been described in the preceding sections and is summarized in the table below. The urgency of referral and evaluation directly relates to the patient's hemodynamic status, acuity, alarm signs, and ability to maintain nutrition.

When to refer to a surgeon	
Emergent, via emergency room	Acute emesis, severe abdominal pain with radiographic evidence of intraabdominal pathology Perforated viscus Acute cholecystitis/appendicitis High-grade bowel obstruction Nonreducible hernia with or without emesis
Urgent	Acute emesis, mild–moderate pain, maintaining hydration Low-grade bowel obstruction Acute cholecystitis/appendicitis Microperforated diverticulitis Chronic emesis with recurrent dehydration Gastric outlet obstruction Chronic cholecystitis Newly diagnosed mass
Nonurgent	Chronic emesis over months, primarily painless Hiatal hernia or reflux Biliary colic, biliary dyskinesia, or chronic cholecystitis Reducible hernia Chronic partial obstruction/adhesions Chronic mesenteric ischemia (referral to vascular surgeon directly)
Nonurgent referral to otolaryngology (ENT)	Emesis with vestibular symptoms Vertigo, Meniere's disease, labyrinthitis Patients with abnormal Dix–Hallpike maneuver or weber and Rinne hearing tests Patients with inner ear or head and neck pathology on CT/MRI head
When to refer to a gastroenterologist for endoscopic evaluation	
Emergent, via emergency room	Acute emesis with evidence of gastrointestinal bleeding
Urgent	Acute bilious emesis, mild–moderate pain, maintaining hydration Inflammatory bowel disease Nonperforated diverticulitis

(continued)

When to refer to a gastroenterologist for endoscopic evaluation	
Nonurgent	Chronic emesis with or without mild abdominal pain Concerns for ulcer disease or reflux, nonbilious emesis Nonbilious emesis or regurgitation concerned for esophageal dysmotility or stricture Nonbilious partially digested food with history or medication consistent with gastroparesis confirmed by nuclear medicine gastric emptying test Bilious emesis with blood per rectum, rule out colon malignancy

Suggested Readings

1. Tome J, Kamboj AK, Sweetser S. A practical 5-step approach to nausea and vomiting. Mayo Clin Proc. 2022;97(3):600–8. https://doi.org/10.1016/j.mayocp.2021.10.030. PMID: 35246289
2. Anderson WD 3rd, Strayer SM. Evaluation of nausea and vomiting: a case-based approach. Am Fam Physician. 2013;88(6):371–9. Erratum in: Am Fam Physician. 2013 Dec 1;88(11):728. Erratum in: Am Fam Physician. 2014 Feb 1;89(3):152. PMID: 24134044
3. Frese T, Klauss S, Herrmann K, Sandholzer H. Nausea and vomiting as the reasons for encounter in general practice. J Clin Med Res. 2011;3(1):23–9. https://doi.org/10.4021/jocmr410w. PMID: 22043268; PMCID: PMC3194022
4. Bohner H, Yang Q, Franke C, Verreet PR, Ohmann C, the Study Group Acute Abdominal Pain. Simple data from history and physical examination help to exclude bowel obstruction and to avoid radiographic studies in patient with acute abdominal pain. Eur J Surg. 1998;164:777–84. https://doi.org/10.1080/110241598750005435. Reviewed/Revised Jan 2022 | Modified Dec 2023

7 Vomiting in Children

Sophia M. V. Schermerhorn, Joseph Lee,
and Romeo C. Ignacio Jr

S. M. V. Schermerhorn · J. Lee
Department of Surgery, Naval Medical Center San Diego,
San Diego, CA, USA

R. C. Ignacio Jr (✉)
Department of Surgery, University of California San Diego School of
Medicine, La Jolla, CA, USA
e-mail: r1ignacio@health.ucsd.edu

G. P. Kohn et al. (eds.), *The SAGES Manual of Surgical Referral for Primary and Emergency Care*,
https://doi.org/10.1007/978-3-031-92678-5_7

7.1 Neonates and Infants (from Birth to 2 Years of Age)

7.1.1 History and Exam

Emesis in the neonatal period warrants close attention since this can be the first harbinger of a congenitally dysfunctional or obstructed gastrointestinal system. Thorough patient histories should include birth history and gestational age, the existence of any documented congenital abnormalities, feeding patterns, and stooling history. The distinction between bilious and nonbilious emesis is especially important. The presence of biliary emesis warrants thorough investigation in the newborn period as the primary symptom of obstructive pathologies outlined below and generally warrants immediate surgical referral. Furthermore, comprehensive physical examinations should include discernment of any external morphologic abnormalities that may indicate an underlying congenital syndrome.

Laboratory tests to consider:

- Complete blood count (CBC): hemoglobin/hematocrit, white blood count with differential, and platelets
- Complete metabolic panel (CMP): sodium, potassium, chloride, bicarb, creatinine, BUN, magnesium, phosphorus
- Liver function test (LFTs): should include bilirubin (both direct and indirect), transaminases, venous lactate level

7.1.2 Imaging

7.1.2.1 Abdominal Radiography [4]

Abdominal radiography (two views: upright and supine recommended) is an appropriate initial imaging technique for all pediatric patients with emesis [4]. Abdominal radiography can be diagnostic or direct the next appropriate imaging study. Both supine and upright views are preferred for evaluating gas patterns and free air. If an upright view cannot be obtained, the left-lateral decubitus view can be a suitable alternative. The prone view can also be utilized if additional information is needed to look for a rectal gas pattern, which may be absent in the case of obstruction.

7.1.2.2 Upper GI Series [4]

An upper gastrointestinal (UGI) series is a contrast-mediated evaluation of upper gastrointestinal tract anatomy to evaluate sources of proximal intestinal obstruction. Dilute barium is the preferred contrast agent for this study unless there is a suspicion of intestinal perforation. This study allows for the evaluation of the anatomy of the upper gastrointestinal (GI) tract to include the location of the duodenal jejunal junction (DJJ), an important anatomic landmark in the workup for malrotation. Both anteroposterior (AP) and lateral views are important when obtaining a UGI.

7.1.2.3 Contrast Enema [4]

Like the UGI series, a contrast enema is a useful study for evaluating the colon and rectum. The choice of contrast agent differs depending on the indication for the study. When used for diagnostic purposes, a water-soluble contrast agent such as iothalamate meglumine is first used. For therapeutic purposes, other contrast agents such as gastrograffin, a high osmolarity agent, or air can be leveraged depending on the purpose and will be discussed separately.

7.1.3 Differential Diagnosis

- Infectious
  - Neonatal sepsis
- Necrotizing enterocolitis (outside the scope of this chapter)
- Spontaneous intestinal perforation
  - Metabolic disorders
  - Inborn errors of metabolism
- Upper GI obstruction
  - Tracheoesophageal fistula
  - Hypertrophic pyloric stenosis

  - Malrotation with midgut volvulus
  - Duodenal obstruction
  - Jejunoileal atresia
  - Abdominal mass
  - Umbilical hernia (discussed in the *Children* section)
  - Inguinal hernia (discussed in the *Children* section)
- Lower GI obstruction
  - Meconium ileus
  - Colonic atresia
  - Anorectal malformation
  - Hirschsprung's disease
  - Other causes
- Gastroesophageal reflux
- Food allergies (e.g., milk allergy)
- Trauma
- Nonaccidental trauma

Can be managed by PCP	Requires emergency room evaluation (ERE)	Requires ERE + surgical review	Should get outpatient referral to other specialists
Neonates and infants			
Gastroesophageal reflux Food allergies	Neonatal sepsis	Spontaneous intestinal perforation Hypertrophic pyloric stenosis Malrotation with midgut volvulus Duodenal obstruction Obstructive/incarcerated umbilical hernia Obstructive/incarcerated inguinal hernia Trauma Nonaccidental trauma Colonic atresia Hirschsprung's disease Anorectal malformation	Metabolic disorders Inborn errors of metabolism Nonobstructive umbilical hernia (outpatient surgical referral) Nonobstructive inguinal hernia (outpatient surgical referral) Meconium ileus

Can be managed by PCP	Requires emergency room evaluation (ERE)	Requires ERE + surgical review	Should get outpatient referral to other specialists
Children			
Viral infections Urinary tract infection Constipation Anxiety Food allergies	Diabetic ketoacidosis Electrolyte abnormalities Increased intracranial pressure Toxin/poisons	Intussusception Appendicitis Obstructive/incarcerated umbilical hernia Obstructive/incarcerated inguinal hernia Meckel's diverticulum Foreign body ingestion Abdominal mass	Metabolic disorders (medicine) Eosinophilic esophagitis (gastroenterology) Inflammatory bowel disease (gastroenterology) Nonobstructive umbilical hernia (outpatient surgical referral) Nonobstructive inguinal hernia (outpatient surgical referral)
Adolescents			
Psychological Medication side effects Pregnancy Ruptured ovarian cyst Viral gastroenteritis	DKA Ectopic pregnancy Pelvic inflammatory disease Nephrolithiasis Pancreatitis	Ovarian/testicular torsion Small bowel obstruction Appendicitis Cholecystitis Obstructive/incarcerated umbilical hernia Obstructive/incarcerated inguinal hernia	Cyclical vomiting disorder (gastroenterology) Eating disorder (psychiatry) Inflammatory bowel disease (gastroenterology)

Hypertrophic pyloric stenosis	Abdominal ultrasound CMP
Malrotation with midgut volvulus	Lactate CBC Upper GI series
Duodenal obstruction	Lactate CBC Upper GI
Hernia	Clinical exam
Trauma	Pending mechanism—ATLS principles
Nonaccidental trauma	Skeletal series, CPS Other tests pending symptoms and mechanism
Colonic atresia	Contrast enema
Hirschsprung's disease	Contrast enema
Anorectal malformation	Based on exam
Abdominal mass	MRI or CT
Intussusception	Abdominal ultrasound
Appendicitis	Abdominal ultrasound MRI abdomen/pelvis if nondiagnostic CBC
Meckel's diverticulum	CBC Meckel's scan (if bleeding presentation) Abdominal radiography (if obstructive symptoms)
Foreign body ingestion	Abdominal radiography CBC
Ovarian/testicular torsion	Pelvis/testicular ultrasound CBC
Small bowel obstruction	Abdominal radiography CBC CMP Lactate
Cholecystitis	RUQ ultrasound CBC Liver function tests

7.1.4 Surgical Conditions

7.1.4.1 Tracheoesophageal Fistula

Tracheoesophageal fistula (TEF) constitutes a spectrum of malformations arising from the incomplete formation and separation of the trachea and esophagus during foregut development. It exhibits a strong correlation with additional congenital anomalies, including Trisomy 13, 18, and 21 (present in 5–10% of cases) and other VACTERL conditions (up to 50%) [1–3]. Given these potential associations, the recommended diagnostic workup for individuals diagnosed with TEF extends to cardiac and renal ultrasound and radiography of the entire spine [1]. Symptoms of TEF manifest differently depending on the specific malformation type (with detailed classification beyond the scope of this text), potentially featuring regurgitation, difficulty managing secretions, and episodes of coughing and choking. Diagnosis involves the inability to fully pass a small feeding tube, confirmed through radiographic imaging [3]. After TEF diagnosis, the placement of a Replogle tube is advised to suction secretions and prevent aspiration [2]. After diagnosis, the patient should be admitted to the neonatal intensive care unit, and surgical consultation should be obtained.

7.1.4.2 Hypertrophic Pyloric Stenosis

Hypertrophic pyloric stenosis (HPS) is caused by progressive hypertrophy of the circular muscular layer of the pylorus, eventually causing partial or complete obstruction. The peak incidence occurs between 2 and 10 weeks of life [1]. The typical history includes emesis that becomes more frequent and forceful over several days, resulting in progressive dehydration [3]. Emesis is described as a projectile and is nonbilious in character. The hallmark physical exam finding is an "olive-like" mass in the epigastrium [3]. The necessary diagnostic evaluation is based on abdominal ultrasonography measurements with a pyloric muscle thickness greater than 3 mm and length greater than 14 mm ("Rule of Pi – 3.14" as seen in Fig. 7.1) [3, 4]. The typical metabolic abnormality seen on a complete metabolic panel (CMP) is a hypochloremic, hypokalemic metabolic alkalosis, and this derange-

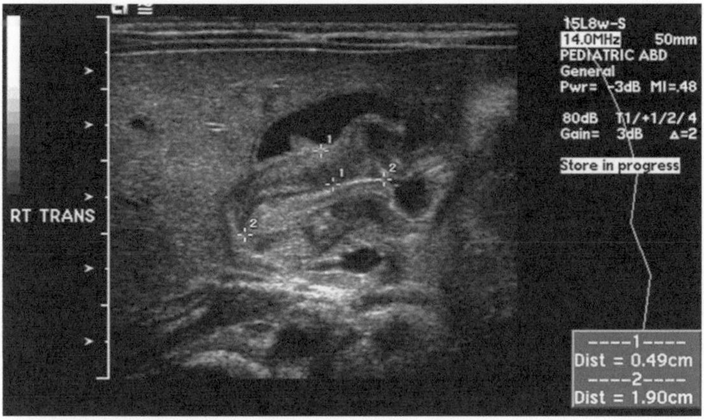

Fig. 7.1 Abdominal ultrasound showing a thickened pylorus with a thickness of 4.9 mm and pyloric length of 19 mm

ment should be corrected before surgical intervention. Therefore, the patient should be given normal saline boluses to correct serum carbon dioxide to less than 30 mmol/L, chloride greater than 100 mmol/L, and normal serum potassium, while pending surgical consultation [3].

7.1.4.3 Congenital Duodenal Obstruction

Congenital duodenal obstruction (CDO) can be caused by both intrinsic lesions such as duodenal stenosis or web and extrinsic lesions such as annular pancreas. Regardless of the source, these lesions lead to a clinical presentation consistent with either partial or complete proximal bowel obstruction. There are many associated syndromes, but the most common are Down syndrome, congenital heart disease, and malrotation, which occur in approximately half of all patients with CDO [1–3]. While the location of the obstruction is variable, 80% of CDO cases are distal to the ampulla, resulting in bilious emesis [2]. The severity of symptoms and the presence of preserved GI function depend on the extent of the obstruction. Workup for suspected CDO starts with an abdominal radiograph (supine and upright views), which may show the classic appearance of the "double bubble sign" (Fig. 7.2) created by

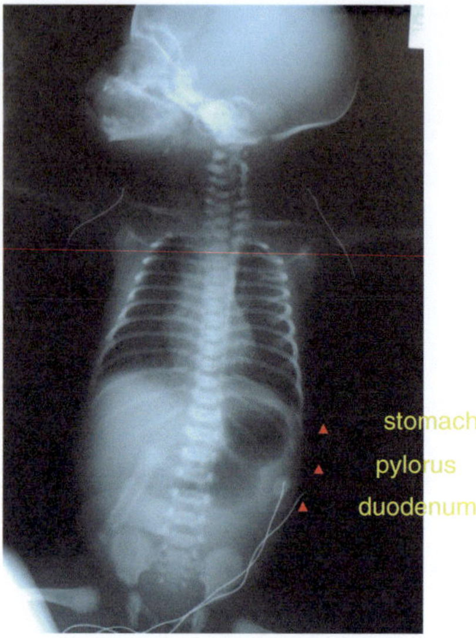

Fig. 7.2 Newborn radiograph showing a double bubble sign

the distal region of the stomach and proximal duodenum and the absence of air distally. If an abdominal radiograph is not diagnostic, a UGI can be performed for evaluation. Importantly, UGI can distinguish CDO from malrotation with midgut volvulus by the location of the duodenojejunal junction (DJJ) [4].

7.1.4.4 Malrotation with Midgut Volvulus

Malrotation arises from the failure of normal herniation and subsequent fixation of the bowel within the fetal abdomen during development. This leads to abnormal connections between the cecum and the right upper quadrant, termed Ladd's bands, and an unusually narrow small bowel mesentery that increases the risk of midgut volvulus. Most symptomatic cases manifest in infancy, presenting with intestinal obstruction due to midgut volvulus, resulting in a clinical tableau of bilious emesis and abdominal distention. Abdominal radiographs often lack specificity, necessitating further investigation with an UGI. A UGI series reveals a DJJ that fails to cross to the left of the midline in malrotation cases. Additionally, midgut volvulus may be characterized by a distinctive “corkscrew” appearance of the contrast or complete obstruction distal to the DJJ [4]. Given the vascular compromise associated with volvulus, malrotation constitutes a genuine surgical emergency, demanding immediate surgical consultation while concurrently ensuring patient resuscitation.

7.1.4.5 Jejunoileal and Colonic Atresia

Unlike duodenal atresia, which is due to failure of the duodenum to recanalize, jejunoileal stenosis or atresia often results from prenatal vascular injury [1]. While classification systems are available for describing the extent and number of diseased segments, the resulting clinical picture is similar regardless of classification. Patients commonly present with bilious emesis and abdominal distention within the first 24 h of life [1]. Patients often fail to pass normal meconium, though a single episode of normal meconium is possible depending on the location of the lesion and its presence should not exclude jejunoileal atresia on the differential. Diagnosis is made with abdominal radiographs alone, with dilated small bowel loops proximal to the lesion(s) [4]. If there is clinical or radiographical evidence of perforation (i.e., calcifications on X-rays), resuscitation should be performed in conjunction with prompt surgical consultation.

The pathophysiology of colonic atresia is like that of jejunoileal atresia and occurs after prenatal vascular injury. The clinical picture is similar to other causes of distal obstruction as already described. After abdominal radiographs have been obtained, contrast enema can distinguish these cases from Hirschsprung’s disease and meconium plug syndrome [4]. Gastrointestinal decompression and intravenous resuscitation should occur while pending surgical consultation.

7.1.4.6 Meconium Ileus

Meconium ileus is a condition limited to patients with cystic fibrosis. Traditionally, meconium ileus was often the first clinical sign of cystic fibrosis, but now this diagnosis is almost exclusively made prenatally due to genetic testing. Meconium ileus is caused by the inspissation of stool in the distal ileum due to the increased viscosity of the meconium from the underlying altered chloride channels [3]. Patients often present within 48 h with bilious emesis and abdominal distention [1]. Abdominal radiographs typically show multiple distended intestinal loops with air-fluid levels, suggesting distal obstruction [4]. Classical descriptions of soap bubbles or ground-glass opacities in the distal ileum may increase clinical suspicion but are neither sensitive nor specific for this diagnosis [3]. Contrast enema will reveal a microcolon or a small caliber colon for the complete length since the stool has never reached the colon. Once the diagnosis is made, contrast enema with gastrograffin can be utilized as a more effective therapeutic agent given the increased osmolarity of the contrast agent [4]. Given the fluid shifts possible with this method, close attention should be given to the hydration and electrolyte status of the patient while performing these enemas [2]. Uncomplicated meconium ileus can often be treated medically with resuscitation and therapeutic enemas. Surgical consultation should be reserved for patients who lack a therapeutic response or for those with complicated meconium ileus. Approximately 40% of patients with meconium ileus present with complications such as volvulus, perforation, and meconium peritonitis. Like patients with any other cause of these complications, these patients should receive adequate resuscitation pending surgical consultation.

7.1.4.7 Meconium Plug

While the pathophysiology of the meconium plug is unknown, it is suspected to be from an immature left colon. Patients present similar to other causes of distal obstruction with bilious emesis and abdominal distention. Abdominal radiographs show nonspecific dilated small bowel and proximal colon. Contrast enema will reveal a normal rectal caliber followed by a small caliber left colon and dilated proximal colon [4]. This is distinct from Hirschsprung's disease (discussed below in the *Infants* section), which typically shows decreased rectal caliber. Often performing the contrast enema with an iso-osmolar contrast agent is enough to relieve the obstruction [2–3].

7.1.4.8 Hirschsprung's Disease

Hirschsprung's disease is caused by the failure of migration of the neural crest cells to form the ganglia of the distal colon [1]. The spectrum of the disease varies depending on the extent of the colon affected but 80% of patients have a transition zone distal to the rectosigmoid junction [1]. The clinical picture is similar to other causes of distal obstruction. Less severe disease may not present until later in life with severe constipation. Abdominal radiograph shows nonspecific bowel dilation. Contrast enema is the study of choice for distinguishing Hirschsprung's disease from other sources of distal obstruction [4]. Diagnosis is confirmed after surgical consultation and rectal biopsy [1].

7.1.4.9 Gastroesophageal Reflux

Gastroesophageal reflux (GER) is the most common cause of emesis, occurring in almost three-quarters of all infants [1]. Despite its frequency, it is rarely pathologic and typically resolves with dietary and feeding schedule changes. Pathologic GER is most often associated with neurologic conditions leading to esophageal, gastric, and small bowel dysmotility and delayed emptying [1]. It can also be caused by structural pathology like hiatal hernias and esophageal atresia. Medical management outside of behavioral changes includes proton pump inhibitors and histamine-2 receptor antagonists. Surgical referral for GER is indicated for failure of medical therapy, structural abnormalities requiring correction, and children with neurologic conditions preventing normal feeding and growth [1].

7.2 Children (Ages 2–12 Years)

7.2.1 History and Exam

As their gastrointestinal system continues to develop, children presenting with emesis can have various systemic etiologies, ranging from metabolic to infectious or obstructive, whether from native anatomy or foreign ingestion. A thorough history should include activity levels and bowel patterns, in addition to their developmental and any previous surgical history. Emesis can commonly be described with terms such as gastric contents, non-bilious/bilious, and nonbloody/bloody. The physical examination should focus on the patient's vital signs (fever, tachycardia, etc.), neurological status, and abdominal exam, evaluating for distension and location of tenderness if elicited.

Laboratory tests to consider:

- Complete blood count (CBC): hemoglobin/hematocrit, white blood count with differential, and platelets
- Complete metabolic panel (CMP): sodium, potassium, chloride, bicarb, creatinine, BUN, magnesium, phosphorus
- Liver function test (LFTs): should include bilirubin (both direct and indirect); transaminases, C-reactive protein (CRP), and erythrocyte sedimentation rate (ESR)
- Urinalysis

7.2.2 Imaging

7.2.2.1 Abdominal Ultrasound [4]

Abdominal ultrasound has been increasingly utilized in the pediatric population as a safe and cost-effective imaging modality. It may be beneficial when the history and examination raise suspicion of appendicitis or intussusception. However, it is important to note that ultrasound is operator-dependent, and challenges may arise in visualizing the appendix, particularly in cases of obesity. Additionally, the technique has a relatively low rate of detecting perforation.

7.2.2.2 Magnetic Resonance Imaging [4]

Abdominal magnetic resonance imaging (MRI) is a promising imaging modality that can be pursued if additional information is indicated based on equivocal ultrasound findings. While this modality does not have associated radiation risks, it does require the child to remain still in the machine for an extended period of time that may pose a challenge to any child and potentially require anesthesia or sedation, especially one presenting with emesis.

7.2.2.3 Computed Tomography [4]

Despite being a preferred radiographic choice in adults, abdominal computed tomography (CT) faces limitations in the pediatric population due to concerns over radiation risks. However, it can still prove valuable in diagnosing complicated appendicitis with abscess or phlegmon. Balancing diagnostic efficacy with radiation exposure becomes imperative when considering CT scans in pediatric cases. If evaluating for an infectious or inflammatory process, intravenous contrast should be administered. Oral contrast should be added with concern for an obstructive process.

7.2.3 Differential

- Metabolic
  - Diabetic ketoacidosis
  - Electrolyte abnormalities
- Infectious/inflammatory
  - *Appendicitis*
  - Gastroenteritis
  - Eosinophilic esophagitis
  - Ulcerative colitis and Crohn's disease
  - Urinary tract infections
- Obstruction
  - Intussusception (see infants)
  - Umbilical hernia
  - Inguinal hernia
  - *Meckel's diverticulum*
  - *Foreign body ingestion*
  - Abdominal mass causing obstruction
- Systemic
  - Increased intracranial pressure (due to mass, infection, or other conditions)
  - Constipation

- Other
  - Toxin/poisons
  - Anxiety
  - Food allergies

7.2.3.1 Acute Appendicitis

Acute appendicitis, the predominant surgical cause of acute abdominal pain in the pediatric population, affects children from toddlers to adolescents. Commencing as vague periumbilical discomfort, the pain gradually localizes to the right lower quadrant (RLQ), accompanied by potential emesis. Additional symptoms such as nausea, low-grade fevers, anorexia, and diarrhea are also common [3]. Key clinical examination findings include palpation tenderness in the RLQ, with additional indicators such as guarding/rebound tenderness, Rovsing's sign, psoas sign, or an obturator sign [3]. White blood cell count with a differential is the most useful laboratory test, while inflammatory markers like CRP and ESR aid in diagnosis.

While many patients can be confidently diagnosed with appendicitis without radiographic studies, children with atypical presentations may benefit from such studies. Ultrasound findings suggestive of appendicitis include a noncompressible, fluid-filled, tubular structure with a wall thickness greater than 6 mm [4]. Other suggestive features include tenderness during the exam, free fluid, appendicolith, increased echogenicity of the periappendiceal fat, or an abscess. When the appendix is visualized, sensitivity is reported to be 100%, specificity 88%, and accuracy 91%. In cases with a nondiagnostic ultrasound study, an MRI can be a useful test with a sensitivity of 96.2% and specificity of 95.7%. Concerns over radiation risks need to be weighed in the use of CT scan imaging in children, despite its sensitivity, specificity, and accuracy of 97%, 100%, and 98%, respectively [1, 4]. Various scoring systems like the Pediatric Appendicitis Score (PAS) and the Alvarado/MANTRELS score aim to predict the likelihood of appendicitis [3]. Despite the benefit of these adjuncts, these scoring systems should not supersede clinical judgment. After the diagnosis of appendicitis is made, the patient should be started on antibiotics and surgical consultation should be made.

7.2.3.2 Meckel's Diverticulum

Meckel's diverticulum (MD) manifests in approximately 1–3% of the population, with the majority of individuals remaining asymptomatic [1, 3]. Those who do experience symptoms often present with signs of obstruction, inflammation, or bleeding [1]. Obstruction can arise when the MD serves as a pathological focal point. In the adolescent population, inflammatory symptoms may mimic those of appendicitis, posing a diagnostic challenge that is often resolved only during surgical exploration when imaging results are inconclusive.

Painless bleeding symptoms tend to manifest in younger children. When addressing bleeding concerns, the technetium 99 m pertechnetate scintiscan (commonly referred to as the Meckel's scan) boasts a sensitivity ranging from 80–95% (Fig. 7.3) [1]. Other imaging adjuncts that may be more readily available include CT and abdominal ultrasound. If bleeding is the chief complaint, CT angiogram can aid in diagnosis. On the other hand, if the

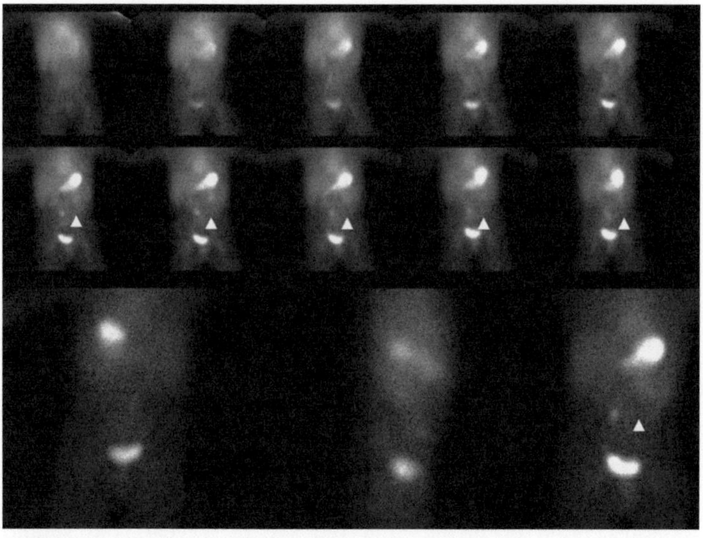

Fig. 7.3 Meckel's scan showing uptake along the right lower abdomen (white arrows)

patient presents with obstructive symptoms, oral contrast can be added when obtaining a CT scan.

7.2.3.3 Foreign Body Ingestion

Children may present following a witnessed ingestion event, but the manifestation of symptoms varies based on factors like age, the size of the swallowed object, and the location of impaction. Surprisingly, up to 50% of patients may remain asymptomatic [1]. Symptomatic cases involving gastric or duodenal foreign bodies often exhibit abdominal pain, nausea, and emesis. Fortunately, about 80–90% of foreign bodies less than 2 cm that reach the stomach typically pass through uneventfully [2]. Intestinal foreign bodies that have passed the gastroduodenal region but become symptomatic, frequently with bilious emesis and abdominal distension, are more likely to require surgical intervention.

Primary diagnostic tools for foreign body ingestion involve plain abdominal radiographs, which are adept at identifying radio-opaque objects like magnets and uncovering potential complications such as obstruction or perforation [4].

While asymptomatic children with small foreign bodies can undergo safe observation with serial radiographs, symptomatic cases indicating suspected or identified complications warrant surgical consultation. Lithium-ion batteries and magnet ingestions are considered true emergencies, mandating immediate surgical intervention. Conversely, the ingestion of sharp objects is less alarming than anticipated, with only 4% of children requiring surgery and a significant 79% requiring no intervention [2, 3].

7.2.3.4 Intussusception

Intussusception is a condition characterized by the telescoping or invagination of one portion of the intestine into another, leading to potential bowel obstruction and ischemia. This condition primarily affects infants and toddlers ages 3 months to 3 years [3]. Intussusception in this age group is typically due to hypertrophied lymphoid tissue, hypothesized to be from viral etiologies. Intussusception occurring after the age of 5 years old should heighten concern for a possible pathologic lead point, such as Meckel's diverticulum or abdominal mass as the root cause of intussusception.

The classic triad of symptoms includes abdominal pain, emesis, and the passage of "currant jelly" stool from a combination of blood and mucus but all three components are only present in a small subset of patients [1]. The imaging modality of choice is an abdominal US with the hallmark finding of the "target sign." [4] Prompt recognition and intervention are essential in managing intussusception to prevent bowel ischemia. In a hemodynamically stable patient, nonoperative reduction may be attempted with pneumatic or hydrostatic enema, with success rates of 80–90% [3]. This can be repeated for an unsuccessful initial attempt or recurrence. Surgical consultation is indicated for persistent or recurrent disease despite multiple reduction attempts, concern for pathologic lead point, more likely in patients over 5 years of age, and hemodynamic instability or concern for perforation.

7.2.3.5 Inguinal Hernia

Congenital inguinal hernias, due to a patent process vaginalis, are a more common occurrence in male patients, with an incidence of 1–5% [3]. This incidence is two to three times higher in preterm infants and is directly proportional to the level of prematurity. Hernias are more likely to be on the right side due to a delay in descent of the right testis compared to the left [3]. Patients typically present with an asymptomatic groin bulge, but the presence of an incarcerated hernia could lead to abdominal pain, emesis, and other obstructive symptoms. Testicular infarction associated with inguinal hernias occurs at an increased rate compared to adults, with an incidence of up to 30% in children under 3 months [1]. The diagnosis of both asymptomatic inguinal hernia and incarcerated inguinal hernia is made clinically.

Incarcerated or strangulated inguinal hernias require urgent surgical evaluation, especially if there is a concern for bowel obstruction. While pending evaluation, an attempt should be made at a reduction with Trendelenburg positioning and sedation if available to allow gravity and a relaxed abdominal wall to assist [1]. If the reduction is successful, patients should be admitted to the hospital, and inguinal hernia repair is often performed during the same admission. By contrast, if reduction is unsuccessful, surgical repair is performed urgently.

7.2.3.6 Umbilical Hernia

Umbilical hernias are common in infants and children due to a lack of complete closure of the umbilical ring. Similar to inguinal hernias, these defects are more common in children born prematurely. Most often, these defects close spontaneously as children age, and surgical consultation for an asymptomatic umbilical hernia is only indicated for children over 4–5 years of age [3]. However, for any patient presenting with clinical signs and symptoms of an incarcerated or strangulated umbilical hernia, urgent surgical consultation is indicated in addition to attempts at reduction as detailed in the "Inguinal Hernia" section.

7.3 Adolescents (Age 12–21 Years of Age)

7.3.1 History and Physical

As adolescents become more physiologically akin to adults, the approach to adolescents with emesis starts to mirror the adult workup for emesis. The history should focus on the chronicity and quality of symptoms in addition to the presence of symptoms outside the gastrointestinal tract. In female patients who have undergone menarche, menstrual history becomes relevant. Finally, social history, such as sexual activity, substance use, and psychological history all become more relevant in the adolescent patient with emesis.

7.3.2 Laboratory Tests to Consider

- Complete blood count (CBC): hemoglobin/hematocrit, white blood count with differential, and platelets
- Complete metabolic panel (CMP): sodium, potassium, chloride, bicarb, creatinine, BUN, magnesium, phosphorus
- Liver function test (LFTs): should include bilirubin (both direct and indirect); transaminases, C-reactive protein (CRP), and erythrocyte sedimentation rate (ESR)

- Urinalysis
- Pregnancy test
- Sexual transmitted infection studies: evaluate for gonorrhea, chlamydia, trichomonas

7.3.3 Imaging

7.3.3.1 Ultrasonography [4]

As an imaging modality without associated radiation, abdominal ultrasonography (US) remains the primary imaging modality utilized in this age group. Ultrasonography can be utilized to evaluate the biliary tree, the genitourinary system, and the appendix in this population.

7.3.3.2 Computed Tomography [4]

As the growth rate of adolescent patients starts to slow, the risk for malignancy due to radiation starts to approach that of adult patients. The risks and benefits of CT imaging must be considered in the diagnostic evaluation. Adding this imaging technique into the workup should be a decision between the provider, the parent, and the patient.

7.3.4 Differential

- Neurologic
  - Increased intracranial pressure
  - Vestibular sources
  - Intoxications/medication effects
- Psychological
  - Eating disorder
  - Cyclical vomiting disorder
- Metabolic
  - Diabetic Ketoacidosis
- Genitourinary
  - Pregnancy
  - Ectopic pregnancy

  - Ovarian or testicular torsion
  - Pelvic inflammatory disease
  - Ruptured ovarian cyst
  - Nephrolithiasis
- Gastrointestinal
  - Viral gastroenteritis
  - Pancreatitis
  - Small bowel obstruction
  - Appendicitis
  - Cholecystitis
  - Hernia
  - Inflammatory bowel disease

7.3.4.1 Ovarian Torsion

Ovarian torsion manifests as an abrupt and intense abdominal pain accompanied by nausea and emesis, arising from the twisting of the ovary on its vascular pedicle and resulting in ischemia. In over half of patients, this is prompted by an enlarged ovary due to an ovarian cyst or ovarian mass. While ovarian torsion is not exclusive to any specific age group, it is most prevalent in reproductive-age women. Ultrasound is the preferred imaging modality to evaluate for this condition, but prompt surgical consultation and interventions should not be delayed if ultrasound is not readily available and the patient has a concerning exam (Fig. 7.4) [4].

7.3.4.2 Testicular Torsion

Testicular torsion arises from the failure of the testis to appropriately anchor itself to the scrotum during its descent from the abdomen in the fetal period. This condition gives rise to the potential for a twisting of the spermatic cord, leading to ischemia of the testis. Patients present with an acute onset of scrotal pain accompanied by nausea and emesis. If suspicion of testicular torsion arises, prompt diagnosis followed by immediate surgical intervention is imperative to maximize the likelihood of preserving testicular function. While testicular ultrasonography can offer valuable diagnostic insights when the clinical picture is unclear,

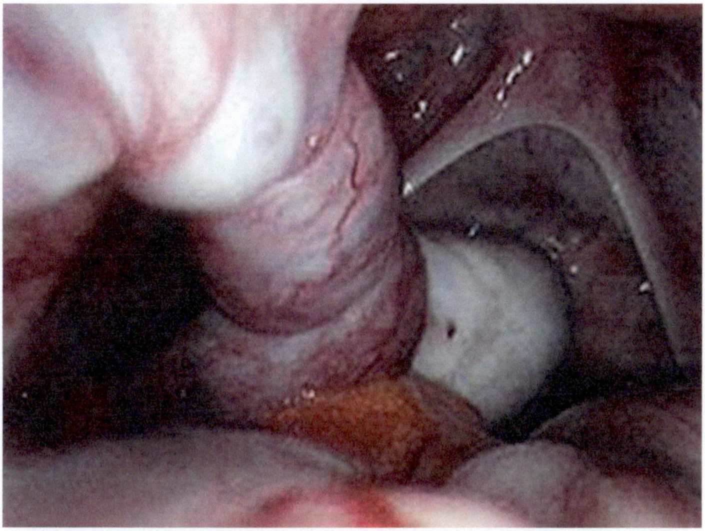

Fig. 7.4 Intraoperative photo demonstrating a left ovarian torsion

any delay in obtaining imaging should not hinder the prompt initiation of surgical consultation.

7.3.4.3 Symptomatic Cholelithiasis/Acute Cholecystitis

The spectrum of disease caused by gallstones affects the pediatric population similarly to the adult population. The most common cause of gallstone formation in neonates and infants is cholestasis from total parenteral nutrition [2]. In the child and adolescents, cholesterol stones have become the most common etiology with the sharp rise in obesity over the past several decades [1]. Hemolytic disease resulting in pigmented gallstones is a rarer source of gallbladder symptoms. Patients present with right upper quadrant pain and emesis similar to adults, although the pain can be difficult to localize in younger children. As in adults, ultrasound is the preferred imaging modality to evaluate the gallbladder wall, the common bile duct, and the presence of stones. CBC, LFTs, and lipase are all useful laboratory adjuncts to evaluate for the severity or presence of cholecystitis, choledocholithiasis, and pancreatitis. Surgical consultation is appropriate for any pediatric patient with an unknown etiology of abdominal pain and identified cholelithiasis, especially if the patient has risk factors, as mentioned above.

7.3.4.4 Inflammatory Bowel Disease

Inflammatory bowel disease occurs in a bimodal distribution, with the first peak between 15 and 30 years of age. While the full extent of this disease process is outside of the scope of this chapter, IBD should be on the differential for any adolescent presenting with weight loss and chronic abdominal pain, bloody bowel movements, and emesis. Laboratory evaluation should include inflammatory markers such as white blood cell count, CRP, and ESR. Radiological evaluations such as abdominal CT and MRI are useful adjuncts, but diagnosis is made based on colonoscopy. Urgent surgical consultation is indicated for any evidence of complicated disease, including obstruction, perforation, fistula formation, abscess, and toxic megacolon. There are other indications for elective surgical intervention that are more nuanced, including a lack of response to medical therapy, that should be discussed between a gastroenterologist and a surgeon.

References

1. About the PedSurgLibrary. In: Hirschl RR, Powell DD, Waldhausen JJ, editors. Pediatric Surgery NaT. American Pediatric Surgical Association; 2023. https://www.pedsurglibrary.com/apsa/view/Pediatric-Surgery-NaT/829001/all/About_the_PedSurgLibrary. Accessed 19 Dec 2023.
2. Puri P, Höllwarth M, E. Pediatric surgery : diagnosis and management. 2nd ed. Cham: Springer; 2023. https://doi.org/10.1007/978-3-030-81488-5.
3. Holcomb GW, Murphy JP, St Peter SD, Ashcraft GJM, KW. Holcomb and Ashcraft's pediatric surgery. 7th ed. Edinburgh: Elsevier; 2020. https://www.clinicalkey.com.au/dura/browse/bookChapter/3-s2.0-C20160026074. Accessed 19 Dec 2023.
4. Walters M, Robertson RL, Blickman JG. Pediatric radiology : the requisites. 4th ed. Philadelphia PA: Elsevier; 2017. http://ezsecureaccess.balamand.edu.lb/login?url=https://www.clinicalkey.com/dura/browse/bookChapter/3-s2.0-C20110086945. Accessed 19 Dec 2023.

Left Upper Quadrant (LUQ) Abdominal Pain

8

Michelle McCarthy
and George Orthopoulos

8.1 Introduction

Left upper quadrant (LUQ) abdominal pain is a frequent presenting complaint encountered by primary and emergency care physicians, serving as a diagnostic challenge that necessitates a thorough understanding of the complex anatomy and multifaceted etiologies associated with this region. Positioned beneath the ribcage and encompassing vital organs such as the stomach and spleen, as well as the small and large bowel, the LUQ is susceptible to a myriad of pathologies that may manifest as pain. Differentiating between gastrointestinal, splenic, and cardiovascular causes demands a systematic approach, combining astute clinical acumen with comprehensive patient assessment.

This chapter seeks to equip primary care physicians with the tools necessary to navigate the intricate landscape of LUQ pain,

M. McCarthy
Lahey Hospital and Medical Center, Department of General Surgery, Burlington, MA, USA

G. Orthopoulos (✉)
Winchester Hospital, Tufts University School of Medicine, Winchester, MA, USA
e-mail: georgios.orthopoulos@lahey.org

G. P. Kohn et al. (eds.), *The SAGES Manual of Surgical Referral for Primary and Emergency Care*,
https://doi.org/10.1007/978-3-031-92678-5_8

offering a comprehensive guide to constructing a robust differential diagnosis. By delving into the anatomy of the LUQ, exploring common pathologies, and emphasizing the significance of a detailed patient history and physical examination, we aim to empower healthcare providers to identify symptoms that warrant urgent surgical consultation.

8.2 Anatomy of the Left Upper Quadrant

The left upper quadrant is a pivotal region in the abdominal cavity, housing a constellation of organs and structures critical to digestion, filtration, and immune function. An appreciation of the intricate anatomy of the LUQ is fundamental for primary care physicians navigating the diagnostic complexities of left upper quadrant pain.

The stomach plays a crucial role in the LUQ symptomatology. Positioned just beneath the diaphragm, the stomach extends across the upper abdomen. Adjacent to the stomach is the spleen, a vital organ with key immunologic and hematologic functions. The spleen's position beneath the left costal margin makes it susceptible to trauma-related injuries. Inferior to the spleen is the splenic flexure of the colon, which may contribute to LUQ pain in instances of colitis, constipation, obstruction, and rarely diverticulitis. Likewise, small bowel etiologies may present with LUQ pain if the affected bowel is near the LUQ.

The pancreas, though centrally located, can radiate pain to the LUQ. Acute and chronic pancreatitis are notable conditions that may present with left upper quadrant discomfort. The left kidney, while predominantly retroperitoneal, may also contribute to LUQ pain when considering its proximity to the abdominal cavity. Conditions such as renal colic or infection may present with referred pain to the LUQ, necessitating consideration in the diagnostic algorithm.

The understanding of LUQ anatomy extends beyond individual organs, emphasizing the interconnectedness of these structures and the need for a holistic approach when evaluating patients presenting with left upper quadrant pain [1].

8.3 Indications for Surgical Consultation

For the seasoned primary care physician, recognizing indications for surgical consultation is paramount in efficiently triaging patients with left upper quadrant pain. While a comprehensive patient history and physical examination are assumed [2], it is crucial to emphasize certain alarm symptoms that signal the need for prompt surgical evaluation.

8.3.1 Sudden Onset and Intensity of Pain

Abrupt and severe LUQ pain can be indicative of acute processes requiring urgent surgical attention. Conditions such as splenic rupture, aortic dissection, or acute mesenteric ischemia may present with a rapid onset of intense pain. In such cases, immediate surgical consultation is warranted to assess the need for emergent intervention.

8.3.2 Hemodynamic Instability

Any signs of hemodynamic instability, including hypotension, tachycardia, or shock, should raise concern for potentially life-threatening conditions such as perforated viscus or vascular emergencies. Early surgical consultation is imperative to evaluate the need for intervention, whether through exploration, embolization, or other surgical measures. In instances of hemodynamic instability, surgical consultation should not be delayed in order to obtain additional imaging.

8.3.3 Peritoneal Signs

Peritoneal signs, such as rebound tenderness, guarding, or rigidity, suggest an acute abdominal process that may necessitate surgical intervention. Conditions such as closed-loop bowel obstructions and mesenteric ischemia may present with these signs, prompting the need for urgent surgical assessment.

8.3.4 Chronic or Recurrent Symptoms

Chronic or recurrent LUQ pain, especially if associated with weight loss, persistent vomiting, or changes in bowel habits, may signify underlying surgical pathology such as malignancy, chronic pancreatitis, or inflammatory bowel disease. Timely surgical consultation following abdominal imaging is essential to determine the appropriateness of surgical intervention for definitive diagnosis and management.

Early recognition of these alarm symptoms and timely surgical consultation can significantly impact patient outcomes by expediting appropriate intervention and optimizing the management of surgical conditions in the left upper quadrant.

8.4 Imaging Modalities for LUQ Pain

In most circumstances, abdominal computed tomography scan (CT scan) with intravenous contrast is the best diagnostic imaging modality that should be obtained prior to or simultaneously with a surgical consultation for LUQ pain. Exceptions include hemodynamic instability of the patient or if obtaining imaging would significantly delay the patient's care. Although less sensitive than a CT scan, an upright chest X-ray can be obtained to evaluate for free air under the diaphragm if there is concern for perforated viscus. Additionally, a CT angiogram may be indicated if the patient's history and symptoms suggest vascular etiology.

8.5 Gastrointestinal Etiologies

8.5.1 Perforated Peptic Ulcer

Common risk factors include a history of peptic ulcer disease, chronic use of nonsteroidal anti-inflammatory drugs (NSAIDs), smoking, advanced age, and infection with *Helicobacter pylori*. Individuals with these risk factors should be closely monitored for symptoms such as sudden and severe abdominal pain, typically beginning in the upper abdomen, and radiating to other areas. The pain is often exacerbated by movement and can lead to rigidity and guarding on examination. Additional signs include rebound tenderness, a "board-like" abdomen, and, in some cases, signs of sepsis such as fever and tachycardia. As a perforated peptic ulcer is a surgical emergency, prompt recognition of these signs and symptoms is crucial for timely intervention and optimal patient outcomes. CT imaging of the abdomen will reveal intraperitoneal free air and inflammation of the gastric wall adjacent to the perforation site.

8.5.2 Perforated Viscus

Common risk factors include prior abdominal surgery, abdominal trauma, inflammatory bowel disease, diverticulitis, and malignancies. The major signs and symptoms of perforated viscus, like perforated peptic ulcer disease or bowel, involve sudden and severe abdominal pain that rapidly intensifies, often spreading across the abdomen. Patients may exhibit symptoms of shock, including hypotension, tachycardia, and respiratory distress. Physical examination typically reveals guarding, rigidity, and rebound tenderness, indicating peritoneal irritation. In some cases, the pain may radiate to the shoulders due to diaphragmatic irritation. Swift recognition of these clinical features is essential for expeditious diagnosis and immediate surgical management to prevent life-threatening complications. CT imaging of the abdomen will reveal free air likely adjacent to the site of bowel perforation.

8.5.3 Small Bowel Obstruction

Small bowel obstruction is characterized by the mechanical blockage of the small intestine, and several risk factors contribute to its development. Common causes include postoperative adhesions, hernias, inflammatory bowel disease, malignancies, and volvulus. Individuals with a history of abdominal surgeries, particularly those involving the small intestine, are at an increased risk. The major signs and symptoms of small bowel obstruction involve the sudden onset of crampy abdominal pain, typically centered around the area of obstruction and abdominal distension [3]. Nausea and vomiting are common, with emesis often becoming bilious as the obstruction progresses. Patients may experience obstipation, the absence of gas and stool passage, and bloating. Swift recognition of these clinical features is crucial for appropriate management, as untreated small bowel obstruction can lead to complications such as ischemia, perforation, and sepsis. CT imaging of the abdomen, preferably with IV and oral contrast, will demarcate the obstructed segment of the bowel and will help differentiate a bowel obstruction from similarly presenting etiologies such as ileus or enteritis. Helpful labwork includes a complete blood count and lactic acid level to evaluate for ischemia.

8.5.4 Incarcerated Hernia

Incarcerated hernias in the LUQ are relatively uncommon but can occur in individuals with specific risk factors. These risk factors include a history of abdominal surgeries, weakened abdominal muscles, and conditions that increase intra-abdominal pressure, such as chronic cough or constipation. Patients who have undergone procedures in the LUQ, like splenectomy, are at an increased risk for LUQ hernias. The major signs and symptoms of an incarcerated hernia in the left upper quadrant involve localized pain, swelling, and tenderness at the hernia site. Strangulation of the hernia contents should be ruled out prior to any reduction attempt by the primary care provider. A complete blood count (CBC) can be checked for leukocytosis, and a basic metabolic panel (BMP) for metabolite abnormalities. In patients presenting with emesis, a hypokalemic, hypochloremic metabolic acidosis may be present. A lactic acid level can also be checked, although this may be falsely normal. An elevated lactic acid level may also result in a metabolic acidosis. A CT scan with

IV contrast will help to determine if the hernia contains bowel and whether the affected bowel's blood supply is compromised. If the hernia is not strangulated, reduction can be attempted at the bedside. If reduction is possible, the patient should be referred to a general surgery clinic for repair of the hernia. If reduction is not possible or if there is concern for strangulation, urgent surgical consultation should be initiated.

8.6 Splenic Etiologies

8.6.1 Splenic Rupture

One of the most critical considerations in the context of LUQ pain is splenic rupture, often associated with trauma or underlying splenic pathology. Trauma, whether due to motor vehicle accidents, falls, or direct blows to the abdomen, is a primary risk factor for splenic rupture. Additionally, individuals with underlying splenomegaly or hematologic disorders, such as infectious mononucleosis, may be predisposed to splenic rupture even with minimal trauma. Major signs and symptoms of splenic rupture include sudden-onset left upper quadrant or abdominal pain, which may radiate to the shoulder due to irritation of the diaphragm. Accompanying symptoms often include hypotension, tachycardia, and abdominal tenderness. In the diagnostic workup, a CBC will indicate the degree of blood loss. If the patient is hemodynamically stable, abdominal CT imaging is crucial for confirming splenic rupture, assessing the severity of injury, and guiding appropriate management. If the patient is unstable, surgical consultation should be initiated without imaging, although providers trained in point-of-care ultrasound may use ultrasound to confirm the presence of hemoperitoneum without causing a significant delay. In cases of suspected splenic rupture, immediate surgical consultation is paramount for timely evaluation and intervention, which may involve splenectomy or other measures to address the ruptured spleen and prevent life-threatening complications.

8.6.2 Splenic Abscess

Splenic abscess is a rare but serious condition associated with specific risk factors. Individuals with compromised immune systems, such as those with diabetes, chronic kidney disease, or underlying hematologic disorders, are at an increased risk for developing splenic abscess. Additionally, patients with a history of infective endocarditis or those who have undergone splenic procedures may be predisposed to this condition. Major signs and symptoms of splenic abscess include persistent fever, left upper quadrant pain, and signs of systemic infection such as chills and malaise. If a splenic abscess is suspected, an abdominal CT scan with IV contrast should be obtained. If imaging reveals an abscess, blood cultures should be obtained to identify the causative microorganisms. The traditional standard treatment of splenic abscesses was splenectomy; however, the utilization of percutaneous drainage by interventional radiology has grown in popularity. The authors continue to recommend surgical consultation for the presence of a splenic abscess, as treatment practices vary by institution, and failure of percutaneous drainage by interventional radiology will necessitate splenectomy.

8.6.3 Splenomegaly Complications

Major signs and symptoms of splenomegaly may include left upper quadrant abdominal pain or discomfort, a feeling of fullness or bloating, and early satiety. An enlarged spleen may be incidentally discovered during a physical examination or imaging studies performed for unrelated reasons. Diagnostic workup typically involves abdominal CT imaging to confirm splenomegaly and assess its size. Blood tests may be conducted to identify the underlying cause, including complete blood cell count, liver function tests, and tests for specific infections. The need for surgical consultation is often based on several factors, including the underlying cause of splenomegaly and the severity of symptoms.

Splenectomy is often considered in cases of certain hematologic disorders, such as idiopathic thrombocytopenic purpura (ITP), hereditary spherocytosis, and autoimmune hemolytic anemia, where the spleen plays a role in the destruction of blood cells. If splenomegaly is associated with a primary or metastatic malignancy affecting the spleen, surgical removal may be considered as part of the cancer treatment strategy. In cases where splenomegaly causes significant symptoms, such as pain, early satiety, or discomfort, and when these symptoms are unresponsive to medical management, splenectomy may be recommended to improve quality of life.

8.7 Vascular Etiologies

8.7.1 Acute Mesenteric Ischemia

Acute mesenteric ischemia (AMI) is a vascular emergency associated with specific risk factors, signs, and symptoms that demand swift medical attention. Risk factors include atherosclerosis, atrial fibrillation, history of embolic events, and hypercoagulable states. Major signs and symptoms of AMI involve severe abdominal pain disproportionate to physical examination findings, often with an abrupt onset. Patients will likely exhibit signs of peritonitis. Other symptoms include nausea, vomiting, and bloody diarrhea. If there is a high degree of suspicion for AMI, providers should obtain abdominal CT angiography (CTA), allowing for visualization of the mesenteric vessels and assessing blood flow. However, abdominal CT scan with IV contrast will indicate regions of bowel ischemia. Laboratory tests, including elevated lactate levels, aid in confirming ischemia. Given the critical nature of AMI, prompt recognition of risk factors and timely consultation with vascular surgery are essential for optimizing outcomes and preventing irreversible bowel damage.

8.7.2 Ischemic Colitis

Ischemic colitis is caused by transient hypoperfusion of the colon. The splenic flexure of the colon is particularly susceptible to ischemia due to its vascular supply, situated at the junction of the middle and left colic arteries with limited collateral blood supply. Individuals with cardiovascular disease, atherosclerosis, and hypertension are at an increased risk for compromised blood flow to this region of the colon. Major signs and symptoms include left upper quadrant abdominal pain, often crampy and severe, accompanied by tenderness on examination. Patients also often report passing stool mixed with blood within 24 hours of the onset of pain. Laboratory investigation will demonstrate leukocytosis and an elevated lactic acid level. Typical abdominal CT scan findings include segmental thickening of the colonic wall and pericolonic fat stranding. Severe cases may also show pneumatosis intestinalis, intramural hematoma, or perforation. If there is suspicion of ischemic colitis, surgery consultation should be sought.

8.7.3 Splenic Aneurysm

Splenic artery aneurysms (SAAs) are relatively rare but potentially serious vascular conditions with specific risk factors. Common risk factors include pregnancy, portal hypertension, liver cirrhosis, and atherosclerosis. Women of childbearing age are particularly at risk, especially during pregnancy. Major signs and symptoms of SAAs may include LUQ pain, which can be severe and sudden if the aneurysm ruptures, leading to hypovolemic shock. Ruptured SAAs require urgent surgical consultation. However, most SAAs are asymptomatic and are incidentally discovered during imaging studies performed for unrelated reasons. For nonruptured SAAs, diagnostic workup necessitates an abdominal CTA to confirm the aneurysm's presence, location, and size. Indications for vascular surgery consultation include [4]

- Symptomatic aneurysms
- Pseudoaneurysms of any size due to the increased risk of rupture
- Any aneurysm identified in a pregnant patient or a woman of childbearing age

- True aneurysms >3 cm or with a demonstrable increase in size from previous imaging studies

Asymptomatic true aneurysms <3 cm in size that have been stable over multiple imaging studies may be observed and monitored annually with abdominal CT angiography or ultrasound studies to assess for aneurysm growth.

8.8 Conclusion

Evaluating left upper quadrant pain in patients demands a comprehensive understanding of various etiologies, ranging from gastrointestinal and splenic causes to vascular pathologies. Primary and emergency care physicians, as key stakeholders in patient care, play a pivotal role in recognizing the indications for surgical consultation. Through this chapter, we have navigated the intricate landscape of LUQ abdominal pain, emphasizing the importance of a systematic approach to differential diagnosis and timely intervention. Surgical consultation is essential for optimizing patient outcomes when addressing gastrointestinal disorders, splenic pathologies, or vascular emergencies. The nuances of each etiology, their specific risk factors, and indications for surgical consideration provide a roadmap for physicians to navigate the complexities of LUQ pain.

Indications Requiring Emergency Room Evaluation:
Physical exam findings
Abrupt and severe LUQ pain
Peritoneal signs on abdominal physical exam
Hemodynamic instability
Changes from prior patient physical exam/history
Patient with known LUQ vascular etiology (e.g., splenic artery aneurysm or splenomegaly) reporting new or increased LUQ pain
Patient with known abdominal hernia who presents with localized pain, swelling, and tenderness at the hernia site
Laboratory findings (in the presence of abdominal pain)
Leukocytosis

(continued)

Indications Requiring Emergency Room Evaluation:
Lactic acidosis
Imaging findings
Upright chest X-ray with free air present under the diaphragm
Note: The presence of critical physical exam findings (listed above) alone is enough to warrant emergency room evaluation. Obtaining laboratory work or imaging studies should only be performed if doing so would not cause an untimely delay in transferring the patient to an emergency room setting. It is often the case that such laboratory work and imaging studies are more expediently obtainable in an emergency room setting.

Indications Requiring Urgent Surgical Consultation:
Patient history
Chronic or recurrent LUQ pain of unknown etiology
Unintentional weight loss
Recurrent vomiting
Abrupt changes in bowel habits (e.g., new-onset constipation or diarrhea, blood in stool, decreased stool caliber)
Imaging studies (should be obtained prior to surgical consultation)
CT abdomen and pelvis with IV contrast
Note: The presence of alarm symptoms within the patient history could signify a possible malignancy. An abdominal CT scan finding of a new mass should be evaluated urgently by a surgeon. Other abdominal CT findings, such as chronic pancreatitis, gastric ulcer, or colitis, can be evaluated in a nonurgent setting by GI medicine.

Indications Requiring Nonurgent Surgical Consultation:
Patient history
Recurrent, but stable LUQ pain due to a known etiology (e.g., reflux, gastric ulcer, diverticular disease)
Physical exam findings
New, nontender and reducible abdominal hernia
Imaging studies (should be obtained prior to surgical consultation)
CT abdomen and pelvis with IV contrast
Note: While many abdominal pathologies do not require emergency or urgent surgical intervention, patients should be offered nonurgent consultation with a surgeon to discuss possible elective surgical options for their condition.

References

1. Townsend CM, Beauchamp RD, Evers BM, Mattox KL. Sabiston textbook of surgery. 19th ed. Saunders; 2012.
2. Yew KS, George MK, Allred HB. Acute abdominal pain in adults: evaluation and diagnosis. Am Fam Physician. 2023;107(6):585–96. Accessed 30 Dec 2023. https://www.aafp.org/pubs/afp/issues/2023/0600/acute-abdominal-pain-adults.html.
3. Jackson P, Cruz MV. Intestinal obstruction: evaluation and management. Am Fam Physician. 2018;98(6):362–7. Accessed 30 Dec 2023. https://www.aafp.org/pubs/afp/issues/2018/0915/p362.html.
4. Chaer RA, Abularrage CJ, Coleman DM, et al. The Society for Vascular Surgery clinical practice guidelines on the management of visceral aneurysms. J Vasc Surg. 2020;72(1):3S–39S. https://doi.org/10.1016/J.JVS.2020.01.039.

9 Right Upper Quadrant (RUQ) Abdominal Pain

Brittany Wheelock, Colin Bohannan, and Danielle S. Walsh

9.1 Introduction

Abdominal pain in the right upper quadrant (RUQ) is a common complaint for which the underlying pathology can be chronic or acute, mild or severe, and relatively benign or a threat to life. The RUQ contains elements of the hepatobiliary, pancreatic, intestinal, renal, and musculoskeletal systems, all of which could lead to the perception of RUQ pain. Therefore, clinicians must work through the broad differential of causes with a systematic approach utilizing history, examination, laboratory assessment, and radiographic assessment to elucidate the underlying cause.

9.2 History and Examination

The onset, persistence, severity, and timing of pain and associated symptoms provide critical clues to the problem's severity and urgency. Association with meals, activity, time of day, and other symptoms can assist in narrowing the differential diagnosis.

B. Wheelock (✉) · C. Bohannan · D. S. Walsh
University of Kentucky, Lexington, KY, USA
e-mail: bnwh231@uky.edu

G. P. Kohn et al. (eds.), *The SAGES Manual of Surgical Referral for Primary and Emergency Care*,
https://doi.org/10.1007/978-3-031-92678-5_9

Medical history, prior surgical intervention, travel history, and familial disorders are also relevant. Examination should begin with inspection for visible anomalies, such as hernias, followed by palpation of the area. Tenderness over ribs and costal cartilages is common with musculoskeletal disorders. Tenderness below the ribs, especially at McBurney's point, is more suggestive of hepatobiliary disorders. Murphy's sign, in which inhalation while pressing over the expected location of the gallbladder leads to acute pain, highly suggests gallbladder inflammation. Intestinal ulcer disease and pancreatic disease may have more midline tenderness while both pancreatic and renal disease may prove more posterior or flank in location.

9.3 Laboratory Assessment

Because many disorders present similarly, the laboratory evaluation of RUQ pain must be complete and thorough. A comprehensive chemistry panel provides insight into renal function, hydration status, and glucose levels, which may be impacted by pancreatitis. Liver function tests (LFTs) inclusive of aspartate aminotransferase (AST), alanine transaminase (ALT), total and direct bilirubin, and alkaline phosphatase are part of the hepatobiliary evaluation. Total protein and albumin can be suggestive of nutritional status, hepatic function, and renal function. Amylase and lipase give insight into pancreatic disorders. A complete blood count (CBC) can help guide the diagnosis by noting anemia, sometimes caused by hemolysis that can lead to bilirubinate gallstones, and leukocytosis may indicate infection. A urinalysis can further differentiate renal disorders. If initial results suggest a hepatic cause, gamma-glutamyltransferase (GGT), a sedimentation rate, and hepatitis panels may be helpful as second-tier studies.

9.4 Imaging

Ultrasound (US) is the diagnostic imaging modality of choice for RUQ abdominal pain. This provides the optimal visualization of the gallbladder and biliary tree along with the liver above it, medial pancreas, and posterior kidney. Though Doppler imaging added to the US can provide information on the vasculature in the area, it is not generally ordered for patients on the initial assessment, it may be indicated for those with known thrombotic or hepatic disorders. Second-line imaging for hepatobiliary and pancreatic disorders is magnetic resonance cholangiopancreatography (MRCP). Because MRCP sequences should be specifically selected based on the specific question to be answered, it may be best for MRCP imaging to be delayed until specialists have weighed in on the specifics as this imaging is expensive and can be challenging to obtain in many areas. Plain X-ray films have limited value in RUQ pain. While CT scan is more common for other areas of the abdomen, US is prioritized over CT in the RUQ as it identifies stones that may be radiolucent on CT imaging. However, it may be indicated for assessment of a mass, renal disease, or intestinal disorders if additional information is needed after an ultrasound and MRCP is not available or indicated.

9.5 Gallbladder Disease

Gallbladder pathologies are the most common cause for RUQ abdominal pain with symptomatic gallstones as the predominant etiology. Although 10–15% of the population has gallstones, only 5–10% become symptomatic. Asymptomatic cholelithiasis does not warrant surgical attention, but gallstones resulting in biliary colic, pancreatitis, jaundice, ileus, or dilated biliary ducts should be evaluated by a surgeon. Classically, symptomatic cholelithiasis is associated with postprandial pain lasting up to a few hours after meals, often worse with greasy or fatty foods. Pain may also occur at night, waking the sufferer from sleep. At the time of evaluation, patients may not have reproducible pain on examination of the right upper quadrant. The presence of stones and symptoms consistent with symptomatic cholelithiasis warrants an outpatient referral to a surgeon for evaluation for cholecystectomy as the risk of recurrent attacks is 38–50% per year. However, patients with jaundice, fever, severe pain, and emesis may require more urgent assessment in an emergency department. Additionally, an ultrasound with dilation of the biliary tree suggests choledocholithiasis and care should not be delayed in these patients.

Patients with acute cholecystitis may present in conjunction with cholelithiasis accompanied by a sonographic Murphy's sign, gallbladder wall thickening, peri-cholecystic fluid, and stones or sludge in the gallbladder lumen. However, acalculous cholecystitis presents identically but in the absence of stones and sludge. It is important to note that the sensitivity of RUQ ultrasound for acute cholecystitis is only approximately 71%. Leukocytosis may indicate a more urgent surgical referral due to concern for cholecystitis or cholangitis, especially when accompanied by fever and elevated bilirubin. Elevated direct bilirubin and/or elevated LFTs are common in gangrenous cholecystitis, Mirizzi syndrome (blockage of the common bile duct secondary to external compression), or choledocholithiasis. All of these should prompt emergent surgical referral. Additional next steps may consist of MRCP to evaluate for choledocholithiasis, referral for ERCP if suspicion for choledocholithiasis or cholangitis is sufficiently high, or direct cholecystectomy with intraoperative cholangiogram and possible common bile duct exploration.

Consider biliary dyskinesia, a spasm or functional problem of the gallbladder, when symptoms of biliary colic are present but ultrasound imaging shows neither inflammation nor gallstones or sludge. An outpatient hepatobiliary iminodi-acetic acid (HIDA) scan can identify biliary dyskinesia, defined as ejection fraction less than 40% or greater than 80%, and nonurgent referral to general surgery is indicated. Additionally, cholecystokinin (CCK) administration during the HIDA scan can provoke similar RUQ pain and assist in making the diagnosis.

Gallbladder polyps do not typically cause pain, but they may be identified incidentally during the course of workup for RUQ pain or another presentation entirely. Occasionally, polyps may be associated with dyspepsia, RUQ pain, nausea, or vomiting. Polyps can be identified on ultrasound as nonmobile protrusions into the lumen that do not cause acoustic shadowing. While the pathology, appearance, and etiology of gallbladder polyps can be quite complex, identified polyps over 1 cm in diameter warrant cholecystectomy and should be referred to a general surgeon as the risk of malignancy increases in lesions of this size. Asymptomatic polyps smaller than 1 cm should be followed clinically with repeat ultrasound every 3–12 months and referred to a general surgeon if increasing in size.

9.6 Choledochal Cyst

Choledochal cysts are congenital anomalies of the biliary tree, primarily presenting in childhood and less frequently present in adults with pancreatitis or cholangitis. The classically described triad of RUQ abdominal pain, RUQ mass, and jaundice is rarely seen. MRCP is obtained if there is a high suspicion for a choledochal cyst on ultrasound or CT scan. If a choledochal cyst is confirmed, the potential for malignant transformation warrants a nonurgent evaluation by a pediatric or hepatobiliary surgeon. Symptoms requiring hospitalization such as occur with cholangitis, jaundice, and emesis warrant urgent evaluation and surgical consultation.

9.7 Liver Lesions

9.7.1 Infectious

Pyogenic liver abscesses are among the most common infectious liver lesions. Patients typically present with RUQ pain, fever, lethargy, and less commonly, jaundice. A common cause is bacteremia from sources such as endocarditis, dental procedures, or indwelling catheters. They may also be a manifestation of late diagnosis of bowel diseases such as appendicitis, Crohn's, or diverticulitis from bacterial spread to the liver via portal circulation. Other causes of liver abscesses are secondary to *Entamoeba histolytica, Echinococcus granulosus*, and Ascaris, though these are more common after travel from endemic regions. US demonstrates hypoechoic lesion(s) with well-defined borders and variable internal echogenicity. Laboratory evaluation often shows leukocytosis, elevated alkaline phosphatase, and an elevated sedimentation rate.

Treatment for pyogenic abscess is primarily nonsurgical and includes identification and treatment of the underlying cause, IV antibiotics covering for gram-negative and anaerobic organisms for an 8-week course, and consideration of aspiration or drainage by interventional radiology will manage most cases. If initial antibiotic therapies fail, consultation to hepatobiliary surgery for possible resection should be made. Additionally, if the underlying cause for the abscess is identified as a surgical disease (i.e., appendicitis, diverticulitis) consultation with general surgery should be sought.

Amebic abscesses (caused by *Entamoeba histolytica)* are diagnosed with serologic fluorescent antibody testing. Metronidazole 750 mg three times daily for 7–10 days is the treatment of choice and is effective in 95% of cases. Aspiration and drainage are not routinely required unless medical management fails. Surgical evaluation is unlikely to be indicated.

Ascariasis causes biliary obstruction due to adult worms present in the biliary tree, resembling symptoms of symptomatic cholelithiasis, pancreatitis, or cholecystitis, and secondary cholangitic abscesses may be present. Ultrasound may show linear filling defects within the biliary tree. Treatment includes anthelmintics and GI evaluation for ERCP to remove the worms.

Hydatid cysts (secondary to *Echinococcus granulosus)* are the only infectious liver lesion primarily treated with surgical resection. Small, asymptomatic cysts may be treated with albendazole instead of resection. Diagnosis is made with ELISA for echinococcal antigens. Daughter cysts may be present at the periphery of a mother cyst and will be slightly hypodense compared to the calcified mother cyst. Surgical resection of large or symptomatic cysts is indicated due to the increased risk of secondary infection or rupture that can result in anaphylactic shock. Percutaneous drainage is not recommended due to the concern for anaphylaxis, and the patient should be referred to a hepatobiliary surgeon.

9.7.2 Benign

Hemangiomas and noninfectious hepatic cysts are benign liver lesions commonly identified incidentally and do not typically require surgical intervention. After ultrasound, magnetic resonance imaging (MRI) with and without contrast can be diagnostic. A repeat ultrasound to assess hemangioma or cyst size should be considered at 6–12 months. Small, stable lesions require no further follow-up. Enlarging lesions should be reimaged in the same time frame. Very large cysts or hemangiomas (greater than 10 cm) may be symptomatic and should be referred for surgical evaluation or radiology intervention. Cysts with internal septations on US or CT may represent cystadenomas that have the potential to undergo malignant transformation and should be referred for surgical evaluation. The presence of cysts in both the liver and kidneys may signal polycystic disease and prompt gastroenterology and nephrology assessment.

Hepatic adenomas (HA) and focal nodular hyperplasia (FNH) are both benign solid liver lesions. Biphasic CT scans or MRI images with contrast can help distinguish these lesions and guide management. HA is more commonly associated with estrogen exposure and oral contraceptive use and has a risk of both spontaneous rupture with intraperitoneal hemorrhage and potential malignant transformation. Symptomatic lesions or lesions >5 cm should be evaluated for resection. Importantly, these patients should stop oral contraceptive use and alternative forms of contraception should be discussed with primary care providers. FNH can appear similarly on cross-sectional imaging, but it is important to distinguish from HA as the treatment is most commonly reassurance and observation. Follow-up imaging should occur every 6 months until documentation of stability of size and every 1–3 years thereafter. Referral to hepatobiliary surgery can be considered if symptomatic, enlarging, or if malignancy cannot be ruled out.

9.8 Pancreatitis

Acute pancreatitis is a leading gastrointestinal cause of inpatient hospitalization and occurs most commonly due to gallstones or related to alcohol consumption. Diagnosis requires two out of three criteria: pain consistent with pancreatitis, amylase, or lipase greater than three times the upper limit of normal, and CT/MRI imaging consistent with acute pancreatitis. As pancreatitis can be diagnosed from history, physical exam, lab values, and ultrasound, additional cross-sectional imaging should be reserved for patients without a clear diagnosis or those who fail to improve clinically. In patients with gallstone-induced pancreatitis, prophylactic cholecystectomy is generally recommended, and surgical consultation should be obtained. According to the Pancreatitis of Biliary Origin, Optimal Timing of Cholecystectomy (PONCHO) randomized control trial, same admission cholecystectomy is superior to interval cholecystectomy in mild biliary pancreatitis due to decreased mortality and fewer readmissions for biliary complications. In cases of suspected ascending cholangitis in conjunction with pancreatitis, GI should be consulted for urgent ERCP. ERCP in the setting of pancreatitis is otherwise not indicated. Complicated pancreatitis with necrosis and/or infection requires multidisciplinary management with a team of surgeons, gastroenterologists, and interventional radiologists.

9.9 Intestinal Disorders

While intestinal pathology in the RUQ is less common, peptic ulcer disease, gastroesophageal reflux, and appendicitis are all known to cause pain in this region. Peptic ulcer disease, especially of the pyloric channel or duodenum, will commonly present with chronic discomfort and may be accompanied by feeling bloated. In more severe cases, it presents as free air from perforation or intestinal bleeding, which should prompt emergent surgical consultation. Likewise, gastroesophageal reflux can present with burning, especially after meals or on awakening in the morning. Patients with chronic RUQ discomfort and normal hepatobiliary assessment may benefit from a trial of medical therapy for these disorders and/or referral for upper endoscopic assessment.

Although the appendix is commonly located in the RLQ, some patients have the appendix extending superiorly into the RUQ, leading to an atypical pain location. The pain is acute in nature and often followed by development of anorexia, nausea, and emesis. Examination will commonly reveal tenderness, though it can be difficult to elucidate if the appendix is behind the colon. As with classic appendicitis, emergency assessment with comprehensive laboratory studies and imaging is necessary.

9.10 Renal Disorders

The right kidney sits below the liver and behind the hepatic flexure of the colon, leading it to also be a potential source of RUQ pain. Due to its posterior nature, renal pain from stones, pyelonephritis, or other urinary tract obstructions is commonly in the flank or back. Laboratory studies including urinalysis and ultrasonography are commonly diagnostic. While uncomplicated renal disorders are overwhelmingly managed by primary care and emergency room clinicians, complicated or persistent disorders may lead to consideration of urology and/or nephrology consultation. High-grade urinary obstructions or patients with sepsis from pyelonephritis warrant emergency assessment for stabilization and limiting acute renal damage.

9.11 Musculoskeletal Disorders

Disorders of the musculoskeletal system can cause RUQ pain, particularly in younger, active patients. Slipped rib syndrome causes pain around the costal margin that worsens with physical activity. It occurs due to subluxation of the cartilage with irritation of the adjacent intercostal nerve. It can be elucidated on exam hooking the costal margin with the examiner's fingers and pulling upward, leading to the reproduction of the discomfort. When accompanied by tenderness on palpation of the cartilage, costochondritis may also be present. Though initial treatment is expectant and with anti-inflammatory, agents, second-tier treatment may include nerve blocks and physical therapy. Patients with persistent, severe pain may warrant assessment by a surgeon for consideration of a surgical resection.

9.12 Special Considerations of RUQ Pain in Pregnancy

Abdominal pain in pregnancy carries an expanded differential diagnosis and life-threatening etiologies including pre-eclampsia must be ruled out. Due to the gravid uterus pushing the abdominal contents upward in increasing amounts, disorders more commonly causing lower abdominal pain may instead present with upper abdominal pain in pregnancy.

Appendicitis is the most common nonobstetric surgical disease, accounting for two-thirds of surgical emergencies during pregnancy. Nonspecific abdominal pain caused by appendiceal dilation and associated symptoms of nausea and vomiting in early appendicitis may be confused with normal symptoms of pregnancy. Later in gestation, the appendiceal tip may shift cranially due to the size of the gravid uterus, resulting in right flank or right upper quadrant pain. Suspected appendicitis in pregnant patients should be evaluated with ultrasound to avoid ionizing radiation to the fetus from CT scan. If inconclusive, MRI should be considered. Leukocytosis may be identified but is an unreliable diagnostic tool, particularly in the third trimester, as leukocytosis can be a normal finding at this stage in pregnancy. If clinical presentation and imaging studies are consistent with acute appendicitis, surgical intervention with appendectomy is indicated and safe in every trimester of pregnancy. Nonsurgical management with antibiotics in pregnancy is associated with increased likelihood of negative outcomes, including fetal loss; thus, urgent surgical consultation is warranted.

Acute cholecystitis is the second most common indication for nonobstetric operative intervention during pregnancy. Historically, surgery for gallbladder disease was reserved for the second trimester. However, updated guidelines from the Society of Gastrointestinal and Endoscopic Surgeons (SAGES) offer strong recommendations that laparoscopy offers similar benefits compared to laparotomy in pregnant and nonpregnant patients and that laparoscopic surgery is safe in all trimesters when indicated.

Likewise, the American College of Obstetrics and Gynecologists (ACOG) published consensus guidelines stating that medically indicated surgery should not be denied to a patient regardless of trimester as this can adversely affect both the fetus and the mother. Therefore, women in any stage of pregnancy with suspected biliary colic or acute cholecystitis should be referred to a surgeon for a discussion of risks and benefits, with concurrent OB consultation.

Pre-eclampsia typically arises after 20 weeks of gestation and is characterized by severe hypertension. Additional symptoms include blurred vision, abdominal pain (including in the RUQ), hyperreflexia, and edema. Patients with suspected pre-eclampsia should have a urinalysis sent to evaluate for proteinuria and be urgently referred to OB.

Finally, HELLP syndrome (hemolysis, elevated liver enzymes, and low platelets) most commonly occurs in the third trimester or immediately post-partum as RUQ pain, nausea, vomiting, and fatigue. These symptoms have a significant overlap with biliary causes of RUQ pain and clinical manifestations of HELLP. The Tennessee classification for diagnosis of HELLP syndrome requires evidence of hemolysis, elevated liver enzymes, and platelets <100,000. CBC demonstrating normal platelets and normal blood smear may be reassuring in the short term and LFTs rechecked 4 days after cholecystectomy to assure resolution.

9.13 Summary

RUQ pain is a common presentation to both primary care practices and emergency rooms. Due to its diverse causes, a comprehensive assessment inclusive of broad laboratory testing is necessary in most patients (Fig. 9.1). Ultrasonography remains the imaging study of choice due to its superiority in assessment of the biliary system. Surgical consultation is commonly indicated for both emergent and less urgent disorders.

Urgency of surgical or gastroenterology evaluation

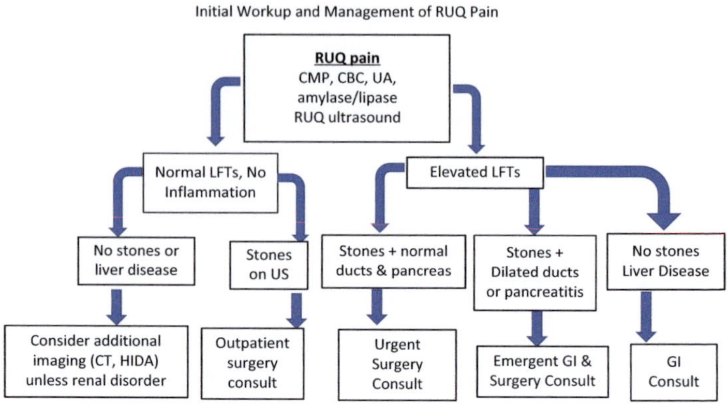

Fig. 9.1 Suggested decision tree for the workup of RUQ pain

PCP management	Asymptomatic cholelithiasis Focal nodular hyperplasia Hepatitis Hemangioma Less symptomatic pyogenic or Amebic abscess Ascariasis, GI consult for possible ERCP Urinary tract infection without sepsis or obstruction
ED presentation	Sudden acute abdominal pain or peritonitis Signs and symptoms of sepsis Oral intake intolerance Concern for cholecystitis, biliary tree obstruction, or severe pancreatitis Urinary obstruction Intestinal disorders with perforation or bleeding
Urgent	Chronic cholecystitis Mild, noninfected pancreatitis Infected necrotizing pancreatitis without improvement Liver abscess without sepsis Complicated urinary infections Concern for malignancy
Nonurgent	Symptomatic cholelithiasis Biliary dyskinesia Choledochal cyst Liver cysts or cirrhosis Hepatic adenoma Hydatid cysts Intestinal disorders without perforation or bleeding

Suggested Reading

1. Russo GK, Zaheer A, Kamel IR, Porter KK, Archer-Arroyo K, Bashir MR, Cash BD, Fung A, McCrary M, McGuire BM, Shih RD, Stowers J, Thakrar KH, Vij A, Wahab SA, Zukotynski K, Carucci LR. ACR appropriateness criteria® right upper quadrant pain: 2022 update. J Am Coll Radiol. 2023;20(5 Supplement):S211–23.
2. Tenner S, Baillie J, DeWitt J, Vege SS, American College of Gastroenterology. American College of Gastroenterology guideline: management of acute pancreatitis. Am J Gastroenterol. 2013;108(9):1400–15; 1416. https://doi.org/10.1038/ajg.2013.218. Epub 2013 July 30. Erratum in: Am J Gastroenterol. 2014 Feb;109(2):302.

10 Periumbilical Pain

Emily J. Baker and Geoffrey P. Kohn

Abbreviations

AAA	Abdominal aortic aneurysm
AXR	Abdominal X-ray
CRP	C-reactive protein
CTAP	Computed tomography abdominal and pelvis, with intravenous contrast
ER	Emergency room
FBE	Full blood examination (also known as CBC, Complete Blood Count)
RIF	Right iliac fossa (also known as RLQ, right lower quadrant)
BMP	Basic metabolic panel (also known as Chem-7 or Urea/Electrolytes/Creatinine)
US	Ultrasound
WCC	White cell count

E. J. Baker (✉)
Eastern Health, Melbourne, VIC, Australia

G. P. Kohn
Monash University, Melbourne, VIC, Australia

Melbourne Upper GI Surgical Group, Melbourne, VIC, Australia

Monash University, Eastern Health Clinical School, Melbourne, VIC, Australia

G. P. Kohn et al. (eds.), *The SAGES Manual of Surgical Referral for Primary and Emergency Care*,
https://doi.org/10.1007/978-3-031-92678-5_10

10.1 Introduction

Patients commonly present to the primary care provider or the emergency room (ER) with periumbilical pain. A spot diagnosis can often be made, for example, in the case of an umbilical hernia; however, others require extensive workup due to the vague non-specific associated signs and symptoms. The range of conditions and the spectrum of severity of each can complicate the referral process. This chapter will cover the common surgical conditions presenting with periumbilical pain, with the aim to help the primary care or ER physician decide who can be managed expectantly, who needs an outpatient surgical referral, and who needs immediate surgical assessment.

Periumbilical pain is pain which is localized or referred to the area around the umbilicus. It may be related to pathology of the skin, the abdominal wall, or intra-abdominal contents (Table 10.1). The majority of uncomplicated presentations related to skin and abdominal wall pathology can be managed in the community or sent to surgical outpatients for nonurgent review. There are a few exceptions that will be covered in more detail below. Periumbilical pain related to intra-abdominal pathology is more nuanced due to the embryological origins of viscera. Midgut structures, that is, the appendix, jejunum, or ileum, refer to the periumbilical area and may present as vague, dull, crampy, burning pain that is poorly localized and typically in the midline due to stretching or inflammation of hollow organs or the capsule of solid organs. In contrast, the parietal peritoneum is innervated by both somatic and visceral afferent nerves. Therefore, when the parietal peritoneum is irritated by noxious stimuli, it is perceived by the patient as localized, sharp pain. Guarding and rebound tenderness over this site is referred to as "peritonitis" and is a sign of progressing pathology, for example, periumbilical pain that migrates to the right iliac fossa (RIF, also referred to as the right lower quadrant, RLQ) as seen in acute appendicitis.

A systematic approach to the initial assessment of a patient presenting with periumbilical pain includes a detailed history about the time course, character of the pain, and any associated

Table 10.1 Sources of periumbilical pain

Location	Urgent	Nonurgent	Nonsurgical—consider medical referral
Skin	Abscess Deep postoperative wound collection Infected urachal cyst	Superficial postoperative wound infection	Cellulitis Herpes zoster
Abdominal wall	Hernia—irreducible +/− signs of obstruction Rectus sheath hematoma	Hernia—reducible Divarication recti	
Intra-abdominal	Infective—appendicitis, Meckel's diverticulitis Obstruction—small or large bowel Vascular—AAA, mesenteric ischemia, ischemic gut Inflammatory—complication of inflammatory bowel disease, that is, stricture		Infective—gastroenteritis Irritable bowel disease Chronic constipation

symptoms. A review of past medical and surgical conditions and a focused abdominal examination is imperative.

An acute onset (hours to days) or an acute change to chronic periumbilical pain is often more concerning than chronic pain (>6 weeks), a rapid onset being more indicative of an underlying surgical pathology and may help decide timing around investigations. The nature or character of the pain gives clues to the underlying pathology. Colicky pain with a short, frequent cycle of 2–3 minutes suggests small bowel pathology such as subacute or complete small bowel obstruction, depending on associated symptoms. Vague central abdominal pain that migrates to RLQ is classic for acute appendicitis, while any pain that is disproportionate to the clinical picture should raise the concern for bowel ischemia. Pain may be associated with oral intake, for example, the postprandial periumbilical pain often reported in patients with mesenteric ischemia or medial arcuate ligament syndrome. A change in pain, that is, increased intensity or severity, or from general to localized, or from intermittent to constant, should raise suspicion for progressive surgical pathology. Pain management is important, and any pain not resolved with simple analgesia or reduction of a lump should be referred for surgical review.

- Associated signs and symptoms
  - Infective: fever, nausea, vomiting, new diarrhea
  - Obstructive: new constipation or obstipation
  - Skin changes: erythema, necrosis, pus, or discharge
  - Loss of appetite and loss of weight

As with any clinical presentation, an appreciation of a patient's history, current medications, and social history will help narrow the possible differential diagnosis. The following are some targeted questions.

- History
  - Known inflammatory bowel disease, cardiovascular disease, peripheral vascular disease, diabetes mellitus, known malignancy
  - Previous abdominal surgery
- Medications: type and last dose
  - Anticoagulants
  - Beta-blockers
  - Oral hypoglycemic agents and insulin
  - Immunosuppression
- Social history
  - Smoking and alcohol intake
  - Mobility and functionality
  - Social supports: especially if a medical enduring power of attorney is required for decision-making

Physical examination: key signs

- Does the patient look well or unwell?
- Is the patient septic?: fever, tachycardia, hypotension, tachypnoea
- Abdominal signs: distension, tenderness to palpation, rebound tenderness, guarding, rigidity, periumbilical lump—reducible or irreducible

Initial management

- Analgesia
- Blood tests: complete blood count, basic metabolic panel, liver function, lipase, blood cultures, and C-reactive protein if febrile
- Antibiotics: if sepsis is suspected or confirmed
- Imaging: computed tomography abdomen pelvis (CTAP) with IV contrast, ultrasound (US), abdominal X-ray (AXR)

Any patient with periumbilical pain and any of the below signs or symptoms requires immediate referral to surgical service through ER::

- Severe sudden-onset pain associated with a periumbilical lump +/− obstructive gastrointestinal symptoms suggests incarcerated/strangulated hernia.
- Pain out of proportion to the clinical presentation suggests visceral ischemia, and in the presence of a palpable and pulsatile midline abdominal mass, a compromised abdominal aortic aneurysm (AAA).
- Obstructive gastrointestinal symptoms: gradual to acute onset of cramping abdominal pain, nausea and vomiting, new inability to pass flatus suggest a small bowel obstruction.
- Hemodynamic instability: tachycardia, hypotension, and tachypnoea.

- Sepsis: febrile, chills or rigors, flushed appearance, and lethargy.
- Abdominal distension, marked tenderness to palpation, guarding, and rebound tenderness or rigidity.

Patients with Red flag signs and symptoms should be sent to the ER for immediate assessment by the surgical service. A verbal handover via phone of your concerns to the ER Admitting Officer +/− the on-call surgical doctor prior to the patient's arrival can help reduce delays through triage. It is not advisable to arrange radiology or pathology investigations prior to referral for patients with Red flag symptoms as this may result in delays in assessment and treatment that can be otherwise avoided by simultaneous assessment and management by the surgical team at the hospital.

Referral process

- Written letter or phone call to on-call surgical team
- Include surgical concern, relevant history, and investigations done to date
- Immediate referrals: keep the patient fasted, assist in transport (such as by ambulance), withhold anticoagulants and oral hypoglycemic agents

Below is a nonexhaustive list of possible differential diagnosis and initial management for periumbilical pain (Table 10.2). Note that if any of these presentations are accompanied by the Red flag signs and symptoms above, the patient should be urgently referred to the ER for surgical review and management.

Chronic or nonurgent surgical conditions that can be referred to the surgical outpatient clinic with appropriate investigations carried out in the community for review with a surgeon (Table 10.2).

Table 10.2 Differential diagnosis and initial management

Condition	Time course	Risk factors	Examination	Investigations prior to referral	Initial management	Referral
Urgent surgical review: refer to the emergency room						
Infective: appendicitis, Meckel's diverticulitis. Periumbilical shifting to right lower quadrant pain. Associated with nausea, vomiting, diarrhea, possible fevers, loss of appetite.	Hours to days	Known Meckel's diverticulum	Tenderness at McBurney's point. Guarding and rebound tenderness suggest peritonism and require urgent surgical review.	Pathology: FBE—raised WCC, raised CRP. NB: may be normal. Imaging: US: helpful in younger patients, not always diagnostic. CTAP scan is more sensitive + specific—not essential if suspecting appendicitis.	Analgesia Withhold anticoagulant/ antiplatelet therapy (with specialist advice) and oral hypoglycemic agents Fast the patient	General surgeon

(continued)

Table 10.2 (continued)

Condition	Time course	Risk factors	Examination	Investigations prior to referral	Initial management	Referral
Bowel obstruction: (small or large bowel) gradual to acute onset of cramping abdominal pain, nausea and vomiting, new constipation or obstipation.	Hours to days	Previous abdominal surgery or intra-abdominal infections, hernia, abdominal malignancy, previous SBO, Inflammatory bowel disease	Abdominal distension and tympanic percussion, tenderness.	Pathology: FBE: raised WCC, BMP: reduced renal function, hypokalemia, raised CRP. Imaging: CTAP: dilated bowel loops with identifiable transition point. AXR: dilated bowel loops with air fluid levels.	Antiemetics and analgesia, withhold anticoagulant/ antiplatelet therapy (with specialist advice) and oral hypoglycemic agents Fast the patient	General surgeon

Irreducible hernia: painful periumbilical lump, irreducible.	Hours	Previous midline abdominal surgery, obesity	An irreducible hernia with tenderness, erythema, or signs of bowel obstruction.	Pathology: nil required for referral unless comorbidities present. Imaging: CT or US demonstrating an abdominal wall defect, typically with characterization of the contents, size of defect normal or thinned with a blue tinge.	Antiemetics and analgesia, withhold anticoagulant/antiplatelet therapy (with specialist advice) and oral hypoglycemic agents Fast the patient	General surgeon

(continued)

Table 10.2 (continued)

Condition	Time course	Risk factors	Examination	Investigations prior to referral	Initial management	Referral
Deep postoperative wound complication: increasing umbilical pain, +/− fever, sweats, chills. Swelling may not be evident for deep infections, erythema.	Days to weeks postoperatively	Recent surgical wound, immunocompromised, diabetic, obese, smoker	Focally tender, erythema, possible palpable lump. There may be active hemopurulent discharge from the wound and wound dehiscence.	Pathology: FBE—WCC and CRP will be raised. Imaging: CT: subcutaneous collection, define the size, character, possible communication with the abdominal cavity. US: subcutaneous collection, define the size, character.	Analgesia, antibiotics	General surgeon for incision and drainage and contact the initial operative surgeon/team

Rectus sheath hematoma: acute-onset central abdominal pain and palpable abdominal mass. +/− nausea, vomiting, fevers, chills.	Hours	Trauma, anticoagulation/ antiplatelet therapy, age > 60 years, pregnancy, respiratory illness, cirrhosis, coagulation disorders, hypertension, renal disease	Palpable abdominal wall mass, tenderness and guarding, nonspecific signs of anemia such as syncope, weakness, dyspnea.	Pathology: FBE— reduced hemoglobin or hematocrit (may remain normal initially), coagulation studies, Imaging: CT with IV contrast.	Analgesia Withhold anticoagulant/ antiplatelet therapy (with specialist advice)	General surgeon +/− interventional radiology
Umbilical abscess: increasing umbilical pain, swelling, discharge +/− fever, sweats, chills.	Days	Recent surgical wound, piercing, immunocompromised, diabetic, obese, smoker	Focally tender erythematous irreducible umbilical lump, +/− sloughy/ necrotic overlying skin, hemopurulent discharge.	Pathology: raised WCC and CRP. Imaging: not required.	Simple skin infections can often be managed with a course of oral antibiotics and analgesia However, referral is suggested if symptoms persist	General surgeon for incision and drainage

(continued)

Table 10.2 (continued)

Condition	Time course	Risk factors	Examination	Investigations prior to referral	Initial management	Referral
Chronic mesenteric ischemia: periumbilical or epigastric pain, radiates to the back. Dull, cramping, postprandial pain. Weight loss and adapted eating patterns.	Hours to months	Smoking, atherosclerosis, peripheral vascular disease, age > 60 years	Nonspecific abdominal findings.	Imaging: CTAP angiography		Vascular surgeon

Nonurgent surgical review: refer to the outpatient clinic						
Superficial postoperative wound infection: increasing umbilical pain, erythema, wound discharge.	Days	Recent surgical wound, piercing, immunocompromised, diabetic, obese, smoker	Focally tender erythematous, hemopurulent discharge. No associated lump/abscess.	Pathology: FBE: raised WCC and CRP. Imaging: not required.	Simple skin infections can often be managed with a course of oral antibiotics and analgesia However, referral is suggested if symptoms persist	General surgeon for wound review

(continued)

Table 10.2 (continued)

Condition	Time course	Risk factors	Examination	Investigations prior to referral	Initial management	Referral
Urachal abnormalities: recurrent umbilical infections / discharge +/– infraumbilical/ suprapubic pain associated with abnormal appearance of the umbilicus. +/– hematuria / dysuria. Loss of appetite, nausea / vomiting. Umbilical lump.	Days to years, may present in childhood or adulthood	Failure of a section of the urachus to seal off during fetal development	Discharge or pus from the umbilicus, infraumbilical tenderness. Umbilical lump.	Pathology: WCC and CRP will be raised in active infection; however, it may be normal. FBE, BMP, Urinalysis may be positive for infection and /or blood Imaging: CTAP or renal tract US will show urachal remnant. Or possible metastatic disease.	Simple skin infections can often be managed with a course of oral antibiotics However, referral is suggested if symptoms persist Analgesia	General / pediatric surgeon or urologist for further assessment and management as there is a wide differential

Uncomplicated hernia: painful periumbilical lump, may be reducible or nontender irreducible lump.	Hours to years	Previous midline abdominal surgery, obesity	A reducible periumbilical lump, minimal tenderness, intact overlying skin. An irreducible hernia with minimal tenderness.	Pathology: nil required for referral unless comorbidities present. Imaging: CTAP or US demonstrating an abdominal wall defect, typically with characterization of the contents, size of defect normal or thinned with a blue tinge.	Analgesia	General surgeon

- Uncomplicated symptomatic hernia: ideally a brief referral letter explaining the time course, symptoms, and impact on daily living that the patient is experiencing.
- Periumbilical lumps may be secondary to a congenital urachal disorder, that is, patent urachus, urachal polyp, or granuloma. Alternatively, they can represent advanced underlying malignancy; a "Sister Mary Joseph's nodule" is a metastatic deposit at the umbilicus.

Conditions that do not require surgical referral (Table 10.3):

- Uncomplicated gastroenteritis: a condition often referred to the ER with the suspicion of appendicitis, especially in young patients who initially present with nausea/vomiting and diarrhea and vague abdominal pain.
- Asymptomatic hernia.

Management of the patient with periumbilical pain without red flag signs or symptoms, and with no clear diagnosis able to be made clinically, should undergo general investigations in the community and be managed expectantly in the first instance. A summary of the recommended surgical referral pathway is listed in Table 10.3.

Table 10.3 Summary of referral pathway

Location of pathology	Urgent: referral to ER for surgical review	Nonurgent: referral to surgical outpatients	Nonsurgical: consider medical referral
Key features	Hemodynamic instability, sepsis, sudden severe pain, intestinal obstructive symptoms	Hemodynamically stable, no sepsis, minimal pain	Hemodynamically stable, no sepsis, minimal pain
Skin	Abscess Deep postoperative wound collection Infected urachal cyst	Superficial postoperative wound infection (no associated abscess) Urachal abnormalities	Cellulitis Herpes zoster
Abdominal wall	Hernia: irreducible +/– signs of obstruction Rectus sheath hematoma	Hernia—reducible Divarication recti	
Intra-abdominal	Infective: appendicitis, Meckel's diverticulitis Obstruction: small or large bowel Vascular: AAA, mesenteric ischemia, ischemic gut Inflammatory: complication of inflammatory bowel disease, i.e., stricture		Infective: gastroenteritis Irritable bowel disease Chronic constipation

Suggested Reading

1. Lamm R, et al. Diagnosis and treatment of appendicitis: systematic review and meta-analysis. In: SAGES Guidelines. 2023. Available via https://www.sages.org/publications/guidelines/diagnosis-and-treatment-of-appendicitis-sr-and-meta/
2. Struller F, Weinreich FJ, Horvath P, Kokkalis MK, Beckert S, Königsrainer A, Reymond MA. Peritoneal innervation: embryology and functional anatomy. Pleura Peritoneum. 2017;2(4):153–61. https://doi.org/10.1515/pp-2017-0024. PMID: 30911646; PMCID: PMC6328075.
3. Tendler D, Lamont J, Smeds M. Chronic mesenteric ischemia. In: UpToDate. 2022. Available via https://www.uptodate.com/contents/chronic-mesenteric-ischemia?sectionName=Vascular%20imaging&search=rectus%20sheath%20hematoma&topicRef=290&anchor=H353596&source=see_link#H23493586.

11 Left Lower Quadrant (LLQ) Abdominal Pain

Kareem Marwan

Acute left lower quadrant (LLQ) pain can be the presenting symptom for surgical and nonsurgical conditions. The latter as well as chronic presentations are beyond the scope of this chapter. A non-exhaustive list of the differential diagnoses (Table 11.1) to consider should be on the mind of the primary care or emergency physician.

K. Marwan (✉)
Colorectal & Robotic Surgeon, Melbourne, VIC, Australia
e-mail: kmarwan@gmail.com

G. P. Kohn et al. (eds.), *The SAGES Manual of Surgical Referral for Primary and Emergency Care*,
https://doi.org/10.1007/978-3-031-92678-5_11

Table 11.1 Differential diagnoses of acute LLQ pain

Surgical	Nonsurgical
General surgical: Diverticulitis Complicated: perforation, phlegmon formation Acute groin conditions: Complicated (incarcerated or strangulated) inguinal hernia Inflamed lymph node Groin abscess Complicated (Incarcerated or strangulated) abdominal wall hernia (Spigelian, incisional) Other abdominal wall conditions: Rectus sheath hematoma Cellulitis or abscess Abdominal malignancy: Colorectal cancer (obstructing) Advanced abdominal malignancy *Urological:* Ureteric stone Other acute obstructive uropathy (e.g., blood clot, tumor) Testicular torsion *Gynecological:* Ectopic pregnancy Ovarian torsion	*Medical/gastroenterology:* Acute colitis (infective, IBD, indeterminate) Constipation *Primary care / renal medicine* Urinary tract infection (UTI) *Gynecology* Endometriosis Ovarian pathology (ovarian cysts, tumors) Tubal pathology (salpingitis, pelvic inflammatory disease [PID])

11.1 History and Examination

As it is well beyond the scope of this chapter to go through each of the conditions listed, a practical approach guided by important factors in both history and examination will be used here. The following focused questions should guide the workup.

11.1.1 Is It Truly an Isolated LLQ Pain?

It is not uncommon for the patient to describe a "left lower" abdominal pain, which in fact is flank pain, or groin pain that is perceived from and/or extending to the left lower quadrant. Examination of the loin is important. Dysuria, loin to groin pain, and a tender renal angle are indicative of an obstructive ureteric pathology. Similarly, an incarcerated hernia may present with generalized "soreness" in the left lower quadrant. Groin and scrotal examination may reveal a complicated hernia or a torted left testicle; the latter may present with scrotal and left lower quadrant pain.

11.1.2 Are There Associated Symptoms?

Associated gynecological symptoms could point toward ovarian torsion or a pregnancy complication such as ectopic pregnancy.

Associated gastrointestinal symptoms could guide the diagnosis: mucous and/or bloody diarrhea may be associated with colitis. Diverticulitis usually presents with a "stitch" like pain in the left lower quadrant and is more often associated with constipation than diarrhea. Previous similar known attacks of diverticulitis may help confirm the diagnosis clinically.

Persistent vomiting may indicate an obstructive process in bowel or urinary tract.

General or systemic manifestations such as fatigue, fever, and loss of appetite usually accompany infective processes; while unexplained weight loss and anemia may be signs of chronic disease or occult malignancy.

11.1.3 Abdominal Examination?

Perhaps the most important question to answer is:

Does the patient have an acute abdomen?

An acute abdomen warrants prompt surgical referral irrespective of the cause.

A patient presenting with LLQ pain yet who examines as generalized tenderness with peritonism (guarding and rebound tenderness) may indicate a quickly evolving surgical pathology such as perforated bowel (diverticulitis, colitis, cancer), bleeding from a ruptured ectopic pregnancy, or other less common pathology.

Localized surgical pathology that irritates the peritoneum locally will give rise to *localized peritonitis,* often made obvious by localized tenderness, guarding, and rebound tenderness in the LLQ. Examples include acute uncomplicated diverticulitis, perforated contained diverticulitis, and early complicated ectopic pregnancy.

11.2 Workup

An important question to ask is whether any investigation is required at all. For the purpose of surgical referral, a clinically obvious incarcerated abdominal wall hernia, testicular torsion, an abdominal wall abscess, or an abdomen with generalized peritonitis are all time-critical conditions and require no further investigations. This is even more crucial if the intended investigation would delay surgical management.

Routine blood tests should be performed and will provide basic information. Raised inflammatory markers (leukocytosis and C-reactive protein) often indicate an inflammatory or infective process; however, these should not be relied on to exclude such conditions as they may be normal, particularly early in the presentation. A urine or blood pregnancy test is very relevant in a female patient in the reproductive age group. Anemia or iron depletion may indicate a more chronic underlying process such as inflammatory bowel disease or occult malignancy.

CT Scan of the Abdomen and Pelvis, with IV Contrast While not the simplest investigation to obtain, it is the most informative though its delay is often the cause of delayed management. Modern CT scanners deliver much less radiation compared to older ones, and the concern around radiation dose should not obviate its use when appropriately indicated.

If the history and examination are clearly in keeping with a gynecological pathology, a pelvic ultrasound may be the ideal initial scan.

Ultrasound Abdominal, pelvic, or both can be very informative if used in the correct indication. If readily available, a prompt scrotal Doppler ultrasound can confirm early testicular torsion; a pelvic ultrasound can identify an ectopic pregnancy or ovarian torsion.

Table 11.2 Quick guide to essential workup prior to surgical referral

	CT abdomen / pelvis[a]	Abdominal ultrasound	Pelvic ultrasound	Groin ultrasound
Diverticular disease	✓	○	×	×
Inguinoscrotal	✓	×	×	✓
Abdominal wall	✓	✓	×	×
Abdominal malignancy	✓	○	○	×
Urological	✓	✓	○	×
Gynecological	✓	○	✓	×

[a]CT of the abdomen and pelvis is most informative with intravenous (IV) contrast. In select cases, noncontrast CT is more specific, such as for diagnosis of urinary tract stones and abdominal wall hernia. Allergy to contrast should also be considered

✓ Useful and / or diagnostic

○ Of limited benefit

× Not useful

Table 11.2 provides a quick guide to pre-referral imaging workup.

11.3 Management

11.3.1 When to Refer to Surgeons?

Acute LLQ abdominal pain that proves to be of surgical nature should be referred to the relevant surgical service.

11.3.2 When Not to Refer to Surgeons?

A clear nonsurgical diagnosis (Table 11.1) can be either referred to the relevant specialty or managed by the primary care physician depending on local expertise and available resources.

Table 11.3 outlines a quick guide to the urgency of referrals or nonreferral in some of the most frequently encountered presentations of LLQ pain.

Table 11.3 A guide to managing different urgency levels for LLQ pain presentations

	Emergent	Urgent	Nonurgent	Other
Diverticular disease	Acute severe diverticulitis Acute complicated diverticulitis (e.g., perforation, peritonitis) Any with significant acute pain requiring narcotics	Subacute presentations or chronic complication (e.g., colovaginal fistula, colovesical fistula)	Chronic diverticular pain without evidence of diverticulitis	Mild diverticulitis in immunocompetent patients. Refer to text p5.
Inguinoscrotal	Testicular torsion Incarcerated or strangulated hernia Abscess	Large groin hernias and/or difficult reduction (incarcerating)	Reducible groin hernias	N/A.
Abdominal wall	Incarcerated or strangulated hernia Abdominal wall abscess Rectus sheath hematoma with severe pain	Symptomatic abdominal wall hernias, with clear signs of intermittent incarceration or intermittent bowel obstruction	Reducible abdominal wall hernias	Mild infections, small abscesses, hematomas can be managed by the PCP.

	Emergent	Urgent	Nonurgent	Other
Abdominal malignancy	Causing severe pain Causing bowel obstruction Requiring time-critical management[a]	Incidental finding of GI, urological, or gynecological cancer	N/A	Cases where a medical oncologist input is required, e.g., hematological malignancies, palliative care, etc.
Urological	Obstructive uropathy Causing severe pain	Other subacute causes of obstructive uropathy[b]	Other urological conditions[b]	
Gynecological	Ectopic pregnancy Ovarian torsion Causing severe pain	Significant endometriosis[c, d]	Other gynecological conditions[d]	

Emergent: requires presentation to the emergency department
Urgent: requires urgent referral to the relevant surgical specialty
Nonurgent: requires nonurgent referral to the relevant surgical specialty
Other: can be managed by the primary care physician or referred to other specialties such as GI medicine and oncology
[a]As is the case of abdominal imaging showing impending bowel obstruction on a Friday night, with otherwise minimal symptoms
[b]Specialist urologist input required
[c]Specialist gynecologist input required
[d]When symptoms are thought to be clearly secondary to significant endometriosis

11.3.3 Management of Selected Surgical Conditions by the Primary Care Physician

Current SAGES practice recommendations support the management of mild uncomplicated diverticulitis in immunocompetent patients in the outpatient setting. Furthermore, a trial of non-antibiotic therapy can be considered with appropriate follow-up in select patients [1].

Bowel rest by downgrading the oral intake to clear fluids, with or without oral antibiotics providing gram-negative and anaerobic cover, as well as adequate pain relief should suffice as the mainstay of initial conservative management. A patient who shows little to no response to this approach should be referred to surgeons without further delay.

Diverticular pain without clear CT evidence of diverticulitis may be managed in a similar fashion as above.

Simple antibiotic management of early stages of localized LLQ infection (cellulitis) without systemic manifestations is not unreasonable.

Reference

1. Francis NK, Sylla P, Abou-Khalil M, Arolfo S, Berler D, Curtis NJ, Dolejs SC, Garfinkle R, Gorter-Stam M, Hashimoto DA, Hassinger TE, Molenaar CJL, Pucher PH, Schuermans V, Arezzo A, Agresta F, Antoniou SA, Arulampalam T, Boutros M, Bouvy N, Campbell K, Francone T, Haggerty SP, Hedrick TL, Stefanidis D, Truitt MS, Kelly J, Ket H, Dunkin BJ, Pietrabissa A. EAES and SAGES 2018 consensus conference on acute diverticulitis management: evidence-based recommendations for clinical practice. Surg Endosc. 2019;33(9):2726–41. https://doi.org/10.1007/s00464-019-06882-z. Epub 2019 June 27. PMID: 31250244; PMCID: PMC6684540.

Right Lower Quadrant (RLQ) Abdominal Pain

12

Noah Jordan and Danielle S. Walsh

12.1 Introduction

Right lower quadrant (RLQ) abdominal pain is one of the more common locations for urgent assessment, particularly since the public are aware of its association with appendicitis. While appendicitis is the most common diagnosis, the similarity of symptoms and presentations to a diverse assortment of disorders in the intestinal, urinary, gynecologic, and lymphatic systems requires the evaluating clinician to remain unbiased and consider a broad differential diagnosis with each patient. Using a consistent assessment algorithm inclusive of history taking, physical examination, broad laboratory studies, and radiographic assessment can minimize the risk of misdiagnosis (Table 12.1).

N. Jordan · D. S. Walsh (✉)
University of Kentucky, Lexington, KY, USA
e-mail: danielle.walsh@uky.edu

G. P. Kohn et al. (eds.), *The SAGES Manual of Surgical Referral for Primary and Emergency Care*,
https://doi.org/10.1007/978-3-031-92678-5_12

Table 12.1 Evaluation summary

History	
	Onset, duration, location, migration, and radiation of pain
	Associated symptoms, including fever, chills, nausea, vomiting, anorexia, diarrhea, constipation, blood in the stool or urine, dysuria, respiratory system changes, and new onset of bulges or masses
	Travel history, dietary history, medications, and exposure to sick contacts
	Prior surgery and medical disorders
	In women: pregnancy, menstrual cycles, sexual activity
Physical exam	
	Inspection for distention or any other abnormalities
	Evaluation location, softness, bowel sounds, percussion, and masses, with focus on peritoneal findings
	Perform special tests for suspected appendicitis if indicated
	Selective pelvic and rectal examinations
Laboratory	
	All: complete blood count, comprehensive chemistry, amylase/lipase, CRP/ESR, urinalysis
	Selective: β-hCG, respiratory panel, gastrointestinal panel, stool studies, STD testing
Imaging	
	Plain films: constipation, intestinal obstruction, free air, pulmonary disorders with referred abdominal pain
	Abdominal ultrasound: appendicitis, mesenteric adenitis, hepatobiliary, pancreatic, renal obstruction
	Pelvic ultrasound: gynecologic pathology, pregnancy
	CT scan: bowel and urinary pathologies
	MRI: if patient has contradiction to radiation exposure

12.2 History

When assessing a patient with RLQ pain, a comprehensive history is essential for developing a differential diagnosis and determining those who may need urgent surgical referral. It is crucial to inquire about the onset, duration, inciting events, and nature of the pain, as well as its location, including any radiation and migration of the pain. Patients should be questioned about the presence or absence of associated symptoms such as fever, chills, nausea, vomiting, anorexia, diarrhea, constipation, blood in the stool or urine, dysuria, respiratory system changes, and new onset of bulges or masses in the area. Note whether emesis is bilious, bloody, or neither. A travel history is important to identify potential travel-related illnesses, gastroenteritis, or other less common conditions. Evaluating the dietary history can reveal recent changes that may have contributed to the pain. Women should be asked about the potential for pregnancy, menstrual cycles, and prior gynecologic disorders. Finally, documenting the patient's medical and surgical history is essential prior to surgical referral as this information can enhance diagnosis and provide valuable insights for surgical assessment.

12.3 Physical Examination

Inspection and palpation are crucial in the evaluation of right lower quadrant pain. As part of a standard physical examination, take note of the patient's status prior to touching them. Patients with peritonitis lay very still as motion induces pain. In contrast, those with crampy pain from intestinal spasms tend to writhe or move frequently to find comfort. The neck, oropharynx, and lungs should be evaluated due to the common presence of mesenteric adenitis in the RLQ in association with strep throat, pneumonia, and even viral respiratory infections.

A detailed abdominal assessment is needed. Begin with visual inspection inclusive of the genitalia and groins, noting the presence or absence of distension, prior surgical scars, and bulges, masses, or potential hernias. Ask the patient to press their own abdomen and localize the site of maximal pain and tenderness. Percuss for tympany as is found with gas-filled bowel and fluid waves as is found with ascites. Then begin palpation, noting masses, hernias, the softness or firmness of the abdomen, and peritoneal signs that occur with testing for rebound or shaking the bed. Look for special signs that provide valuable insights, particularly in cases of appendicitis. Tests such as tenderness at McBurney's point, the psoas sign, and the obturator sign are effective methods for evaluating peritoneal inflammation commonly associated with appendicitis. Ischemic bowel will commonly have pain out of proportion to the physical exam findings.

A rectal examination with guaiac testing is essential in the presence of diarrhea and patient reports of blood in the stool or melena. In females, a bimanual pelvic examination is important to evaluate for possible gynecologic pathologies as the cause of right lower quadrant abdominal pain. However, this is commonly deferred in prepubertal and never sexually active adolescents in favor of imaging.

12.4 Laboratory Studies

Because of the diversity of organ systems that can cause RLQ pain, a broad screening using laboratory testing is employed. With the exception of patients in which the diagnosis is readily apparent, such as an incarcerated right inguinal hernia in a child, these screening labs serve to not only guide the remaining diagnostic workup, they also serve as the foundation for what is needed for proceeding with safe surgical intervention. Laboratory studies that may assist in the diagnosis of right lower quadrant pain include

- Complete blood count (CBC) with differential cell counts: for the assessment of infectious causes, anemia, and potential hematologic/lymphatic contributors.
- Comprehensive chemistries: useful to assess electrolyte disturbances, nutritional status, hepatobiliary causes, and renal contributors.
- C-reactive protein (CRP) and/or erythrocyte sedimentation rate (ESR): sensitive laboratory values for inflammation.
- Pancreatic function with an amylase and/or lipase.
- Urinalysis: assessment for urinary tract infection, proteinuria, or hematuria.

More selective testing can be considered in the following circumstances:

- β-hCG testing in women of childbearing age for assessing of pregnancy: testing can be via urine or serum.
- Respiratory panel testing or more selective tests for infectious organisms such as Covid-19, influenza, *Streptococcus*, and RSV in the setting of outbreaks, exposure, or the right presentation.
- Gastrointestinal panels and stool studies with patients in whom there is concern for food-borne illness, antibiotic-induced diarrhea, or exposure to others with the same.
- Testing for sexually transmitted diseases (STDs) may be indicated based on a combination of history, examination, and index of suspicion.

12.5 Radiographic Studies

The best radiographic modality for evaluation of RLQ pain is dependent on suspected pathology. Plain films are not needed in most patients, but it should be considered first line in the setting of bilious emesis with concern for bowel obstruction, peritonitis when free air is anticipated and for which extremely urgent intervention is expected (precluding cross-sectional imaging), suspected constipation as the underlining cause for pain, foreign body ingestion, and possible referred abdominal pain from a pulmonary disorder. The American College of Radiology guidelines recommend abdominal and pelvic ultrasound as the first line for the evaluation of suspected appendicitis and the evaluation of gynecologic pathology. CT scans are commonly employed if studies if ultrasonography proves indeterminant or body habitus precludes accurate assessment. If a renal source is expected, as with a kidney stone, the study is usually without contrast. For most patients, the CT scan will be performed with Intravenous contrast, especially for suspected appendicitis, diverticulitis, and enteritis. Oral contrast may be added to IV contrast when assessing for intestinal obstruction as occurs in adhesive disease, volvulus, and similar. MRI is used infrequently in the standard evaluation of RLQ pain due to the lack of urgent accessibility and cost, but it may be used in specific cases when avoidance of radiation as in pregnant patients, children, and inflammatory bowel disease.

12.6 Differential Diagnosis

12.6.1 Gastrointestinal Causes

12.6.1.1 Appendicitis

Appendicitis is caused by inflammation of the appendix, which can be precipitated by an obstructing fecolith or primary wall inflammation. Appendicitis classically presents as periumbilical pain that migrates to the right lower quadrant and becomes gradually worse with the development of focal right lower quadrant peritonitis. Patients with appendicitis tend to present with less than 72 hours of pain, often within 24 hours. They may have low-grade fevers and progress to anorexia, nausea, and vomiting usually after the onset of pain. Diarrhea can be present but is more common with perforated appendicitis than early appendicitis. An appendix on or near the ureter or bladder can lead to dysuria and WBCs in the urinalysis with an absence of urinary bacteria. Patients who have perforated appendicitis may have a temporary relief of pain at the time of perforation before having more generalized peritonitis from abdominal contamination. Appendicitis is traditionally treated with acute surgical intervention to prevent complications such as perforation. However, a growing body of evidence supports successful management of early appendicitis with immediate initiation of antibiotics alone. Criteria for trial of nonoperative management of appendicitis remain less well defined and should only be selected in conjunction with a surgeon to facilitate rapid transition to surgical intervention in those who do not respond appropriately to antibiotics.

12.6.1.2 Gastroenteritis

Gastroenteritis is caused by viral, bacterial, or parasitic infection leading to inflammation of the intestines. Pain with gastroenteritis can vary widely, as may the predominant symptoms, including changes in stooling function, nausea, and vomiting. A cramping, dull pain may come and go with the peristalsing movement of the intestines. Gastroenteritis pain may also present as a generalized discomfort or sharper focal pain. Gastroenteritis is typically a self-limited disease. Treatment of gastroenteritis is typically supportive measures with a focus on hydration. Bloody diarrhea is a more concerning feature and should prompt more emergent assessment and supportive care.

12.6.1.3 Diverticulitis

Diverticulitis more commonly presents with left-sided abdominal pain due to diverticular inflammation in the descending and sigmoid colon. However, diverticula may also occur in the cecum leading to inflammatory RLQ pain. Though more common in children than adults, Meckel's diverticulitis may also mimic acute appendicitis and present as RLQ pain. Though recent years have seen a shift toward nonoperative management of classic left-sided and sigmoid diverticulitis, patients with symptomatic diverticula should have urgent surgical assessment.

12.6.1.4 Inflammatory Bowel Disease, esp. Crohn's Disease

Inflammatory bowel disease is another pathology that can present with RLQ pain. Crohn's disease will more commonly present this way as the terminal ileum is the typical point of maximal inflammation and enters a fixed cecum in the RLQ. Patients with inflammatory bowel disease tend to have long-standing abdominal pain that varies in intensity and flares intermittently. Patients will also have other symptoms, including constipation and/or diarrhea and bloody stools. Inflammatory bowel disease is a multisystem disease and may cause concurrent joint pain, skin, and/or eye complaints. Suspected inflammatory bowel disease can be evaluated via CT scan, which will show bowel wall thickening and inflammation or definitive diagnosis can be made via colonoscopy and tissue sampling. Gastroenterology will be a pertinent referral in these patients' long-term care and surveillance.

12.6.1.5 Intestinal Obstruction

Bowel obstructions occur far more commonly in patients with prior abdominal surgery, though tumors and congenital disorders can also precipitate obstruction. Adhesive bands are particularly adept at leading to internal hernias and volvulus. Obstruction pain can be variable in intensity early on, can be less focal, and may have a worsening with bowel peristalsis. Obstructions that go on to ischemia lead to more continuous pain with increased severity. Patients develop progressive intolerance of oral intake and abdominal distention, with more distal obstructions leading to greater distension. If a bowel obstruction is suspected, CT imaging with oral and IV contrast is an important next step in the evaluation as well as surgical referral for prompt evaluation and management. A closed-loop bowel obstruction can cause ischemia with life-threatening complications.

12.6.1.6 Mesenteric Adenitis

Mesenteric adenitis can be the great imitator for appendicitis, especially in children. Mesenteric adenitis is caused by inflammation of the mesenteric lymph nodes usually in the setting of recent illness or sick contacts. Streptococcal pharyngitis is particularly notable for inducing both mesenteric adenitis and acute appendicitis. Patients with mesenteric adenitis typically report GI-related symptoms of gastroenteritis that preceded the pain, which is the inverse of the common appendicitis sequence. The pain tends to be self-limited and improved with supportive care. While mesenteric adenitis may be differentiated via history, definitive diagnosis is through imaging showing enlarged lymph tissue with a normal-appearing appendix. Surgical referral is not necessary if imaging is diagnostic.

12.6.2 Genitourinary Causes

12.6.2.1 Nephrolithiasis (Kidney Stones)

Patients with nephrolithiasis tend to present with sharp or stabbing back pain that may also cause pain in the stone-specific side of the abdomen. Nephrolithiasis commonly causes radiation of pain along the course of the ureter into the groin. Patients may also experience hematuria and urinary symptoms. While some stones may pass spontaneously, others require the care of a urologist for management.

12.6.2.2 Urinary Tract Infection

Urinary tract infections may cause RLQ pain accompanied by urinary symptoms such as urgency and frequency. Urinalysis is often diagnostic, though imaging to assess for obstruction or persistent inflammation of the urinary tract can be helpful in patients who do not respond to antibiotics or appear more toxic.

12.6.2.3 Ectopic Pregnancy

Ectopic pregnancy is a serious diagnosis that should be considered in women of childbearing age presenting with lower abdominal pain. Patients may also experience vaginal bleeding or spotting or more vague symptoms of nausea and vomiting. If suspected, this should be urgently evaluated with pelvic ultrasound, with emergent referral to a gynecologist if positive.

12.6.2.4 Ovarian Cyst or Torsion

Ovarian cysts are common in females and can occur as early infancy due to maternal hormones, in any age due to tumors, and most commonly in women of childbearing age. Variable abdominal pain from cysts presents most commonly at the time of ovulation—2 weeks into a typical 28-day cycle. Ovarian cysts usually are self-limited but may be removed if they are large or continue to be symptomatic. Cysts can also become a lead point for ovarian torsion. Ovarian torsions present as sudden sharp lower abdominal pain that is unrelenting and may cause acute nausea and vomiting. Both cysts and torsions are emergently evaluated via pelvic ultrasound with focus on cyst size, presence of fluid vs solid components, and Doppler blood flow to the adnexa. Prompt gynecologic surgical referral for possible preservation of the ovary is indicated.

12.6.3 Other Causes

12.6.3.1 Hernias

A variety of hernias may cause RLQ pain. An inguinal hernia typically presents with groin pain but may have pain that radiates to the RLQ or down into the genitalia. If a patient has prior surgical scars, especially in the RLQ, an incisional hernia is a consideration. A Spigelian hernia is a less common hernia largely in older adults and is caused by protrusion of abdominal contents between the lateral edge of the rectus abdominis muscle medially and the semilunar line laterally. If a hernia is the suspected cause of the patient's pain, physical examination can commonly identify it and should include notation of whether it is reducible, incarcerated, or strangulated (incarceration with ischemia). Acutely incarcerated and strangulated hernias require urgent surgical referral due to the risk of progression to bowel obstruction and necrosis. Reducible hernias are more commonly managed in the elective, outpatient setting.

12.7 Indications for Referral

Though some causes of RLQ, such as mesenteric adenitis, reducible hernia, and gastroenteritis, can undergo a trial of outpatient management, the vast majority of patients with RLQ pain require same-day examination, laboratory assessment, and imaging. Those presenting to a primary care office can be assessed for the few nonemergent diagnosis, such as reducible hernias and adenopathy in nontoxic patients, but the need for bloodwork and radiographic studies to work through the broad differential above commonly leads patients to be evaluated in an emergency room. A delay in diagnosis for many of the common disorders can lead to serious injury to the patient and poor outcomes. Outpatient medical offices contacted with potentially life-threatening symptoms should encourage patients to call for emergent transport directly to an emergency room; these symptoms include unremitting severe and acute pain, known pregnancy, hemodynamic

Table 12.2 Emergencies for referral

Indications for emergent surgical referral for right lower quadrant pain
Acute onset of pain that inhibits activities of daily life
Emesis with inability to maintain hydration or transition to bilious
Bloody emesis, diarrhea, or urination
Diarrhea with inability to maintain hydration
Inability to urinate or marked decrease in urination
Hemodynamic instability
Findings of peritonitis or an incarcerated hernia on examination
Pain out of proportion to abdominal examination findings
Suspicion for appendicitis
Pregnancy

instability, description of peritonitis, severe diarrhea, and repeated emesis, especially if bilious or bloody (Table 12.2).

Most emergency rooms will promptly consult the appropriate surgeon specialist for further assessment and management. Outpatient but timely referral to a surgeon can occur for pain of a more chronic and/or intermittent nature, subacute diverticulitis, mildly symptomatic hernias that can be reduced, and adenopathy. Urologic-based disorders such as stones, hematuria, dysuria, hydronephrosis, and recurrent urinary tract infections may be amenable to urgent but not emergent assessment by a urologist and/or nephrologist, though symptomatic urinary obstruction requires emergent assessment. Gynecologic emergencies, such as ectopic pregnancy, tubo-ovarian abscess, and ovarian torsion, are commonly managed through the emergency department in conjunction with a gynecologic surgeon. Gastroenterologists often partner with surgeons for the management of nonischemic colonic volvulus, enteritis, and inflammatory bowel disease. They also perform nonacute colonoscopy in patients with diverticulitis or in the assessment of colonic disorders, including masses, strictures, and bleeding. Finally, the full spectrum of intestinal, urologic, gynecologic, and other abdominal disorders in a child or adolescent may be managed by a pediatric surgeon, depending on local resources and norms.

12.8 Conclusion

RLQ pain is a common complaint requiring urgent to emergent assessment with a comprehensive history, examination, laboratory assessment, and radiographic imaging. It commonly requires the involvement of a surgeon or surgical specialist for timely intervention as delay can lead to increased morbidity and mortality. Patients presenting to the outpatient clinician should be encouraged to proceed with a comprehensive evaluation unless a clearly nonemergent cause is identified on examination.

Suggested Reading

1. Cartwright SL, Knudson MP. Evaluation of acute abdominal pain in adults. Am Fam Physician. 2008;77(7):971–8.
2. Lotfollahzadeh S, Lopez RA, Deppen JG. Appendicitis. [Updated 2024 Feb 12]. In: StatPearls [Internet]. Treasure Island (FL): StatPearls Publishing; 2024 Jan-. Available from: https://www.ncbi.nlm.nih.gov/books/NBK493193/.
3. Vaghef-Davari F, Ahmadi-Amoli H, Sharifi A, Teymouri F, Paprouschi N. Approach to acute abdominal pain: practical algorithms. Adv J Emerg Med. 2019;4(2):e29. https://doi.org/10.22114/ajem.v0i0.272. PMID: 32322797; PMCID: PMC7163264.
4. For Diagnosing appendicitis in children >5 years old:pARC Score: www.mdcalc.com/calc/10201/pediatric-appendicitis-risk-calculator-parc.

Groin Pain Syndrome (Formerly Known as Sportsman's Hernia)

13

Chrys Hensman

13.1 Changes to Taxonomy, Investigations, and Pathology

It is critically important that correct terminology is used to describe the many pathological conditions that may present as groin pain syndrome (GrPS); terminology such as sportsman's hernia that has been used in the past has been replaced by the term GrPS following consensus meetings in Manchester, Doha, and Italy [1].

Chronic groin pain is a common and complex problem among athletes but can also occur in the general population. This condition used to be known to most as "sportsman's hernia." Due to the complex anatomical aspects of the groin and adjacent structures, many conditions can present as groin pain. It is also known as inguinal disruption according to the latest consensus.

C. Hensman (✉)
Monash University, University of Adelaide, Swinburne University, LapSurgery Australia, Dandenong North, VIC, Australia
e-mail: chensman@lapsurg.net.au

G. P. Kohn et al. (eds.), *The SAGES Manual of Surgical Referral for Primary and Emergency Care*,
https://doi.org/10.1007/978-3-031-92678-5_13

Groin pain is a common symptom in athletes, accompanied by a very complex nomenclature that makes diagnosis and treatment challenging. Despite the publication of three consensus statements, rejected terms are still widely used in the literature. Healthcare professionals dealing with groin pain should be careful when examining the literature since the use of various terms in different ways may lead to false conclusions, thus making evidence-based practice difficult.

13.2 Diagnosis

Good history and clinical examination are important and the cornerstone to diagnose GrPS, but mainly to also to rule out other differential diagnoses and associated injuries that can also present as chronic groin pain. Diagnosis and decision for surgical intervention for GrPS are on clinical grounds.

Practice Point 1
The common presentation is groin pain, not exclusively worsened by exercise, in male athletes but also described in females.

Practice Point 2
The use of specialized diagnosis tests and/or decision for intervention is mainly based on clinical grounds.

- **What constitutes an emergency requiring ER presentation?**

The red flag symptoms and signs are the following and require escalation of the referral on for specialist opinion; these include but are not exclusive of

- Systemic symptoms such as fever, chills, and loss of appetite.
- Radiological investigation indicates serious pathology such as osteitis pubis or major hip pathology.

What requires urgent surgical review?

- Worsening symptoms with immobility and systemic symptoms outlined above indicative of sepsis or infection requires escalation of the referral process.

What requires nonurgent surgical review?

- It is appropriate to refer on to the nonsurgical option if after a period of conservative measures of 4–6 weeks there is a lack of improvement or worsening of symptoms.

What features would mean that the condition can be managed by the primary care physician (PCP)?

- In the setting where clinical examination and radiological investigation does not reveal any significant pathology, it is appropriate for the PCP to continue management with input from a physical therapist.
- The management by the PCP will include general advice on activity, rest, and avoidance of aggravating triggers combined with simple analgesics such as paracetamol, and where safe and there is no contraindication, the judicious use of nonsteroidal anti-inflammatory agents for a short period of time (2–4 weeks) may be prudent.

Imaging modalities such as ultrasound of the groin, hip, and pelvis and MRI of the groin and hips utilizing a specific MRI protocol to investigate GrPS are best discussed with the radiological service you use. Rarely nuclear medicine bone scans, when osteitis pubis is suspected, may have their roles to help achieve diagnosis and look for other causes of groin pain.

Practice Point 3

The investigation by ultrasound of the groin, pelvis, and hips, MRI of the abdomen, pelvis, and hips and groins by the use of a specific GrPS, MRI protocol (best discussed with your preferred provider) may help with diagnosis and exclude other causes of pain but clinical examination and careful physical evaluation of symptoms must always be corelated to special investigations And are as important as imaging.

Recommended treatment for sportsman's hernia, to begin with, is essentially a trial of conservative treatment that includes physiotherapy, sports rehabilitation, and medications for symptomatic pain relief.

- A short period of conservative management may be indicated, in pragmatic terms a period of 2–4 weeks, when the clinical findings and imaging do not indicate serious pathology.
- Review process after this time frame is prudent to gauge progress and assess if referral on for further assessment may be required.

Surgical intervention can be discussed if there is a failure of conservative treatment when specific pathology is found on special investigations. Recommended surgery is open or laparoscopic hernia repair with mesh. However, as this is a complex and still a poorly understood problem, a multidisciplinary approach is recommended to optimize the patient's outcome.

Practice Point 4

GrPS is mostly treated in a multidisciplinary approach and in the first instance involves sports rehabilitation and involvement of a sports physician and physiotherapist and pain medication.

- Surgical treatment may be indicated when specific pathology such as hip pathology is pinpointed. Ultrasound-directed intervention may also be helpful when tendinitis is identified as an etiology.

As there is still limited evidence on this topic, more studies are required in order to come up with strict guidelines or protocols to recommend a systematic approach to GrPS (sportsman's hernia).

Reference

1. Bisciotti GN, Zini R, Aluigi M, Aprato A, Auci A, Bellinzona E, Benelli P, Bigoni M, Bisciotti A, Bisciotti A, Bona S, Brustia M, Bruzzone M, Canata GL, Carulli C, Cassaghi G, Coli M, Corsini A, Costantini A, Dallari D, Danelli G, Danesi G, Della Rocca F, De Nardo P, Di Benedetto P, Di Marzo F, Di Pietto F, Eirale C, Ferretti A, Fogli M, Foglia A, Guardoli A, Guglielmi A, Lama D, Maffulli N, Manunta AF, Massari L, Mazzoni G, Moretti B, Moretti L, Nanni G, Niccolai R, Occhialini M, Panascì M, Parra MF, Pigalarga G, Randelli F, Sacchini M, Salini V, Santori N, Tenconi P, Tognini G, Vegnuti M, Zanini A, Volpi P. Groin pain syndrome Italian consensus conference update 2023. J Sports Med Phys Fitness. 2024;64(4):402–14. https://doi.org/10.23736/S0022-4707.23.15517-4. Epub 2023 Dec 21. PMID: 38126972.

Melena

14

Rodolfo J. Oviedo

14.1 Background

The word melena comes from the Greek *melas* or *melaina*, for the color black. It represents the external manifestation of acute or chronic upper gastrointestinal bleeding (UGIB) or lower gastrointestinal bleeding (LGIB) from a variety of possible etiologies that ultimately express themselves with bleeding per rectum. While the first assumption from the clinician could be of LGIB only, the most common source of melena is UGIB. This may cause delays in diagnostic protocols and in treatment algorithms based on the erroneous assumption that melena must be specific to the lower GI tract. Melena is simply a sign that the stool contains old blood, or blood that has been collected throughout the GI tract during its passage in the lumen over an extended period of time or from a distance with respect to the anal canal that is not compatible with fresh, red blood per rectum, which is known as hematochezia. It is

R. J. Oviedo (✉)
Department of Surgery, Nacogdoches Medical Center,
Nacogdoches, TX, USA

University of Houston Tilman J. Fertitta Family College of Medicine,
Houston, TX, USA

Sam Houston State University College of Osteopathic Medicine,
Conroe, TX, USA

G. P. Kohn et al. (eds.), *The SAGES Manual of Surgical Referral for Primary and Emergency Care*,
https://doi.org/10.1007/978-3-031-92678-5_14

important to mention that melena can be seen with or without hematemesis, which is an external manifestation of UGIB consisting of vomiting fresh blood or coffee-grounds emesis fluid. When melena is associated with concomitant hematemesis, usually the prognosis is worse, and it requires a more expeditious diagnostic and treatment algorithm implementation. While hematemesis has long been regarded as a medical and potential surgical emergency, melena is equally as important as hematemesis for the reasons listed above, and an ABC approach is also required to diagnose its etiology and treat it. This ABC approach refers to the resuscitation protocol that focuses on protecting the *airway*, ensuring that *breathing* is taking place, and securing access to the *circulatory* system via intravenous cannulation and fluid resuscitation, which usually begins with crystalloid and which may require blood products. The most important aspect when treating a patient who is experiencing melena is to follow these basic resuscitation tenets and eventually reach a phase in the treatment algorithm that will require an endoscopic evaluation before considering advanced radiographic diagnostic or therapeutic modalities, which are not considered the gold standard and might not be widely available at all centers.

14.2 Rationale for Surgeon Referral

Referral to a surgeon will depend on the availability of resources and the context of the environment in which the patient is being seen. For example, the workplace could be an academic or urban center where gastroenterologists may be available versus a rural or community practice where surgeons typically perform endoscopy for diagnostic and therapeutic purposes given the lack of availability of gastroenterologists, or simply due to the philosophy of care that has become the norm within that environment. In either case, referral to a surgeon must be ensured if the process of acute UGIB or LGIB expressed as melena cannot be stopped by conventional measures and if endoscopy must be performed due to lack of stabilization of the hemoglobin and hematocrit with or without hemodynamic compromise. Nevertheless, if the cause of melena is chronic GI bleeding from an upper or lower GI source, a surgeon can still be consulted. Referral can be arranged due to the need to perform an endoscopic evaluation that may diagnose a malignant process or a benign type of pathology that may eventually lead to massive and acute GI bleeding if not controlled at an early stage. It is essential to understand that before obtaining advanced radiographic studies such as a nuclear tagged red blood cell scan or a computerized tomography (CT) angiogram, or even a visceral angiogram, all of which have powerful diagnostic and/or therapeutic potential, the gold standard continues to be the performance of an upper gastrointestinal endoscopy or esophagogastroduodenoscopy (EGD) first based on the principle that the most common source of melena is an UGIB source. Then, a colonoscopy is the second diagnostic and potentially therapeutic maneuver after an EGD has been performed and after a mechanical bowel prep has taken place, for completion purposes and especially if an EGD does not show a good enough reason to suspect that the upper GI tract is the source of the bleeding. Both the EGD and the colonoscopy can be performed by a gastroenterologist or a surgeon, but in many communities, especially in smaller cities or towns, or in rural areas, primary care professionals (PCPs) are able to perform these life-saving procedures with efficiency and expertise. This is particularly relevant in many communities where specialist referral may be logistically challenging. However, regardless of which specialist performs the endoscopy, the most important aspect of understanding when to refer a patient to a surgical specialist is the resuscitation outcome. If resuscitation is not adequately achieved, the patient may continue to bleed at a rate that, if not properly addressed and treated, might lead to cardiovascular collapse due to hemorrhagic shock and hypovolemia despite blood product resuscitation and indicated pharmacotherapy.

14.3 Endoscopic Evaluation: How Early?

As mentioned earlier, there are two types of endoscopic evaluation modalities that are relevant in melena: an EGD and a colonoscopy. Typically, the EGD should be performed first and early given the likelihood that the source of hemorrhage, although slow or low-volume, might be from the upper GI tract. Then, a colonoscopy should be performed ideally after 24 hours from presentation and following a mechanical bowel prep, especially if the EGD does not reveal a clear source of bleeding, or a convincing source, at least. Early colonoscopy, in comparison, takes place within the first 24 hours and should be reserved for patients with high-risk features of LGIB such as contrast extravasation on an initial CT scan in the presence of hemodynamic compromise or lack of stabilization of the hemoglobin and hematocrit (H/H). While it has been mentioned that advanced radiographic studies should not take precedence over a proper endoscopic evaluation, many times a CT scan is performed before referral to a surgeon, and in the context of contrast extravasation (leakage) it is reasonable to consider an early colonoscopy depending on the success of administration of the bowel prep and surgeon expertise.

14.4 Potential Sources of Melena

The potential causes of melena can be regarded in terms of their organ of origin. If the oral cavity is the beginning and the ligament of Treitz is considered the end of the upper GI tract, the organs of interest from the upper GI tract are the esophagus, the stomach, and the duodenum. There are also other less frequent sources of acute UGIB that may not have their origin in the lumen of these organs, but which eventually enter their lumen from a different organ or structure. The esophagus has possible etiologies such as esophageal varices, erosive esophagitis, malignancy, infectious esophagitis, Mallory–Weiss tear, or black esophagus (due to ischemia). The stomach may be the source of acute UGIB due to peptic ulcer disease (PUD), gastric varices, malignancy, or a Dieulafoy lesion. The duodenum may be the source due to PUD or malignancy. Examples of less frequent causes are an aortoenteric fistula, hemosuccus pancreaticus, and hemobilia. The lower GI tract, in contrast, begins with the ligament of Treitz and ends with the anal canal. In this setting, the small bowel becomes a difficult organ to assess with typical endoscopic modalities and may require a more thorough and dedicated evaluation with balloon enteroscopy after EGD and colonoscopy have been performed and after advanced radiographic studies such as CT angiogram have been obtained. If the colon is the organ of suspicion, causes may include polyps or tumors, both malignant and benign, vascular lesions such as arteriovenous malformations, diverticulosis, hemorrhoids, rectal ulcers, anal fissures, colonic or rectal varices, colitis (ischemic, infectious, or other types), as well as metastatic lesions.

14.5 Patient Evaluation Prior to Surgeon Referral

Along with the resuscitation efforts described above, equally important is the evaluation of the patient's laboratory studies that are relevant to the episode UGIB or LGIB including the complete blood count (CBC), and basic metabolic profile (BMP), along with coagulation studies such as prothrombin time (PT), partial thromboplastin time (PTT), and international normalized ratio (INR). A type and screen (T&S) and a type and cross (T&C) are mandatory in the context of acute UGIB or LGIB to guide the resuscitation efforts with appropriate blood products depending on the acuity of the situation. Other laboratory studies that may prove useful include the hepatic function panel as well as the arterial blood gas (ABG), especially if the patient is experiencing hemorrhagic shock and if tissue perfusion is a concern due to massive intraluminal hemorrhage. However, before considering advanced radiographic studies that may not have a high rate of success at localizing the bleeding lesions, one must be aware of the shock index (SI) score. The SI score is calculated by dividing the patient's heart rate by the systolic blood pressure. This is an easy assessment tool that, if greater than 1, may indicate the need for a CT angiogram due to the presence of hemodynamic instability from GI bleeding (whether upper or lower). In this context, SI > 1 justifies a CT angiogram. If positive, the bleeding source can be treated endoscopically via EGD or colonoscopy, or sometimes radiographically with a visceral angiogram and embolization. If the CT angiogram is negative, or if the SI score is <1, endoscopy is still performed as the preferred diagnostic and therapeutic modality. Table 14.1 describes the key steps in the clinical decision-making process when evaluating and treating a patient with melena. Table 14.2 introduces the most important evaluation maneuvers that are necessary prior to consulting a surgical specialist.

Table 14.1 Key features of the clinical decision-making process when evaluating and treating patients with melena

Features of emergency presentation	Criteria for urgent surgical review/consultation	Criteria for nonurgent surgical review—consultation	Conditions for management by PCP versus referral to GI medicine
Hemodynamic instability	Hemodynamic instability	Hemodynamic stability	Hemodynamic stability
Need for significant blood product transfusion without improvement (>4 units of PRBC) over the first 24 hours	Inability to respond to massive transfusion protocol	Appropriate response to blood transfusion	Appropriate response to blood transfusion
Acute/surgical abdomen	Acute/surgical abdomen	Abdominal pain (without peritonitis)	No abdominal pain and resolution of melena

Table 14.2 Diagnostic testing maneuvers prior to consultation with a surgical specialist

Physical exam and clinical maneuvers	Laboratory studies	Radiographic studies
Thorough or focused abdominal physical exam (depending on patient's instability)	CBC	Chest X-ray
If possible, proctoscopy/anoscopy exam	BMP	Abdominal X-ray
Large bore peripheral IV lines with isotonic crystalloid fluids	PT, PTT, INR	CT abdomen/pelvis (unless an acute/surgical abdomen prohibits it)
Blood product transfusion (possible need for massive transfusion protocol)	Hepatic function panel, amylase, lipase	CT abdomen/pelvis angiogram (in cases when surgical consultation cannot be obtained immediately, and only if the patient's hemodynamics allow it)

14.6 Summary and Treatment Algorithm

Figure 14.1 illustrates a practical approach to the diagnostic work-up for melena and the indications for surgeon referral with endoscopic intervention or possible surgery. After initial assessment and resuscitation with the ABC approach, IVF and blood product resuscitation along with laboratory studies evaluation will be followed by referral to a surgical specialist. This is crucial when such efforts do not lead to resolution of the hemorrhagic process and if the hemoglobin and hematocrit and cardiovascular status of the patient continue to decompensate. Surgical judgment regarding the need for an operation after UGI endoscopy is not the subject of this chapter, but it should be discussed by the surgeon with the referring physician depending on the endoscopic findings and the rate of success of intraluminal therapeutic intervention in controlling the source of bleeding with a nonsurgical approach.

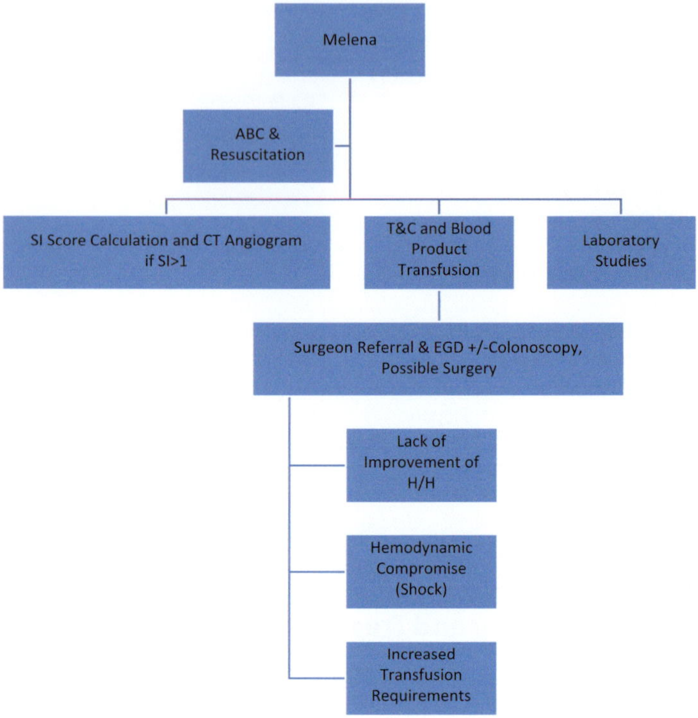

Fig. 14.1 Practical algorithm for the diagnostic workup and management of melena

Selected Readings

1. Morgenthal CB, Richards WO, Dunkin BJ, Forde KA, Vitale G, Lin E, SAGES Flexible Endoscopy Committee. The role of the surgeon in the evolution of flexible endoscopy. Surg Endosc. 2007;21(6):838–53. https://doi.org/10.1007/s00464-006-9109-4. Epub 2006 Dec 16. PMID: 17180263.
2. Barkun AN, Almadi M, Kuipers EJ, Laine L, Sung J, Tse F, Leontiadis GI, Abraham NS, Calvet X, Chan FKL, Douketis J, Enns R, Gralnek IM, Jairath V, Jensen D, Lau J, Lip GYH, Loffroy R, Maluf-Filho F, Meltzer AC, Reddy N, Saltzman JR, Marshall JK, Bardou M. Management of nonvariceal upper gastrointestinal bleeding: guideline recommendations

from the international consensus group. Ann Intern Med. 2019;171(11):805–22. https://doi.org/10.7326/M19-1795. Epub 2019 Oct 22. PMID: 31634917; PMCID: PMC7233308.

3. Aoki T, Hirata Y, Yamada A, Koike K. Initial management for acute lower gastrointestinal bleeding. World J Gastroenterol. 2019;25(1):69–84. https://doi.org/10.3748/wjg.v25.i1.69. PMID: 30643359; PMCID: PMC6328962.
4. Triantafyllou K, Gkolfakis P, Gralnek IM, Oakland K, Manes G, Radaelli F, Awadie H, Camus Duboc M, Christodoulou D, Fedorov E, Guy RJ, Hollenbach M, Ibrahim M, Neeman Z, Regge D, Rodriguez de Santiago E, Tham TC, Thelin-Schmidt P, van Hooft JE. Diagnosis and management of acute lower gastrointestinal bleeding: European Society of Gastrointestinal Endoscopy (ESGE) guideline. Endoscopy. 2021;53(8):850–68. https://doi.org/10.1055/a-1496-8969. Epub 2021 June 1. Erratum in: Endoscopy. 2021 June 17; PMID: 34062566.
5. Oakland K, Chadwick G, East JE, Guy R, Humphries A, Jairath V, McPherson S, Metzner M, Morris AJ, Murphy MF, Tham T, Uberoi R, Veitch AM, Wheeler J, Regan C, Hoare J. Diagnosis and management of acute lower gastrointestinal bleeding: guidelines from the British Society of Gastroenterology. Gut. 2019;68(5):776–89. https://doi.org/10.1136/gutjnl-2018-317807. Epub 2019 Feb 12. PMID: 30792244.

Rectal Bleeding 15

Lawrence Cetrulo

Abbreviations

AVM	arteriovenous malformation
CTA	computed tomography angiogram
IBD	inflammatory bowel disease
IV	intravenous
MRE	magnetic resonance enterography
NEC	necrotizing enterocolitis
NPO	nothing per os
US	ultrasound

15.1 Introduction

Rectal bleeding is a broad description of a problem that can range from a life-threatening emergency to a common occurrence common enough that it becomes a normal part of a patient's life. The vast majority of patients with rectal bleeding that does not result in hemodynamic instability do not need emergent evaluation by a surgical team. Even in the setting of significant rectal bleeding,

L. Cetrulo (✉)
University of Washington – Northwest Hospital, Seattle, WA, USA

G. P. Kohn et al. (eds.), *The SAGES Manual of Surgical Referral for Primary and Emergency Care*,
https://doi.org/10.1007/978-3-031-92678-5_15

consultation of both the surgical team and the gastroenterology team should occur at the same time. Many of these emergency situations can be managed well with endoscopy. In the hemodynamically unstable patient, interventional radiology should also be consulted. In the stable emergency room patient and in the outpatient primary care setting, the outpatient evaluation can happen at a time of convenience to the patient.

Any patient with rectal bleeding should have consideration for a referral for endoscopic evaluation to rule out a potential malignancy, especially in adults 45 and over.

In the pediatric population, the surgical consultation in the emergency room should play an important role in the workup and evaluation. Many of the conditions will not require surgery to resolve, but early involvement of the surgical team can help expedite the most important imaging studies that would be necessary for a safe surgical procedure.

15.2 Pediatric

The etiology of pediatric rectal bleeding can range from benign (infectious, constipation) to severe pathologies that require emergent surgical evaluation. The most important factors to assess are the child's hemodynamic status and clinical exam.

15.2.1 Differential (Pediatric)

- **Anal fissure**
  - In a child with a history of constipation and exam notable for anal fissure, surgical treatment is rarely needed. Symptoms usually improve with medical management.
  - Initial treatment should include stool softeners such as polyethylene glycol (macrogol), Sitz baths daily, and topical analgesics such as lidocaine ointment. Use of calcium channel blockers is increasing in pediatric care but is poorly studied.

  - *Primary care/ED*: Refractory fissure after 6–8 weeks of maximal medical therapy should lead to referral to pediatric surgery.
- **Bleeding Meckel's diverticulum**
  Common congenital anomaly due to incomplete vitelline duct obliteration. Patients are mostly asymptomatic but may present with painless rectal bleeding. A small subset of patients may present with vague gastrointestinal complaints as well. It should be noted that obstruction is the most common presenting symptom of a symptomatic Meckel's before bleeding. Initial workup should include screening for symptoms of anemia.
  - *Primary care*: outpatient Meckel's diverticular scan
  - *ED*: outpatient Meckel's diverticular scan
  - *Consult*: outpatient pediatric surgery referral if scan is positive
- **Bleeding due to IBD (in older children)**
  Presentation in the pediatric patient is variable, as some will have extraintestinal symptoms only. A careful history and physical screening for dermatologic, musculoskeletal, hepatic, ocular, and hematologic symptoms is paramount in addition to the typical weight loss, abdominal pain, rectal bleeding, and diarrheal symptoms.
  - *Primary care/ED*: outpatient diagnostic workup and gastroenterology referral for endoscopic evaluation and disease management.
  - *Consult*: pediatric surgery consult in the ED for acute complications of IBD such as acute bowel obstruction, and refractory unstable bleeding. Otherwise, outpatient referral.
- **Intussusception**
  This is caused by the telescoping of bowel, most commonly at the ileo-colic junction, caused by inflamed Peyer's patches secondary to a recent infection (often upper respiratory). Maintain a high index of suspicion for intussusception in those with a history of lymphoma as well. It happens most commonly in infants and children between 3 months and 3 years of age. They often present with colicky abdominal pain, emesis, and rectal bleeding that is "currant jelly-like."

  - *Primary care*: Immediate ED transfer.
  - *ED*: Obtain abdominal ultrasound (US), look for target sign. Resuscitation is required before almost all surgical procedures. To expedite surgical treatment, initiate fluid resuscitation prior to surgical consultation.
  - *Consult*: Radiology for air enema reduction; pediatric surgery.
- **Volvulus**
  Volvulus occurs due to congenital anomalies of intestinal rotation and fixation. It commonly occurs in the first few weeks of life but may happen at any age. Infants presenting with acute-onset abdominal distention, pain, bilious vomiting, and bloody stools need urgent escalation of care—especially in the setting of hemodynamic instability.
  - *Primary care*: Immediate ED transfer
  - *ED*: Labs, resuscitate. Imaging such as stat upper GI or abdominal X-ray (may show double bubble sign) will help determine urgency of an operation. Make sure of patient nothing per os (NPO) status and try to help ensure that family is present for consent purposes.
  - *Consult*: Start pediatric surgery.
- **Necrotizing enterocolitis**
  A serious illness that primarily affects neonates, in particular preterm infants, due to bacterial destruction of the intestinal wall. Important risk factors include prematurity, low birth weight, and high osmotic strength formula feeding. Symptoms include acute-onset abdominal pain, vomiting, diarrhea, bloody stools, and distention. Exam findings include distention, tenderness, and severe cases may present with abdominal wall erythema and discoloration.
  - *Primary care*: Immediate ED transfer
  - *ED*: Abdominal X-ray to rule out perforation. Look for signs of pneumatosis intestinalis and portal venous air.
    - *Initial management*: NPO, nasogastric tube placement, broad-spectrum antibiotics with enteric and anaerobic coverage, and resuscitation.
  - *Consult*: Start pediatric surgery consult.

15.2.2 Differential (Adult)

The differential for adult rectal bleeding is broad—it ranges from benign conditions (infection, trauma) to serious diagnoses such as cancer. History and physics are important. A thorough anorectal exam with digital palpation is paramount to establishing an accurate diagnosis. Having familiarity with bedside anoscopy is crucial in diagnosis for surgical causes and should be available in the ED setting. In-office anoscopic exam is encouraged. *For all patients meeting the requirement for screening colonoscopy, timely referral for colonoscopy is strongly recommended.*

In hemodynamically unstable patients in the ED, rapid consultation should occur depending on the level of workup. Interventional radiology or vascular surgery consultation should also be considered in the unstable patient as angiographic bleeding control can be considered. In the stable patient, it is preferred to have imaging if the bleeding is severe. A computed tomography angiography (CTA) protocolled to GI bleeding [intravenous (IV) contrast on a particular arterial phase, and no oral contrast] should be obtained rapidly.

- **Anal fissure**
  Commonly caused by trauma from constipation or sexual practices. First line of therapy is medical management with aggressive constipation treatment. Consider surgical intervention only after refractory symptoms despite maximal lifestyle and medical management.
  - *Primary care/ED*: Thorough rectal exam, including DRE, to rule out underlying mass. Of note, balancing patient comfort is important in working with patients with anal fissure. DRE can worsen pain and cause repeat tearing.
  - *Consult*: Outpatient referral to general or colorectal surgery for the consideration of Botox injection versus sphincterotomy if symptoms remain refractory after maximal medical therapy in 6–8 weeks.

- **Hemorrhoids (Internal and/or External)**
  Hemorrhoids are normal vascular cushions within the anal canal, a point that should be considered when patients report having hemorrhoids in the ED or outpatient setting. They provide bulk to facilitate continence. When hemorrhoids prolapse due to increased abdominal pressures such as pregnancy, chronic straining from constipation, and COPD, patients can experience pruritus, bleeding from superficial excoriation, pain, burning, and mucous discharge. Important differentials to consider include anorectal and/or colon cancer in the right age groups or those with significant personal/family risk factors.
  A thorough rectal examination is important for these patients, especially in the outpatient setting. It can often avoid the need for surgical consultation. Discussion of bathroom habits including duration of time spent both on the toilet total and time straining, some type of common nomenclature such as the Bristol stool chart to describe the quality of the patients' stools, and cleaning habits. If pruritus is a major presenting symptom, it is especially important to address these issues before surgical consultation. Over wiping, using hydrocortisone-containing compounds, and use of suppositories can often worsen symptoms long term and increase the frequency of rectal bleeding.
  – *Primary care/ED*: Thorough rectal exam, including DRE to rule out underlying mass. Anoscopic evaluation can help determine hemorrhoid location and grading.
  – *Consult*: Outpatient referral to general or colorectal surgery for banding vs excision if symptoms remain refractory after maximal medical therapy in 6–8 weeks. ED evaluation only if there is concern for external hemorrhoid thrombosis.
    - A patient presenting with less than 72 h of anal pain and clinical findings suggestive of a thrombosed external hemorrhoid should have urgent surgical consultation. Rarely, internal hemorrhoids can create a significant level of rectal bleeding. Especially in a patient on chronic anticoagulation, internal hemorrhoids can cause rapid bleeding. Rectal packing with gauze can help temporarily reduce the bleeding until the surgical team can evaluate the patient.

- **Rectal prolapse**
  Tends to occur in older, female individuals, associated with weakened pelvic floor. Symptoms will include incontinence, protrusion, and mucous discharge or bleeding. The exam will show full thickness, circumferential intussusception of the rectal mucosa. Unlike other common causes of rectal bleeding, the treatment for rectal prolapse is surgical, although aggressive avoidance of constipation remains an important strategy to improve symptomatic control. **Polyethylene glycol (also known as Macrogol) should be the primary stool softener to use in all adult patients.**
  - *Primary care*: Thorough rectal exam with Valsalva maneuver to confirm the presence of rectal prolapse. No indication for ED evaluation if not acutely incarcerated/strangulated.
  - *ED*: When evaluating a patient with acutely incarcerated prolapse, attempt manual reduction over a warm cloth. Apply granulated sugar on the prolapsed tissue and re-attempt reduction in 15–20 min. In the setting of incarceration/irreducible prolapse, these maneuvers will still help reduce the size of the prolapse.
    - To optimize success, pain control and anxiolytics can be considered. Patient positioning is important in this disease process as well. Having the patient in the lateral decubitus position with their knees up to their chest can optimize success rates.
  - *Consult*: Outpatient colorectal surgery referral unless incarcerated and cannot be reduced.
- **Arteriovenous malformation (AVM)**
  These are rare, abnormal connections between the arterial and venous systems in the small bowel or colon. They can cause occult, chronic lower GI bleeding, which may lead to significant and symptomatic anemia. Note that when it occurs in the colon, it can result in rapid, arterial bleeding. Acquired lesions usually occur in older individuals, commonly in the ascending colon. Congenital lesions typically impact younger patients and are large in size. Diagnosis is made endoscopically, although some can be seen on contrasted CT scan. Given

advancements in endoscopic treatment of GI bleeds, surgical intervention is rarely required.

- *Primary care*: Referral for endoscopic evaluation first with surgical evaluation following if endoscopic management fails.
- *ED*: CTA abdomen/pelvis with and no oral contrast in those presenting with rectal bleeding, anemia, and no additional findings on physical exam.
  - In any bleeding patient, a CTA protocolled for GI bleeding will be of significant benefit.
- *Consult*: If CT confirms an AVM in a stable patient, outpatient GI referral is recommended. Surgical consult is usually indicated in the setting of clinically significant, ongoing bleeding that has been resistant to endoscopic treatment. Resuscitation and potential blood transfusions should be initiated early and in the emergency setting in a patient with acute findings. Reversal of anticoagulation should be considered as there is significant overlap in the patient population presenting with AVM and those on anticoagulation.
  - Consultation can be placed early so that the surgical team is aware of the patient but should not occur prior to GI involvement.

- **IBD (Crohn's/ulcerative colitis)**

  In the setting of a patient presenting with toxic megacolon from recalcitrant UC, prompt surgical consultation and intervention is required. This can present with rectal bleeding. Basic lab studies, including CBC, coagulation panel, type, and screen, and IV fluid resuscitation should be initiated immediately.

  - *Primary care/ED*: Colonoscopy for tissue diagnosis of IBD and trial of targeted treatment. If referring for surgical resection, consider obtaining CT abdomen/pelvis with IV contrast.
  - *Consult*: Surgery consult for acute complications of IBD such as acute bowel obstruction, and refractory unstable bleeding. Otherwise, outpatient colorectal surgery referral would be appropriate.

- **Malignancy (anorectal, colonic)**
  For all patients presenting with rectal bleeding, especially in conjunction with anemia, constitutional symptoms, and significant risk factors, malignancy should be high on the differential. Early presentations may include vague abdominal discomfort, changes in stool habits, signs and symptoms of anemia, and unintentional weight loss. Late presentations may include acute bowel obstruction and/or perforation. For the stable patient in
  - *Primary care*: For the stable patient, urgent referral for colonoscopy is paramount. If malignancy is found, staging CT chest/abdomen/pelvis with IV contrast should be obtained in conjunction with oncology and surgical referral.
  - *ED*: If stable, obtain completion staging CT including CT chest/abdomen/pelvis with IV contrast with outpatient referral.
  - *Consult*: General surgery/colorectal surgery if patient is presenting with an acute perforation or obstruction. For new diagnoses of cancer, urgent outpatient surgical referral is sufficient.

Conclusion The differential diagnosis in a patient with rectal bleeding is extensive. When appropriate, surgical consultation should occur early in the process as part of a multidisciplinary approach to manage these often-complex patients. However, many of the diseases discussed above do not require emergent surgical evaluation. Outpatient workup is often the most appropriate path for benign anorectal pathologies. Anal fissures, hemorrhoids, and even diverticular bleeding can resolve with nonsurgical management. This is true for the adult population, but in the pediatric population there is more of an acute role for the surgical team. There are many conditions that require surgical intervention for resolution.

15.3 Pediatric Conditions Causing Rectal Bleeding

	Emergent surgical eval	Urgent surgical eval	Nonurgent/ outpatient surgical eval	PCP/GI no surgical evaluation needed	Outpatient imaging	ED evaluation imaging
Anal fissure	None needed	None needed	Outpatient evaluation if failed 6–8 weeks of management from PCP/GI	Outpatient eval	None	None
Meckel's diverticulum	None needed	If evidence of bowel obstruction	If no anemia, outpatient evaluation if diagnosis is confirmed	PCP to manage and order Meckel's scan	Meckel's diverticulum scan	Meckel's diverticulum scan
IBD	If evidence of perforation, peritonitis, refractory bleeding, or hemodynamic instability	None needed	Outpatient workup if stable in ED	GI primarily should manage this condition	Colonoscopy	CT abdomen/ pelvis with IV contrast if suspicious for complicated IBD (stricture, perforation, fistula)

	Emergent surgical eval	Urgent surgical eval	Nonurgent/outpatient surgical eval	PCP/GI no surgical evaluation needed	Outpatient imaging	ED evaluation imaging
Intussusception	None needed	Urgent surgical evaluation, do not wait to initiate fluid resuscitation prior to surgical consult	If air-contrast enema resolves volvulus, nonurgent ED consult is appropriate	ED evaluation from surgery needed	ED evaluation from surgery needed	Abdominal US
Volvulus	Emergent evaluation for peritonitis	Urgent evaluation if hemodynamically stable and no peritonitis, but needs urgent evaluation	Emergent or urgent evaluation needed	Emergent or urgent evaluation needed	ED evaluation from surgery needed	Abdominal X-ray, upper GI series preferred
NEC	Emergent evaluation needed when this diagnosis is made	None	None	None	ED evaluation from surgery needed	Abdominal X-ray

15.4 Adult Conditions Causing Rectal Bleeding

	Emergent surgical eval	Urgent surgical eval	Nonurgent/outpatient surgical eval	PCP/GI eval, no surgery needed	Outpatient imaging	ED evaluation imaging
Anal fissure	None needed	None needed	Outpatient evaluation appropriate	Outpatient evaluation with GI appropriate	Colonoscopy in those with concerning symptoms, or those meeting screening criteria	None; outpatient colonoscopy if appropriate
Hemorrhoids	None needed	For acute thrombosis within 72 hours urgent surgical eval, for refractory bleeding urgent surgical eval	For all other stable patients, outpatient evaluation appropriate	GI outpatient evaluation appropriate	Colonoscopy in those with concerning symptoms, or those meeting screening criteria	None; outpatient colonoscopy if appropriate
Rectal prolapse	If evidence of acute strangulation/ischemia emergent eval	None needed	For stable patients seen in outpatient PCP/GI office, refer to outpatient colorectal surgery. For stable ED patients, outpatient evaluation appropriate	GI evaluation outpatient	Colonoscopy, MR defecography if available	None; outpatient colonoscopy

	Emergent surgical eval	Urgent surgical eval	Nonurgent/ outpatient surgical eval	PCP/GI eval, no surgery needed	Outpatient imaging	ED evaluation imaging
AVM	None needed	For refractory bleeding, urgent consult	Rarely need outpatient surgery for stable patients	GI primary management of this condition	None	CTA abdomen/ pelvis to rule out other sources of bleeding
IBD	If evidence of acute perforation and peritonitis emergent consult appropriate	If bowel obstruction present, urgent surgical consultation in ED is appropriate	If clinically stable in ED and no obstruction symptoms present, outpatient surgical evaluation is appropriate	GI should primarily manage stable chronic patients	Colonoscopy, CT abdomen/pelvis with IV contrast if suspicious for complicated IBD	CT abdomen/ pelvis with IV contrast if suspicious for complicated IBD; outpatient colonoscopy
Malignancy	If evidence of perforation or peritonitis	If obstruction is present urgent surgical consult is appropriate	Stable patient can follow up with surgery outpatient	GI in ED evaluation for colonoscopy when obstruction is absent	CT abdomen/ pelvis with iv contrast for evaluation of primary tumor. CT chest for metastatic work up Colonoscopy for tissue diagnosis	CT abdomen/ pelvis with iv contrast for evaluation of primary tumor; CT chest for metastatic workup

Suggested Readings

1. https://fascrs.org/ascrs/media/files/Education/2023-Anal-Fissures-CPG.pdf
2. https://fascrs.org/getattachment/Healthcare-Providers/Education/Clinical-Practice-Guidelines/2022-AnorectalAbscess_FistulainAno_RectovaginalFistula-CPG.pdf?lang=en-US
3. https://fascrs.org/getattachment/Healthcare-Providers/Education/Clinical-Practice-Guidelines/2021-Ulcerative-Colitis-CPG.pdf?lang=en-US
4. https://fascrs.org/ascrs/media/files/downloads/crohns-CPG-2020.pdf
5. https://fascrs.org/ascrs/media/files/downloads/Clinical%20Practice%20Guidelines/cpg_management_of_hemorrhoids.pdf

Change in Stool Caliber 16

Brittany E. Levy and Danielle S. Walsh

16.1 History Taking for Stool Changes

Query of stool habits can be strained, even in the patient–physician relationship due to societal connotations of discussing bowel habits. Therefore, specific and targeted history-taking questions are necessary to properly delineate important diagnostic information for both benign and malignant colorectal diseases. Scoring systems for colorectal and small bowel diseases such as irritable bowel syndrome, inflammatory bowel syndrome, and colon cancer exist, and while the individual questions differ, the overarching themes are similar. Pertinent aspects include abdominal pain (and location), abdominal distention, frequency and consistency of stooling, presence of blood, and effect of stooling habits on the quality of life. A Bristol Stool Chart can assist in the assessment of stool consistency. A discussion of these topics is necessary to understand the underlying causes of changes in stool caliber as the coinciding symptoms may provide insight into the etiology.

Changes in stool caliber classically are associated with colon and rectal cancer, possibly related to the relative narrowing of the colon secondary to a mass obstructing the lumen. However, this symptom alone is not sufficient for the diagnosis of colon cancer

B. E. Levy · D. S. Walsh (✉)
University of Kentucky, Lexington, KY, USA

G. P. Kohn et al. (eds.), *The SAGES Manual of Surgical Referral for Primary and Emergency Care*,
https://doi.org/10.1007/978-3-031-92678-5_16

as more commonly thin stools are associated with loose stools and diarrheal illness. Therefore, further investigation is warranted to identify associated symptoms. Narrow stools associated with anemia, abdominal cramping, obstructive symptoms, and tenesmus do require further evaluation for colorectal cancer, including laboratory and endoscopic investigation.

Stool caliber changes associated with inflammatory bowel disease can be better investigated using scoring systems such as the Pediatric Ulcerative Colitis Activity Index (PUCAI) score or the Mayo score Disease Activity Index (DAI) for ulcerative colitis for children or adults, respectively. For patients scoring significantly on these scoring systems, further investigation for their stool changes should be pursued toward a diagnosis of inflammatory bowel disease. This includes laboratory evaluation, stool studies, endoscopic, and radiographic evaluation.

Irritable bowel disease can be scored using the Irritable Bowel Severity Scoring System and is often a diagnosis of exclusion after malignancy, inflammatory bowel disease, chronic constipation, or acute diarrheal illness have been ruled out via history, laboratory, or endoscopic evaluation. This scoring system ranges from 0 to 500, and those scoring above 75 indicate a diagnosis of irritable bowel syndrome to differing degrees of severity (mild, moderate, severe).

In addition to the above-discussed chronic diseases known to impact bowel caliber, acute or chronic changes can occur with acute illness and constipation. Acute diarrheal illnesses from common gastroenteritis pathogens may present as a much more acute onset often with a patient history of sick contacts, ingestion of at-risk meals, or recent travel. These pathogens can usually be identified via stool studies. Chronic constipation can also present as changes in stool caliber, which are typically reversed with changes in bowel regimen and antidiarrheal medications. Untreated constipation can lead to diverticular diseases. Diverticulitis, especially when recurrent, can lead to stricturing disease and cause a narrowing of stool caliber. Conversely, when acute diverticulitis flares, loose stool may occur along with acute-onset abdominal pain.

16.2 Laboratory Evaluation

Laboratory evaluation for a change in bowel habits should include standard blood work including a complete blood count to evaluate for leukocytosis, anemia, and microcytic anemia. Additionally, evaluation of albumin levels may provide diagnostic value for inflammatory bowel disease as it is classically a protein-losing enteropathy. For acute intestinal flares, enteritis, and diverticulitis, C-reactive protein (CRP) may be useful. If concern for diverticular disease or colon cancer is strong, a computed tomography scan of the abdomen and pelvis with oral and intravenous contrast may be useful for diagnosis and classification. The above history-taking and scoring systems will then provide differing algorithms for further evaluation. If clinical concern for colon cancer arises, obtaining a carcinoembryonic antigen (CEA) may be of benefit.

Stool studies are useful both in inflammatory bowel disease and for the characterization of an acute diarrheal illness. If concerned about inflammatory bowel disease, a stool calprotectin or stool lactoferrin can be obtained and will be useful moving forward for trending. Gastrointestinal pathogen multiplex PCR panels can be helpful for community-acquired or travel-related diarrheal illness for pathology identification of causative viruses, bacteria, and parasites.

Chronic constipation and irritable bowel disease have limited laboratory evaluation for diagnosis. A plain X-ray of the abdomen can be effective for assessing stool burden in constipation and guiding effective management. Irritable bowel disease is often a diagnosis made after other workup has excluded inflammatory bowel disease and other more concerning disorders.

16.3 Referral Patterns for Common Pathologies

Identification of the above pathologies and their diagnostic algorithm will directly relate to the appropriate specialist referral. If concerned about an underlying colon or rectal cancer following laboratory studies and a computed tomography scan, prompt referral to a gastroenterologist or colon and rectal surgeon is needed for endoscopic evaluation and cancer care. If concern for obstructive symptoms related to the acute change in stool caliber, the patient may require emergency care and surgical evaluation.

Diverticular disease will also require referral to a colon and rectal surgeon for the evaluation and management of chronic strictures or surgical intervention. Laboratory evaluation and timely computed tomography scan are appropriate prior to referral. If a patient is found to have complicated diverticular disease, inpatient treatment may be necessary for antibiotic administration and/or surgical intervention.

Inflammatory bowel disease is largely managed by gastroenterology subspecialists, and only after the failure of medical management, acute perforation, or other life-threatening manifestations of uncontrolled disease is surgical intervention necessary. Emergency evaluation and emergency surgical intervention may be necessary for patients with hemodynamic instability, perforation, or toxic megacolon.

Similarly, irritable bowel disease and chronic constipation can often be managed with medical management by gastroenterology subspecialists. Acute diarrheal illnesses are frequently self-limiting and uncommonly require antimicrobials for treatment. Severity of symptoms may guide the need for laboratory studies and stool studies. However, patients may require emergency medical evaluation and treatment for dehydration, systemic illness, or significant blood in the stool. Patients should follow up with a primary care provider for resolution of symptoms within 14 days and to ensure no other changes in bowel habits are present after the resolution of their diarrheal illness.

Assessing stool caliber change

Possible causes:
  Colon cancer
  Diverticulitis
  Constipation
  Inflammatory bowel disease
  Irritable bowel disease
  Infectious enteritis

(continued)

<table>
<tr><td colspan="2">Diagnostic laboratory evaluation:
CBC
Albumin levels
CRP
CEA (if concern for colon cancer)</td></tr>
<tr><td colspan="2">Management approaches:</td></tr>
<tr><td>Emergent/urgent</td><td>Outpatient</td></tr>
<tr><td>Obstructive symptoms
Rectal bleeding
Peritonitis
Acute/severe systemic illness</td><td>Chronic nature
Heme detected in stool
Weight loss without malnutrition
Mild/nonspecific abdominal pain</td></tr>
</table>

Suggested Readings

1. Borhan-Manesh F. "Low caliber stool" and "pencil thin stool" are not signs of colo-rectal cancer. Dig Dis Sci. 2009;54(2):208–11. https://doi.org/10.1007/s10620-008-0356-1.
2. Coakley KM, Davis BR, Kasten KR. Complicated diverticular disease. Clin Colon Rectal Surg. 2021;34(2):96–103. https://doi.org/10.1055/s-0040-1716701.
3. Dotson JL, Crandall WV, Zhang P, et al. Feasibility and validity of the pediatric ulcerative colitis activity index in routine clinical practice. J Pediatr Gastroenterol Nutr. 2015;60(2):200–4. https://doi.org/10.1097/MPG.0000000000000568.
4. Travis SP, Schnell D, Krzeski P, et al. Reliability and initial validation of the ulcerative colitis endoscopic index of severity. Gastroenterology. 2013;145(5):987–95. https://doi.org/10.1053/j.gastro.2013.07.024.

17 Constipation

Lindsay T. Bryant, Danielle S. Walsh, and Eric J. Rellinger

17.1 Pediatric Constipation

17.1.1 Introduction

Constipation is a common gastrointestinal complaint and frequent cause of abdominal pain in children that afflicts approximately 12–18% of all children and is commonly remedied with lifestyle, dietary, and over-the-counter medications. Diagnostic criteria for functional constipation were refined by the Rome Foundation and diagnostic criteria are met when at least two criteria describing stool frequency, hardness, size, incontinence episodes, rectal stool burden on physical exam, or volitional stool retention are present [1, 2]. Diarrhea may also be reported in the setting of constipation and lead to pseudoincontinence secondary to loose stool leaking around hard, impacted stool. Initial management of functional constipation treatment is focused on reassurance and fecal elimination through counseling on dietary, activity, and behavioral modifications or use of laxative medications to achieve symptom relief. Functional constipation is a diagnosis of exclusion and necessitates thoughtful evaluation looking for alarm symptoms

L. T. Bryant · D. S. Walsh · E. J. Rellinger (✉)
University of Kentucky, Lexington, KY, USA
e-mail: Eric.Rellinger@uky.edu

G. P. Kohn et al. (eds.), *The SAGES Manual of Surgical Referral for Primary and Emergency Care*,
https://doi.org/10.1007/978-3-031-92678-5_17

that may necessitate more thorough or expedited subspecialty evaluation. Anatomic causes of constipation (including Hirschsprung's disease, anorectal malformation, and anal stenosis) encompass a small proportion of children with constipation who benefit from early pediatric surgical referral. Nonanatomic constipation refractory to laxative trials benefit from pediatric gastroenterology referral. Select children refractory to conservative management strategies may benefit from specialized bowel management programs or surgical referral.

17.1.2 Differential Diagnosis

Initial evaluation of children presenting with constipation should identify alarm signs and symptoms to exclude alternative diagnoses or identify children with secondary causes of constipation that may benefit from specialized therapeutic strategies. Obstipation, refractory emesis, abdominal distension, acute-onset symptoms, and fevers raise concern for obstruction, and early pediatric surgery referral is appropriate. Rectal bleeding may herald underlying intestinal ischemia in the setting of surgical emergencies such as necrotizing enterocolitis, intussusception, midgut volvulus, but may also be seen with less ominous etiologies such as an anal fissure or cow's milk allergy. Hirschsprung's disease, anorectal malformation, and anal stenosis are congenital/anatomic disorders that most commonly present as newborn distal intestinal obstruction but less frequently present in delayed fashion with constipation as a dominant symptom. Alarm features may also prompt further investigation into underlying neurogenic, myogenic, endocrine/metabolic, or inflammatory causes of secondary constipation.

17.1.3 History

Obtaining a thoughtful patient history is helpful in identifying children who may benefit from early subspecialty referral/consultation (Table 17.1). Delayed passage of meconium (24–48 h),

Table 17.1 Clinical features that guide initial management and referral for constipation

What constitutes an emergency requiring ER presentation?	Failure to maintain hydration Acute-onset abdominal pain Severe abdominal pain Obstipation Rectal bleeding Refractory emesis Bilious or feculent emesis Fevers
What requires urgent surgical referral?	Signs of sepsis Involuntary guarding/peritonitis Obstipation Bilious or feculent emesis Concern for perforated viscus Large-volume rectal bleeding Incarcerated rectal prolapse Children: Concern for Hirschsprung's associated enterocolitis
What requires nonurgent surgical referral?	Children: Concern for an anatomic cause of constipation (i.e., Hirschsprung's disease, anorectal malformation, anal stenosis) Constipation refractory to medical and subspecialty (GI) optimization History of colon resection Consideration of bowel management (depending on regional resources/ expertise) Adult: Constipation refractory to subspecialty optimization Concern for malignancy or inflammatory bowel disease Low-volume rectal bleeding History of colon resection Constipation-associated diseases refractory to conservative management (anal fissure, rectal prolapse, hemorrhoids)

(continued)

Table 17.1 (continued)

What features would mean that the condition can be managed by the PCP?	Absence of alarm features
What features should prompt referral to nonsurgical subspecialties?	Fecal impaction Nonanatomic constipation refractory to laxative trial Rectal bleeding Concern for underlying malignancy or inflammatory bowel disease Concern for underlying metabolic/endocrine dysfunction Children: Failure to thrive

family history of Hirschsprung's disease, Down's syndrome, failure to thrive, chronic abdominal distension, and report of explosive stools raise suspicion for Hirschsprung's disease as an underlying cause of constipation. These historical factors should prompt referral to a pediatric surgeon for consideration of rectal biopsy with or without contrast enema. Family history of cystic fibrosis may be contributory to identifying distal intestinal obstructive syndrome as an alternative diagnosis. Fatigue, dry skin, unexplained weight gain, hair loss, and cold intolerance may be suggestive of hypothyroidism. Medications, including diuretics, calcium-containing medications, opioids, and antidepressants, may provoke or exacerbate constipation. Lower extremity weakness and bladder incontinence may suggest a common neurogenic cause for pelvic outlet obstruction. A thorough social history may also point to psychological factors contributory to stooling difficulties including any history of prior abuse. Restricted diet and a sedentary lifestyle may be suggestive of functional constipation.

17.1.4 Physical Exam

A thorough examination of the abdomen and perineum is critical for the assessment of children presenting with constipation.

Severe distension and involuntary guarding are not typical of constipation and should prompt consideration of alternative diagnoses. A thorough perineal examination is helpful in identifying anatomic causes of constipation that benefit from pediatric surgical referral. Physical exam alone is sufficient for identifying anorectal malformations and anal stenosis. Anorectal malformations result from an abnormal position of the anal opening outside of the anal sphincter muscle complex. The location of the anal sphincter complex is frequently heralded by an anal dimple at the site of hyperpigmented skin within the midline of the perineum. Anal stenosis is far less common and is characterized by a normally positioned anal opening that is small in caliber. The diagnosis of anal stenosis is based upon the size of the anal opening determined by the passage of Hegar dilators. The normal anus size increases with age and is ~12 mm in term newborns. Due to its association with Currarino's triad, exam findings concerning anal stenosis should prompt further investigation into the presence of a presacral mass and sacral defects. Large presacral masses may be palpable on digital rectal exam. Passage of explosive stools with rectal stimulation or tight anal canal may also be suggestive of Hirschsprung's disease. Large sacral dimples and midline lower back hair tufts and hemangiomas can be associated with underlying neural tube defects, while lower extremity motor deficits should prompt further investigation for spinal abnormalities that may provide a unifying neurogenic cause.

17.1.5 Studies to Consider Prior to Subspecialty Referral

Laboratory evaluation can frequently be avoided in the absence of alarm features. Basic metabolic panel with calcium, complete blood count, C-reactive protein, blood lead levels, thyroid function tests, urinalysis with culture, or celiac screening panel may be considered based upon risk factors. Classically, inflammatory markers (i.e., white blood cell count and C-reactive protein) are not elevated with functional constipation and should prompt further consideration of alternative diagnoses, particularly when considering constipation as a potential explanation for new-onset abdominal pain.

Lifestyle modification and/or laxative trial is a reasonable first step for treating constipation. An abdominal radiograph may be a helpful adjunct if these efforts are not efficacious or there is clinical concern for rectal fecal impaction (Table 17.2). Noting the pattern of stool burden on these films can help guide next steps in therapeutic escalation. Large rectal stool burdens may benefit from the initiation of enemas or rarely manual disimpaction under sedation. A lateral decubitus view can be helpful and sensitive for the assessment of free air if there are any concerning exam features including fevers, abdominal tenderness, leukocytosis, or ill-appearance that may suggest an alternative cause for presentation or complication of severe constipation such as a stercoral ulcer or megacolon. Computed tomography of the abdomen and pelvis with IV contrast may be a useful adjunct if the history, imaging, and exam raise concerns for a small, large bowel obstruction, or complications of severe constipation such as stercoral perforation. Due to radiation exposure concerns, early referral/consultation with a pediatric surgeon may obviate the need for cross-sectional imaging in children with obstructive symptoms.

17.1.6 Whom to Refer/Consult

In the absence of alarming features, lifestyle modification, laxative trials, and/or short course of enema administration are an

Table 17.2 Initial workup and management prior to consider before surgical referral for constipation

Laboratory tests	Complete blood count Basic metabolic panel
Radiographic studies	Plain film of the abdomen and pelvis
Initial management	If ill-appearing, obtain IV access and start resuscitation If refractory emesis, consider nasogastric decompression

appropriate first step prior to subspecialty referral. Children with exam or historical features concerning potential congenital/anatomic causes of constipation previously described should prompt pediatric surgical consultation. Children with non-anatomic constipation refractory to laxative trials benefit from referral to a pediatric gastroenterologist for consideration of advanced laboratory testing, endoscopy, physiologic imaging studies, or biofeedback trials. In rare instances, children may benefit from surgical evaluation after demonstrating failure of conservative multimodal strategies. Depending upon regional resources, pediatric surgeons may offer enrollment in a specialized bowel management program or consider benefits of surgical procedures including botox injections, antegrade continence enemas, sigmoid resection, stoma creation, and/or sacral nerve stimulators.

17.2 Adult Constipation

17.2.1 Introduction

Adult constipation is one of the most prevalent gastrointestinal complaints impacting roughly 10–20% of adults. The Adult Rome IV criteria define adult functional constipation as having at least two of the following:

> Fewer than three spontaneous bowel movements per week, straining in over 25% of defecation attempts, lumpy or hard stools in at least 25% of defecation attempts, a sensation of anorectal obstruction or blockage in at least 25% of defecation attempts, a sensation of incomplete defecation in at least 25% of defecation attempts, and the need for manual maneuvering to defecate in at least 25% of defecation attempts.

Irritable bowel syndrome with constipation, opioid-induced constipation, and functional defecation disorders are other subtypes of Rome IV constipation disorders. Paradoxical diarrhea may also be present in rectal fecal impaction or irritable bowel syndrome mixed type. Similar to children, constipation is a frequent presenting symptom in adults, and initial evaluation emphasizes thorough history-taking and physical examination to guide the need for further laboratory or imaging studies. Many alarm signs and symptoms overlap between adults and children, but the differential disease burden in adults can alter next diagnostic and/or therapeutic efforts.

17.2.2 Differential Diagnosis

The increased incidence of colorectal cancer, inflammatory bowel disease, medication use/substance abuse, and associated chronic medical conditions broadens the differential diagnosis of adults presenting with constipation. Obstipation, abdominal distension, severe abdominal pain, and emesis raise concern for small bowel obstruction as an alternative diagnosis, with adhesive bowel disease, malignancy, hernias, and inflammatory bowel disease being the most common etiologies. Large bowel obstruction is most commonly secondary to colorectal cancer in adults; however, diverticular disease, inflammatory bowel disease, sigmoid volvulus, and extrinsic malignant compression are also important considerations. Secondary constipation due to chronic medical diseases, including hypothyroidism, hyperparathyroidism, diabetes mellitus/insipidus, abnormal musculature, medication/drug use, anxiety/depression, myogenic, and neurogenic causes, is also more common in adults, and concerning clinical features may guide further diagnostic evaluation. Functional defecation disorders, including dyssynergic defecation and inadequate defecatory propulsion, have also been identified in over half of all adults with constipation and guided history and physical exam may prompt early subspecialty referral, physiologic testing, and early implementation of biofeedback therapy.

17.2.3 History

Alarm symptoms help identify adults who benefit from early subspecialty referral (Table 17.1). Acute changes in bowel habits, obstipation, severe abdominal pain, fevers, and emesis are concerning features that raise concern for obstruction. Constitutional symptoms, unintentional weight loss, changes in stool caliber, and rectal bleeding may be associated with colorectal cancer and inflammatory bowel disease. Family history of colorectal cancer or inflammatory bowel disease and prior endoscopic findings may also prioritize next diagnostic steps. Review of prescribed medication and recreational drug use are key historical contributors with opioids, calcium channel blockers, and antidepressants being common contributors to constipation. Obtaining a psychosocial history can also be beneficial in determining whether the constipation is related to major depressive disorder, anxiety disorder, or somatization disorder. Excessive straining, digital evacuation maneuvers, or history of sexual abuse or trauma may prompt early referral to assess for functional defecation disorders or irritable bowel syndrome with constipation that may benefit from specialized multidisciplinary treatment approaches including biofeedback. Refractory and debilitating constipation symptoms should also prompt gastroenterology referral.

17.2.4 Physical Exam

A complete physical exam focusing on identifying alarm signs is a key step in evaluating adults with constipation (Table 17.1). Abdominal distension, tympany, unexplained ascites, palpable masses, and involuntary guarding are concerning abdominal exam features that should escalate early diagnostic testing and subspecialty referral. Lymphadenopathy raises suspicion for malignancy. External anal exam may reveal (1) signs of chronic constipation (fissures or hemorrhoids), (2) masses, or (3) signs of perianal Crohn's disease (induration/abscesses, fissures, fistulae, or skin tags). Rectal prolapse may be solicited with a Valsalva maneuver. Direct rectal exam should be performed in willing patients without severe anal pain or immunocompromise. Presence of a mass, stricture, or gross blood may be noted on digital rectal exam and can drastically alter management strategies. Hard, firm stool in rectal vault may guide prompt enema challenges or manual stool evacuation to relieve rectal impaction. Meticulous digital rectal exam may also be useful in soliciting paradoxical anal contraction or perineal descent that can be highly predictive in screening for functional defecatory disorders.

17.2.5 Studies to Consider Prior to Specialty Referral

Lifestyle modification and a laxative trial is the appropriate first step prior to laboratory or imaging studies. Lack of response to initial treatments may prompt laboratory evaluation with a basic metabolic panel with calcium and a complete blood count (Table 17.2). The results may raise concern for alternative diagnoses or secondary causes of constipation. Elevated leukocyte count and C-reactive protein are suggestive of an acute inflammatory/infectious process and should prompt further consideration of alternative diagnoses. Hypercalcemia may be associated with both hyperparathyroidism and malignancy. Thyroid function and celiac panels can be helpful in identifying secondary causes of constipation but may be deferred in the acute care setting. Fecal occult blood test may prompt further investigation into colorectal cancer and inflammatory bowel disease.

Clinical features concerning intra-abdominal catastrophe, such as peritonitis and signs of sepsis, should prompt early surgical referral to guide expeditious workup and intervention. Plain abdominal radiographs are a useful adjunct to support the diagnosis of constipation and evaluate fecal burden to guide antegrade or retrograde management strategies (Table 17.2). Computed tomography of the abdomen and pelvis with IV contrast is a useful adjunct if concerns for small or large bowel obstruction arise. Local expertise should be engaged to help determine the utility of advanced functional imaging studies for patients suffering from refractory constipation (defecography, colonic transit studies, or anorectal manometry). A nonoperative trial may be utilized in conditions such as partial bowel obstruction and complete small bowel obstruction. A change to operative management would be warranted by leukocytosis, signs of strangulation, signs of peritonitis (fever, abdominal rigidity, guarding), and lack of clinical improvement after 48–72 h.

17.2.6 Whom to Refer/Consult

In the absence of alarming clinical features, lifestyle modifications focused on improving fluid intake, physical activity, and fiber supplementation (20–35 g/d) can be a helpful, low-cost strategy. Lack of response should prompt a therapeutic trial of antegrade medical management with bulk-forming laxatives, osmotic, or stimulant laxatives. Rectal fecal impaction may be responsible for failure of medical therapy and enemas may offer a useful short-term adjunct. In refractory cases, rectal fecal impaction may require manual disimpaction, and in rare cases endoscopic fragmentation is necessary. Gastroenterology referral is appropriate for patients with constipation refractory to dietary/lifestyle modifications and laxative trials. Advanced diagnostic testing or escalation of therapy to colonic secretogogues and prokinetic agents may be next steps in therapeutic escalation. Identifying alarm symptoms concerning colon cancer and inflammatory bowel disease (weight loss, bloody stools, stool caliber changes, anemia, fecal occult positivity, cachexia) should prompt early referral for endoscopy. A small minority of patients with severe constipation refractory to medical optimization may benefit from surgical intervention, including stoma creation, creation of Malone antegrade continence enema, colectomy, or sacral nerve stimulation. Secondary consequences of constipation (i.e., anal fissure, rectal prolapse, hemorrhoids) may also benefit from surgical referral if severe or refractory to conservative management strategies.

Suggested Readings

1. Benninga MA, Faure C, Hyman PE, St James Roberts I, Schechter NL, Nurko S. Childhood functional gastrointestinal disorders: neonate/toddler. Gastroenterology. 2016:S0016-5085(16)00182-7. https://doi.org/10.1053/j.gastro.2016.02.016. Epub ahead of print. PMID: 27144631.
2. Bharucha AE, Lacy BE. Mechanisms, evaluation, and management of chronic constipation. Gastroenterology. 2020;158(5):1232–1249.e3. https://doi.org/10.1053/j.gastro.2019.12.034. Epub 2020 Jan 13. PMID: 31945360; PMCID: PMC7573977.

3. Hyams JS, Di Lorenzo C, Saps M, Shulman RJ, Staiano A, van Tilburg M. Functional disorders: children and adolescents. Gastroenterology. 2016:S0016-5085(16)00181-5. https://doi.org/10.1053/j.gastro.2016.02.015. Epub ahead of print. PMID: 27144632.
4. Mearin F, Lacy BE, Chang L, Chey WD, Lembo AJ, Simren M, Spiller R. Bowel disorders. Gastroenterology. 2016:S0016-5085(16)00222-5. https://doi.org/10.1053/j.gastro.2016.02.031. Epub ahead of print. PMID: 27144627.
5. Nyam DC, Pemberton JH, Ilstrup DM, Rath DM. Long-term results of surgery for chronic constipation. Dis Colon Rectum. 1997;40(3):273–9. 10.1007/BF02050415. Erratum in: Dis Colon Rectum 1997 May;40(5):529. PMID: 9118740.

Anal Pain and Anal Fissures 18

Andrew Whipkey and Danielle S. Walsh

18.1 Introduction

Anal pain is a common, nonspecific symptom for which patients seek evaluation and treatment. The broad differential includes anal fissure, internal or external hemorrhoid, perianal abscesses or fistulas, rectal or anal malignancy, labial or vulvar malignancy, anorectal sexually transmitted infections, rectal prolapse, and inflammatory bowel disease (IBD). Navigating through this array of diseases quickly and efficiently can pose a challenge for busy clinicians. However, with a thorough history, review of systems, and exam, the most likely diagnosis can usually be ascertained with minimal need for laboratory and radiographic studies. Table 18.1 provides a summary of considerations for the evaluation and management of perianal complaints. While most management is medical, surgical referral should be considered when conservative measures have failed, the diagnosis is uncertain, or the presentation is atypical.

A. Whipkey (✉) · D. S. Walsh
Department of Surgery, University of Kentucky,
Lexington, KY, USA

Markey Cancer Center, University of Kentucky,
Lexington, KY, USA
e-mail: andrew.whipkey@uky.edu

G. P. Kohn et al. (eds.), *The SAGES Manual of Surgical Referral for Primary and Emergency Care*,
https://doi.org/10.1007/978-3-031-92678-5_18

Table 18.1 Summary

What may cause a patient to present to the ED?
Severe anal pain may necessitate nonurgent vs urgent surgical referral
Newly diagnosed anal fissures (most scenarios)
Thrombosed external hemorrhoids
Perianal or perirectal abscess with or without fistulas
Perianal symptoms accompanied by with systemic illness
Acute perianal trauma due to assault or abuse depending on local norms
Ongoing or large volume perianal bleeding
What requires urgent surgical review?
Pathology that would benefit from expeditious assessment or intervention
Thrombosed external hemorrhoids identified within 72 hours of symptom onset
Perianal or perirectal abscesses, with or without associated fistula
Acute perianal trauma due to assault or abuse depending on local norms
Persistent perianal bleeding
What requires nonurgent surgical review?
Patients who fail to improve with conservative management or for whom the diagnosis is uncertain
Anal fissures on conservative management for 6+ weeks requiring additional treatment
Fissure location not posterior midline
Patients with fissure and comorbidities such as HIV and IBD
Suspicion of anal fissure unconfirmed on physical examination and not responding to conservative management
What can be managed by a PCP?
Patients with posterior midline anal fissures warrant a 4-6-week trial of conservative management including
Identification and removal of inciting traumatic factors as indicated
Bowel habit assessment with limiting of prolonged straining
Dietary and fiber supplements
Stool softeners titrated to soft bowel movements
Topical nifedipine ointment
Diazepam (pending prescriber comfort)

18.2 History and Review of Systems

The first step in assessing anal pain is to clarify whether it is dull vs sharp, mild vs severe or spasmodic and intermittent. Dull pain reflects visceral sensation, suggesting location above the dentate line, whereas sharp pain reflects somatic sensation, suggesting location below the dentate line. Spasmodic pain correlates to contraction of the anal sphincter complex.

Anal fissures, which are longitudinal tears in the anal mucosa below the dentate line due to trauma, most commonly have sharp, severe pain exacerbated by the passage of bowel movements and with performing hygiene. Trauma in this context refers to force that stresses the anal canal; once a single or collective force exceeds an individual threshold of tissue integrity, a fissure develops. Further inquiry should ascertain incidences of acute trauma and/or accumulation of chronic low-grade traumas. Lower GI tract instrumentation, such as recent digital rectal examination (DRE), rigid proctoscopy, flexible-sigmoidoscopy, or colonoscopy, can cause acute trauma. Acute injury also includes sexual assault, consensual intercourse, and use of sex toys or other foreign objects that stress the anal canal. Due to their sensitive nature, these topics should be addressed cautiously, with the recognition that some patients and their loved ones may withhold information, especially in the case of children and adolescents. The clinician should take great care to be supportive while ensuring patient safety and obligations to report potential assault of minors and other protected classes.

Though acute traumatic events may or may not be reported, patients more frequently present with symptoms of anal fissures after an accumulation of recurrent, low-grade trauma. Constipation, despite being a common physiologic source of chronic anal trauma, is often denied by patients. To ensure effective query, it is useful to guide the patient through a discussion of bowel habits in general, including duration of time between bowel movements, time spent passing the feces, degree of strain, volume of stool with each passage, stool consistency, and patterns of stool withholding. For instance, patients who work in careers that do not permit easy access to restrooms may voluntarily suppress the act of defecating, leading to large, hard bowel movements. Harder stools require more force to propel through the GI tract than softer stools and cause more trauma. Visual aids, such as the Bristol stool scale, can assist patients in describing their stool consistency. The diameter and length of stool can impact the anal canal with thinner stools less likely to traumatize. High-frequency small bowel movements also pose a risk of trauma as they increase shearing stress on the anal mucosa with repeated defecation.

The clinician should also assess for lower GI bleeding as anal fissures classically cause bright red blood "per rectum," though this is a clinical misnomer in that the pathology is distal to the rectum. The blood can be noticed (1) on stool, (2) in the toilet bowl water, (3) on toilet paper when performing hygiene, and (4) on undergarments/clothing. However, there is virtually always a temporal relationship with bleeding and having had a bowel movement as fissures do not tend to bleed unless they are re-traumatized. Both acute and chronic trauma leading to a fissure can be accompanied by blood. Notably, while small amounts of bleeding can be managed as an outpatient, marked bleeding unresponsive to local management may require referral to an emergency room for urgent assessment.

18.3 Physical Exam

Physical exam alone can be confirmatory of anal fissures. Exam considerations include patient privacy, positioning, visualization, and DRE. The perineal area should ideally be examined in a private room with curtains in front of a closed door. Additionally, patients should be permitted to choose if others are in the room with them, save the clinician performing the exam and a clinical chaperone. Patient relaxation and comfort are also of paramount importance as those who are anxious or uncomfortable are more likely to contract their external sphincter or gluteal muscles, limiting visualization and effectiveness of exam.

The goals of positioning should be good exposure and patient comfort. Prone position with jackknife variation provides arguably the best visualization. However, some prone patients may experience subjective dyspnea and consequent anxiety, leading to muscle contraction that hinders assessment. Another option is to have the patient stand with exposed buttocks and with hips flexed between 45° and 90°; from this position, gentle superolateral traction on each buttock will often permit adequate visualization.

Other options include either a right or left lateral decubitus position with lateral traction of the higher buttock to expose the anus. Positions may be augmented by hip flexion (e.g., "knees tucked") but carry the drawback of inability to apply traction to the lower buttock.

Once positioned, the external exam may reveal the fissure with or without traction maneuvers. Fissure edges may be raised, and granulation tissue may be present depending on chronicity; an acute fissure is more likely to have raw, actively bleeding mucosa. Hemostasis can be achieved through tamponade with gauze products. Classic fissures are located in the posterior midline. The presence of a "sentinel skin tag" is suggestive of a healing subacute fissure. Fissure location should be documented using the anatomic nomenclature of posterior midline, anterior midline, right lateral, or left lateral as clock-based nomenclature depends on patient position.

If the diagnosis of an anal fissure is unclear by visual inspection alone, proceed with gentle palpation. The patient should be warned that this is likely to reproduce significant pain, but it confirms the diagnosis. If neither visual exam nor palpation is diagnostic, perform a careful DRE with gloved hand and judicious use of lubricant. Internal examination should be circumferential pending patient tolerance and should assess for palpable defects in nonvisible anal mucosa with reproduction of pain symptoms. Instances when a clinician ought to defer bedside DRE are during times of severe pain and active bleeding as it may cause further exacerbation.

Thrombosed external hemorrhoids, which appear as raised columns of tissue below the dentate line, can mimic the acute pain of anal fissure. While a fissure is a mucosal tear and commonly has a visible mucosal defect, hemorrhoids occur due to swelling of the blood vessels in the anus with a protrusion of tissue. The two can be difficult to distinguish on exam, though external hemorrhoids with thrombosis have a blue or violet hue with severe pain even in the absence of palpation. Fissures may not be painful until they are palpated. History may also help reconcile exam findings as bowel-habit-associated bleeding is not present with external hemorrhoids. Conversely, internal hemorrhoids are characterized by blood with bowel movements. However, these lesions are classically not painful as they are located above the dentate line. It is possible to have combined internal and external hemorrhoids, but this scenario would likely present with multiple hemorrhoidal columns visible on examination.

Anorectal abscesses and anal fistulas can mimic fissures. Most anal fistulas arise from gland occlusion at the dentate line, resulting in abscess formation, though clinicians should also consider IBD (specifically Crohn disease) in these patients. Examination may reveal a swelling adjacent to the anus with an open drainage site if the fistula tract has managed to discharge through the skin. Anal fistulas do not commonly open in the posterior midline, further helping to distinguish them from fissures. Anorectal abscesses and anal fistulas may be difficult to visualize on examination, however, depending on location, body habitus, and duration of symptoms.

18.4 Adjuncts in Evaluation

While most anal fissures can be diagnosed through history and physical exams, limited adjuncts may be considered prior to expert referral. Anoscopy, an extension of physical exam, is a useful adjunct for evaluating anal mucosa; however, it can exacerbate pain like with DRE and should not be performed in an awake patient with acute symptoms. While this precludes utilization in the primary care setting, anoscopy may be utilized in the emergency room by trained clinicians in conjunction with sedation to aid in the diagnosis of occult anal fissures.

Imaging is not particularly useful in diagnosing anal fissures but may be helpful in diagnosing perianal disease when neither fissures nor hemorrhoids are present. Anorectal or vulvovaginal malignancy may be evaluated with CT. Anorectal abscesses, with or without fistulas, that cannot be identified on examination (e.g., are clinically occult) warrant a CT scan. CT or MRI may also be indicated prior to definitive treatment of fistula-in-ano. If patient history, family history, or examination are concerning for IBD, consider CT or MRI to evaluate for complications such as intestinal strictures, fistulas, perforations, or abscesses. Sedated anoscopy, proctoscopy, flexible sigmoidoscopy, or colonoscopy may be recommended should exam and imaging prove nondiagnostic.

18.5 Conservative Management for Anal Fissure

After the diagnosis of a classic anal fissure, a trial of conservative management should be initiated in the outpatient setting. Management typically includes a combination of lifestyle modifications, such as increasing dietary fiber intake, stool softeners, and topical medications. Stool softeners should be titrated to soft bowel movements. Topical nifedipine ointment may provide benefit as it relaxes the anal sphincter to afford less-traumatizing stool passage; patients should be instructed that this formulation requires compounding, which may lead to minor delays in filling or refilling a prescription. Topical lidocaine therapies can assist with pain but do not promote healing. Another medication to consider is diazepam, which treats and prevents spasmodic pain secondary to anal sphincter spasms; as this is a controlled substance with sedative effects, incorporation of this as part of a treatment regimen for anal fissures depends on patient reliability and prescriber comfort. Aside from diazepam, most treatments for anal fissures are well-tolerated and have low-risk side effect profiles. Thus, depending on clinician comfort, it would be reasonable to initiate conservative management when the diagnosis of anal fissure is highly suspected but not confirmed. If the source of anal canal trauma was identified through history, the clinician should counsel the patient on avoiding the contributing factors. This would include limiting prolonged straining during defecation and avoiding fecal withholding.

18.6 Surgical Referral and Timing

Conservative management should be trialed over approximately 4–6 weeks with reassessment in the primary care setting. If improving, patients may continue conservative management for resolution. Counsel should include that even a single large or hard bowel movement can reinjure the mucosa and require reinitiation of treatment. Patients who fail conservative management warrant outpatient surgical referral as they are candidates for more invasive treatments such as botulinum injection and lateral internal sphincterotomy, both of which may be performed electively under anesthesia. Though symptoms are understandably distressing for patients, anal fissures do not meet the criteria for surgical emergency. In cases of diagnostic uncertainty, outpatient surgical referral should be considered; if needed, a surgeon may schedule an evaluation under anesthesia with anoscopy or other endoscopy to permit adequate assessment.

There are several scenarios in which surgical referral may bypass typical outpatient management practices. Patients with anal fissures resulting from confirmed or presumed nonconsensual trauma (e.g., abuse or sexual assault) are often evaluated in an emergency room setting in conjunction with emergency room clinicians, forensics experts, law enforcement, and others working as a collaborative multidisciplinary team. Evaluation may require anesthesia, depending on a patient's physical and psychological discomfort following the traumatic event(s). Expertise from surgeons (general surgeons or colorectal surgeons in adults, vs pediatric surgeons in children and adolescents) and/or gynecologists may be requested to document exam findings during this evaluation.

Early surgical referral should also be considered when the fissure occurs in a position other than the posterior midline. Anterior midline anal fissures are associated with underlying anal sphincter and/or pelvic floor dysfunction. These patients commonly have long-standing issues with dysmotility, slow-transit, pelvic organ prolapse, etc. Though conservative measures may be initiated, pelvic floor dysfunction is most successfully managed with outpatient multidisciplinary care teams involving gastroenterologists, surgeons, urologists, and/or gynecologists.

Lateral anal fissures also signal underlying conditions including HIV, malignancies, IBD, and tuberculosis and warrant multidisciplinary care. Patients diagnosed with HIV and perianal disease require clinicians with focused training in HIV and infectious diseases, along with ongoing surveillance for anal dysplasia via anal pap smears and/or anoscopy. While conservative measures should be initiated, any consideration of invasive treatment options should be delayed until viral load and CD4 counts are medically optimized. Patients with lateral fissures associated with tuberculosis should also be evaluated by infectious disease experts to ensure quarantine and treatment protocols are followed. These patients may also begin conservative treatment immediately; invasive options should be delayed until the patient has completed tuberculosis treatment.

Fissures associated with IBD are commonly co-managed with gastroenterologists for medical therapy to control their IBD. Surgical management in this population should be delayed until an acute inflammatory episode has resolved or the fissure is deemed an isolated location of IBD activity. Given that IBD patients typically require multiple procedural interventions throughout their lives, early inclusion of a surgeon in the patient's care team is recommended.

Anal and vulvar dysplasia are correlated and termed anogenital dysplasia, with ideal management occurring in conjunction with gynecologists. Surgical evaluation is also warranted when diagnostic evaluation for an anal fissure confirms an alternative perianal pathology, including thrombosed hemorrhoids within 72 h of abrupt onset of pain. These patients may benefit from a timely thrombectomy. Likewise, patients found to have a perianal or perirectal abscess, with or without associated fistulas, warrant timely surgical evaluation as these conditions are unlikely to resolve without intervention.

Acknowledgments Dr. Whipkey's contribution to this publication was supported by the National Institutes of Health through NIH Training Grant T32CA160003. The content is solely the responsibility of the author(s) and does not necessarily represent the official views of the NIH.

Suggested Readings

1. Anal fissure. Stanford Medicine Children's Health. 2024. Available from: https://www.stanfordchildrens.org/en/topic/default?id=anal-fissure-134-174#:~:text=A%20fissure%20is%20caused%20by,not%20the%20same%20as%20hemorrhoids.
2. American Society of Colon and Rectal Surgeons Anal fissure. ASCRS. 2024. Available from: https://fascrs.org/patients/diseases-and-conditions/a-z/anal-fissure
3. Jahnny B, Ashurst JV. Anal Fissures. [Updated 2022 Nov 14]. In: StatPearls [Internet]. Treasure Island (FL): StatPearls Publishing; 2024. Available from: https://www.ncbi.nlm.nih.gov/books/NBK526063/.

Part II

Examination Findings

Breast Disease 19

Sydney Pekarek and Anna Katz

19.1 Introduction

Breast complaints are commonly experienced by patients and account for at least 3% of female primary care visits. One in eight women in the United States are going to develop breast cancer within the course of their life. While pediatric breast masses are much less common, there remains a prevalence of up to 3.2%. For pediatric masses, 95% are found to be benign fibroadenomas. Only 0.02% are malignant. With increasing rates of breast cancer in the adult population, identification and appropriate workup are necessary for appropriate care. Timely care is achievable; however, it requires coordination and cooperation with primary care providers/pediatricians in coordination with breast surgeons, plastic surgeons, medical and radiation oncologists, and genetic specialists. The American Society of Breast Surgeons recommends date between the first biopsy and the first treatment date be less than 60 days. The aim of this chapter is to provide a guideline for the workup of breast complaints as well as when to refer to specialists.

S. Pekarek (✉) · A. Katz
Advocate Medical Group, Park Ridge, IL, USA
e-mail: sydney.pekarek@aah.org; anna.katz@aah.org

G. P. Kohn et al. (eds.), *The SAGES Manual of Surgical Referral for Primary and Emergency Care*,
https://doi.org/10.1007/978-3-031-92678-5_19

19.2 Workup

Common breast complaints include breast masses, mastalgia (breast pain), and nipple discharge. The workup for these complaints should not replace screening recommendations. Firstly, a history and physical exam should be performed. A thorough history should include family history as available, history of genetic syndromes, personal history of previous breast lesions, and any other relevant medical and social history. The prevalence of cancer among women who report breast symptoms is estimated to be less than 10%, and those with breast lumps have a higher risk of malignancy than those with breast pain. With any breast complaint, a complete clinical breast exam should be performed. This can assist in guidance of further workup in addition to clinical history. In the pediatric population, it is important to ensure they feel safe and comfortable throughout this sensitive exam. The breast examination should start with the patient seated with hands positioned on their hips. Visual examination of asymmetry, skin changes such as retraction, erythema, skin thickening, or nipple discharge should raise concern. Finally, thorough examination of lymph nodes, including the supraclavicular, axillary, pectoral, and cervical lymph nodes, should be performed. Next, the patient should be positioned supine with arms stretched above their head. It is important to document the breast exam well, including size, location as distance from areolar edge, consistency, and circumferential location on the breast of any findings. Once a palpable mass is identified, further workup with imaging should be performed. It is important to communicate with imaging colleagues in the area of concern to ensure appropriate workup and evaluation.

19.3 Pediatric

Regarding pediatric breast complaints, identification of suspicious history and physical exam guides further workup. Physical exam in pediatric patients must include the age and associated tanner stage. Breast development begins in utero around the fourth week of gestation. The breast bud forms and tissues continue to develop just deep to the epithelium. Neonates may present with gynecomastia due to maternal estrogen exposure. This should be treated with reassurance and observation as these usually resolve within 2 years of age. There should, however, be close observation due to the possibility of lactation from neonatal gynecomastia. This may lead further to mastitis and abscess development, so close observation of resolution is recommended. If there are concerning signs such as redness, swelling, and erythema, pediatric surgery referral may be indicated. Further breast development begins around age 8–13, which is called thelarche. The developmental stages are determined by Tanner stage. Early development of thelarche may be associated with precocious puberty as early as age 6. This requires further hormone workup and evaluation of precocious puberty. If precocious puberty is not identified, an ultrasound may be obtained (Fig. 19.1). If ultrasound is reassuring, no further workup may be indicated. However, in the absence of precocious puberty or abnormal findings on US, further referral to pediatric surgery for further evaluation and workup may be indicated. Idiopathic premature thelarche, ages 1–3, however, usually regresses and does not require further workup. Observation and reassurance are recommended in these cases.

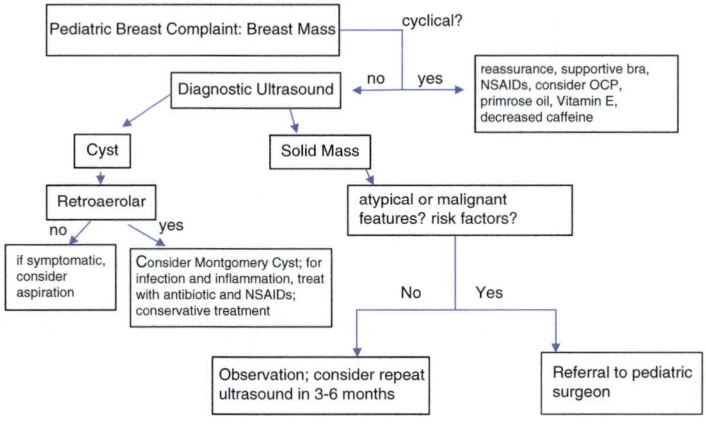

Fig. 19.1 Pediatric breast mass algorithm

History of breast changes with menstrual cycle is the second most common breast lesion and is a normal variant of physiology. This may be treated with reassurance, a supportive bra, and NSAIDS as needed. With high clinical suspicion, ultrasound remains the primary and often only imaging evaluation in the pediatric population. Ultrasound retains a high sensitivity for the detection of lesions in younger, dense breasts with a lack of radiation. Mammography is limited in the pediatric population due to low sensitivity and radiation risks. MRI evaluation is often reserved for disease extent and can further be utilized at the discretion of the treating provider.

Breast cysts are typically well-circumscribed, freely mobile, and will contain fluid on imaging. Most simple cysts regress on their own; however, symptomatic cysts may be aspirated for optimal treatment. Montgomery cysts may present when glands of Montgomery along the areolar become obstructed. These patients may present with painful inflammation or a painless retroareolar mass. Treatment of cysts with concern for infection consists of antibiotics and NSAIDS and may require aspiration, usually under ultrasound guidance. Failure of the above management may prompt surgical referral.

While Breast Imaging Reporting and Data System (BI-RADS) is the gold standard for describing, stratifying, and guiding breast lesion management, its utility in pediatric patients has been questioned. There have been multiple studies demonstrating that BI-RADS overestimates the risk of malignancy in pediatric patients. In general, most small and benign appearing asymptomatic breast masses may be observed alone or followed with ultrasound. Lesions 3–5 cm or those that are growing should be referred to a pediatric surgeon (or general/breast surgeon who cares for pediatric surgical problems) for further evaluation and workup. Other considerations for pediatric surgeon referral include atypical or malignant features, personal history/family history of malignancy, personal history of mantle radiation, genetic mutation/syndrome, or a symptomatic mass.

19.4 Male

Gynecomastia may also occur in boys, either unilateral or bilateral, and presents as retroareolar palpable mass. It often occurs because of estrogen and progesterone as well as leptin, present in fatty tissue. This is treated typically by reassurance and observation as it often regresses within 2 years. If there is no regression, further workup may be indicated, including hormone-level testing. If there is further concern with no obvious hormonal changes, referral to pediatric surgery or plastic surgery may be indicated. Prior to referral, if there continues to be excessive tissue with no identified hormonal cause, US may be indicated as well.

19.5 Adults

Once imaging has been obtained, it is important to interpret results and proceed with further workup when indicated.

For women 30 years or older, following diagnostic mammography, interpretation of radiology assessment is important (Fig. 19.2). All breast imaging must be accompanied by a Breast Imaging Reporting and Data System (BI-RADS) categorization to assist interpretation and direct management. BI-RADS categories are associated with risks of malignancy based on interpretation of the imaging as determined by the American College of Radiology. When reviewing diagnostic mammography, BI-RADS 4 or 5 confers concern for malignancy and diagnostic ultrasound will often be performed followed by a core needle biopsy. These core biopsies can be performed using either stereotactic (mammographic) or ultrasound guidance. Performing diagnostic ultrasound and a core needle biopsy while surgical referral is made optimizes timely diagnosis and intervention. With BI-RADS 1–3, diagnostic ultrasound may be performed. BI-RADS 1, negative imaging, with a high clinical suspicion should proceed to core needle biopsy under palpable guidance and surgical referral. With

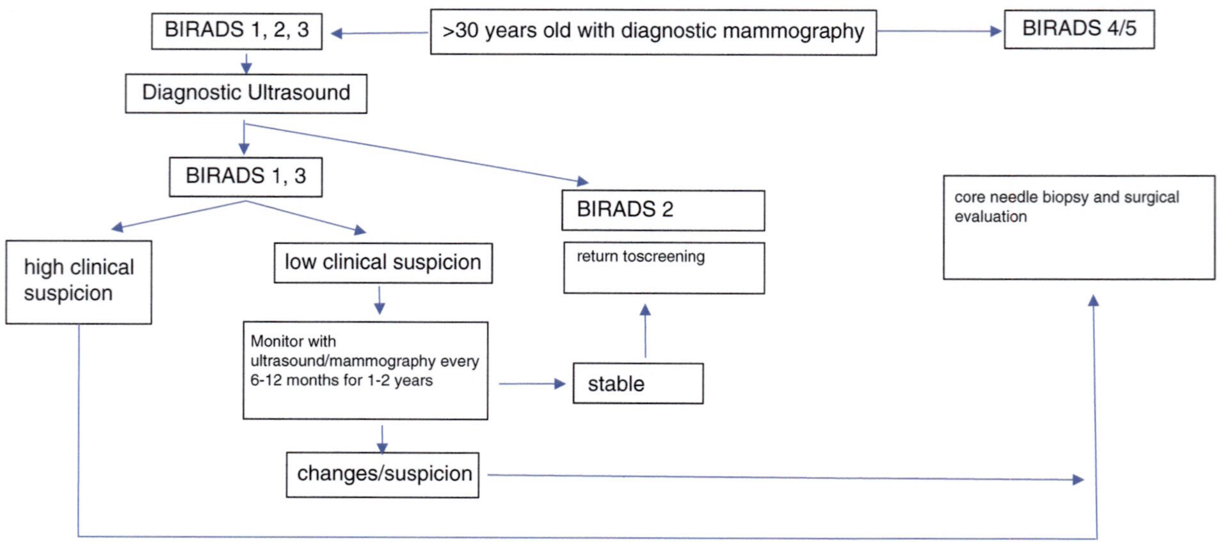

Fig. 19.2 Management of breast lesions in patients >30 y/o, after mammography

low clinical suspicion, monitoring with repeat clinical breast examination followed by repeat ultrasound/mammography every 6 months for 1–2 years can be performed. If stable, the patient can be returned to screening or if change in examination/imaging findings occurs, consider core needle biopsy and referral for surgical evaluation. BI-RADS 2, benign changes, may resume routine screening. BI-RADS 3 findings should be monitored with short-term follow-up commonly at 6, 12, and 24 months using the same imaging modality used to identify the finding.

For women younger than 30 years, clinical breast exam and ultrasound should be performed (Fig. 19.3). Following this, BI-RADS are again used to guide further workup/management. With BI-RADS 1, high clinical suspicion that persists should undergo a diagnostic mammography, core needle biopsy, and referral for surgical evaluation. With low clinical suspicion, this lesion may be monitored with ultrasound and exam every 6–12 months for 1–2 years. With stable imaging, routine screening may resume while any changes in findings prompt biopsy and surgical evaluation. BI-RADS 2 may resume routine screening. BI-RADS 3 with high clinical suspicion should undergo core needle biopsy with surgical evaluation while low clinical suspicion may be monitored with repeat ultrasound every 6–12 months for 1–2 years followed by routine screening. BI-RADS 4/5 requires prompt core needle biopsy and surgical evaluation. Of note, if there is a high clinical suspicion and core needle biopsy is unable to be performed, then surgical referral should occur and surgical excision will need to be considered.

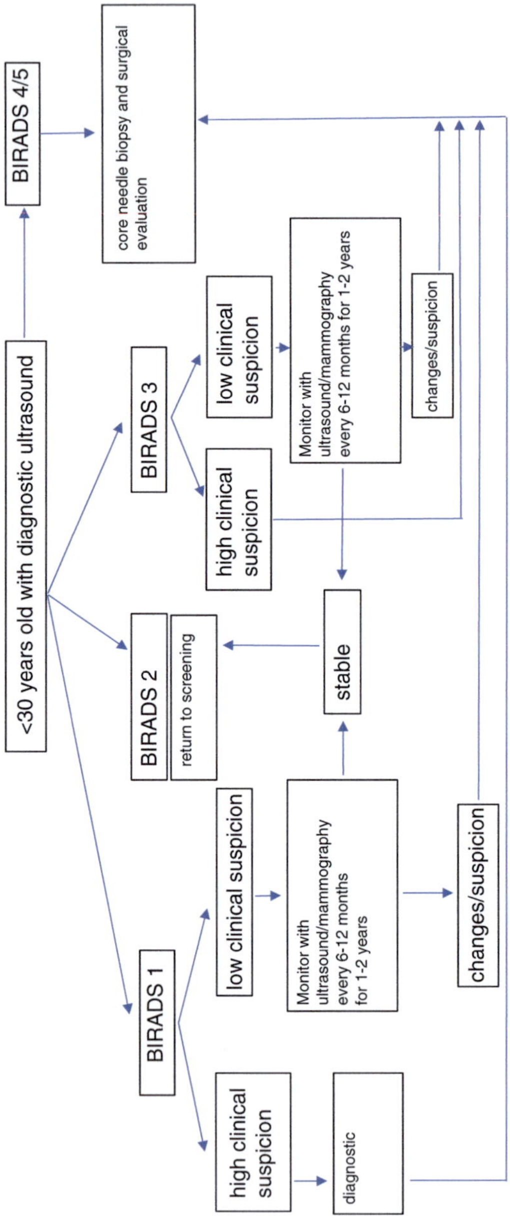

Fig. 19.3 Management of breast lesions in patients <30 y/o, after mammography

19.6 Breast Pain

Breast pain is a common complaint that also presents to primary care settings. Cyclic mastalgia accounts for 2/3 of all breast pain and is most common in ages 20–30 s. This pain tends to be bilateral and may radiate to the axilla. Noncyclical pain may be focal or diffuse and is not associated with menses; this is often in patients who are in their 30–40 s but can occur at any age. Some causes of such pain may be OCP use, hormone therapy, breast trauma, infection, benign tumors, or pain associated with pendulous breasts. All breast pain should be evaluated with a clinical breast exam, and, if a mass is palpated, workup as noted above in addition to surgical evaluation is warranted (Fig. 19.4). If no mass is noted on clinical exam with cyclical history, no imaging is required. Noncyclical pain that is focally located should undergo ultrasound in those under 30 years of age and diagnostic mammography with ultrasound for those aged 30 and greater. Nonfocal and noncyclical pain in patients with no risk factors does not require imaging; however, with patients with risk factors present and over age 40, diagnostic mammography is recommended. There is no evidence that breast pain alone is associated with breast cancer, but it accounts for many referrals to a breast specialist. Treatment of breast pain includes reduction of symptoms and lifestyle modification. First-line treatment includes limiting caffeine intake, dietary modification, ensuring a well-fitting bra, and management of stress/anxiety/depression. NSAIDS may be used as well. Some sources recommend oral vitamin E as well as

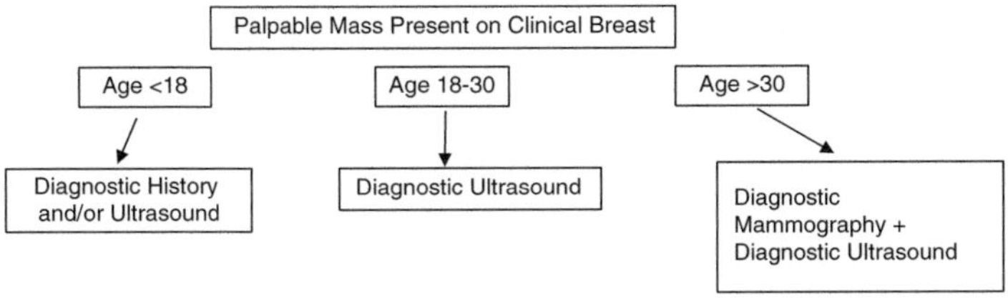

Fig. 19.4 Management of a palpable breast lesion

evening primrose oil supplementation. If conservative management fails, surgical evaluation is warranted.

Infection may be a source of breast pain as well. Mastitis, or inflammation of the breast, may occur in infectious or less commonly granulomatous disease. This most often occurs in patients actively breastfeeding due to decreased bacterial barrier with small breaks in the skin and clogged milk ducts. In nonlactating women, other causes may include metaplasia leading to clogged milk ducts as well. Mastitis can further lead to abscess formation. This is relatively common and occurs at an incidence of 5–10%. For well-appearing women, without signs of abscess, oral antibiotics may be prescribed. If there is clinical evidence on physical exam concerning for abscess, prompt US and surgical evaluation are indicated. Aspiration of breast abscesses may guide antibiotic management and symptom resolution with limited breast tissue deformation. If the patient is not well appearing, the patient should be promptly admitted to the hospital for antibiotics and surgical evaluation. For lactation-associated mastitis, NSAIDS and heat should also be recommended. For prolonged episodes of redness/swelling/induration of skin following the above treatments, imaging should be obtained. Imaging, according to age as noted above, should be obtained followed by prompt surgical evaluation to evaluate for possible inflammatory breast cancer.

19.7 Nipple Discharge

Nipple discharge presents commonly among women; however, underlying malignancy is identified in up to 21% of patients who present with concern for pathologic discharge. All patients who present with galactorrhea should firstly have a human chorionic gonadotropin pregnancy test to rule out pregnancy followed by prolactin and TSH levels. If history and physical exam remain consistent with physiologic discharge, no imaging is indicated. Patients who present with nipple discharge and are over the age of 40 should undergo diagnostic mammography and ultrasound if not performed within the past 6 months. Physiologic discharge should be observed, reassured, and reexamined in short-interval follow-up to assess for resolution. Pathologic discharge, such as spontaneous, unilateral, bloody, serous, serosanguinous, or watery discharge, should be promptly evaluated. Age-appropriate workup should include an ultrasound with/without diagnostic mammography. Following imaging, referral for surgical evaluation is warranted.

19.8 Conclusion

Prompt surgical referral is necessary for suspicious breast lesions. From biopsy diagnosis to the first date of treatment, 60 days or less is associated with better outcomes. Referrals may be placed to a breast surgeon or a general surgeon who specializes in breast care. Some studies suggest that a fellowship-trained breast surgeon or a surgical oncologist has been associated with better cosmetic satisfaction, physical well-being, and adverse radiation effects. Given these reported outcomes, discussion with the patient and options for referral should be provided.

With breast complaints accounting for a significant portion of primary care complaints and rising incidence of new breast cancer diagnoses yearly, it is important for all members of the care team to be educated in the common workup of breast complaints. Timely recognition, imaging, and workup can aid in improved outcomes. Communication amongst care teams and appropriate referral for surgical evaluation will help aid in diagnosing and treating breast complaints.

Thyroid Disease

20

Marina Robson Chase
and William B. Inabnet III

20.1 Introduction

According to the American Association of Endocrine Surgeons, over 100,000 thyroid surgeries are performed annually in the United States. An even greater number of patients will have thyroid conditions requiring routine surveillance or medical management. The primary care provider (PCP) should be comfortable with the initial workup of thyroid disease and have a good understanding of when to refer a patient to an endocrinologist or surgeon for specialty care.

Thyroid disease is managed surgically by surgeons through different training pathways—endocrine surgeons, otolaryngologists, head and neck surgical oncologists, and community general surgeons. Although all of these training pathways have the necessary elements to train thyroid surgeons, studies have shown improved outcomes when patients are managed by a high-volume thyroid surgeon.

In general, evaluation for thyroid disease follows a straightforward workup. Patient history should be taken, including history of

M. R. Chase · W. B. Inabnet III (✉)
Division of General, Endocrine, and Metabolic Surgery, Department of Surgery, University of Kentucky, Lexington, KY, USA
e-mail: william.Inabnet@uky.edu

G. P. Kohn et al. (eds.), *The SAGES Manual of Surgical Referral for Primary and Emergency Care*,
https://doi.org/10.1007/978-3-031-92678-5_20

prior thyroid disease, prior malignancy, exposure to radiation, prior neck surgery, long-term use of medications such as amiodarone or lithium, and family history of malignancy, especially thyroid malignancy. Physical exam may reveal a diffusely enlarged thyroid, palpable thyroid nodules, or a normal thyroid. Preoperative voice quality should be noted. Exam findings according to specific diagnoses are below. Laboratory workup should begin with an assessment of thyroid functional status (hypothyroid, euthyroid, or hyperthyroid). The initial imaging test should be a diagnostic neck ultrasound. Specific diagnoses are discussed in further detail below.

20.2 Goiter

A goiter is an enlarged thyroid gland that can cause aerodigestive compressive symptoms. Goiter can be caused by iodine deficiency (rare in developed countries with iodized salt), multiple benign nonfunctioning nodules, or conditions such as Graves' disease and Hashimoto's thyroiditis that may lead to diffuse enlargement of the thyroid gland over time.

Patients might experience trouble swallowing, a globus sensation in the throat, voice changes including a weak or hoarse voice, trouble breathing when lying flat, a dry cough, and a palpable neck mass. It is important to exclude other etiologies of these symptoms such as gastroesophageal reflux disease, which can cause voice changes and a dry cough, and heart failure, which can lead to orthopnea.

Physical examination will often reveal an enlarged thyroid. The thyroid can be diffusely enlarged or can feel nodular and asymmetric. If the thyroid is significantly enlarged and asymmetric, the trachea may be deviated. The goiter can extend substernally, and the full extent might not be able to be appreciated on physical exam alone. Pemberton's sign is an uncommon physical exam finding in patients with a significantly sized goiter; bilateral arm raise will cause obstruction of venous drainage from the head, leading to facial plethora.

Workup should include a thyroid-stimulating hormone (TSH) level and free T4 (thyroxine) to assess thyroid functional status. Patients with multinodular goiter are typically euthyroid; hyperthyroidism or hypothyroidism warrants further workup as discussed below. Laboratory workup should also include a calcium level, and if elevated, a parathyroid hormone (PTH) level to assess for concomitant hyperparathyroidism. A diagnostic ultrasound should be obtained to assess for nodules concerning for malignancy.

If a patient is euthyroid or hypothyroid without suspicious nodules on ultrasound and does not desire surgery for symptomatic management, the patient does not need to be referred to a surgeon. If there is concern that the goiter is growing rapidly or that symptoms are interfering with quality of life, surgical assessment is appropriate. The primary care provider plays an important role in optimizing the patient for elective surgery, specifically with the management of chronic comorbidities such as hypertension and diabetes. If a patient is referred for surgery, the primary care provider should restrain from making recommendations regarding the extent of surgery (i.e., lobectomy vs. total thyroidectomy); such conversations can lead to misalignment between the patient's and surgeon's respective expectations.

20.3 Hyperthyroidism

The common causes of hyperthyroidism include Graves' disease (an autoimmune condition), single toxic adenoma, and toxic multinodular goiter ("toxic" is synonymous with hyperfunctioning). Thyroiditis can lead to transient hyperthyroidism (discussed below). There are also some less common causes, including amiodarone-induced thyrotoxicosis and iodine-induced hyperthyroidism.

Patients presenting with hyperthyroidism will often complain of tachycardia or palpitations, tremors, GI symptoms such as diarrhea, weight loss, and anxiety. Physical examination may reveal tachycardia, tremor, and tongue fasciculations. Those with

Graves' disease may also present with exophthalmos, pretibial myxedema, and thyroid acropachy, or digital clubbing.

Laboratory testing typically reveals a suppressed TSH and elevated free T4/T3 (triiodothyronine) levels. A low TSH with normal T4 is classified as "subclinical hyperthyroidism" and warrants continued workup and monitoring as it can be indicative of underlying thyroid dysfunction. Patients with Graves' disease will typically have an elevated thyrotropin receptor antibody (TRAb) level, which is an autoantibody that stimulates the TSH receptors, leading to unchecked thyroid hormone production.

A thyroid scintigraphy scan is a radioactive uptake scan that can be helpful to differentiate the etiology of hyperthyroidism. If history, physical exam, and laboratory workup is consistent with Graves', the scintigraphy scan is not mandatory. A patient with Graves' will have diffusely increased uptake throughout the gland, a patient with a toxic adenoma will have increased uptake in a singular nodule with suppression of the uptake of the rest of the thyroid, and a patient with toxic multinodular goiter will have patchy uptake. Thyroid scintigraphy is not indicated for the euthyroid or hypothyroid patient.

Options for the management of hyperthyroidism include radioactive iodine, surgery, and antithyroid medications (methimazole/carbimazole, propylthiouracil). Almost all patients with hyperthyroidism would benefit from a discussion of all three options of disease management; refer to a surgeon unless the patient is well controlled otherwise and not interested in surgery. Patients should also be referred to a thyroid specialist for the management of hyperthyroidism. Ideally, patients should be euthyroid prior to surgery; often beta blockade is necessary prior to surgery for persistent tachyarrhythmias. Accordingly, it is advised that the PCP initiate medical therapy prior to referral.

20.4 Thyroid Nodules and Risk of Malignancy

Thyroid nodules are very common. It is estimated that over 50% of the population will develop a thyroid nodule and that only 5% are malignant. The vast majority of thyroid cancer is well-differentiated thyroid carcinoma (papillary and follicular) that has a very good prognosis. The prognosis is especially good with age under 55; in fact, differentiated thyroid cancer is the only malignancy with age as a criterion in the American Joint Committee on Cancer (AJCC) TMN staging system. Less commonly, patients may have medullary thyroid carcinoma, anaplastic thyroid carcinoma, thyroid lymphoma, or metastases from another primary malignancy.

Patients may present with a palpable, nontender nodule. Alternatively, a thyroid nodule might be discovered incidentally when cross-sectional imaging is performed for a different indication, such as a chest CT or a carotid artery duplex. The American College of Radiology recommends further workup with a dedicated thyroid ultrasound for any nodule with suspicious features on imaging, nodules greater than 1 cm in size for patients under 35 years of age, and nodules greater than 1.5 cm for patients 35 years of age or older.

Physical examination should include assessment of the thyroid gland, preoperative voice quality, and the lymph nodes of the central and lateral neck from the clavicles to the mandible.

Workup should include assessment of thyroid functional status with TSH and T4, as well as calcium and, if elevated, PTH, to assess for concomitant hyperparathyroidism. Every patient with a thyroid nodule should undergo a diagnostic neck ultrasound in order to risk-stratify and determine the need for biopsy. Thyroid biopsy is performed with fine needle aspiration (FNA), typically under ultrasound guidance. The American Thyroid Association and American College of Radiology both have biopsy criteria according to nodule ultrasound characteristics and size with similar diagnostic utility. Biopsies can be performed by radiologists, endocrinologists, or surgeons. Surgeon-performed in-office biopsy is increasingly common.

Patients should be referred to a surgeon prior to biopsy. Certain pathologies will require molecular testing for further guidance of malignancy risk, and this can be obtained at the same time as initial biopsy when indicated. However, if after shared decision-making between patient and surgeon, surgery is indicated due to patient symptoms, patient preference, or concern of inconclusive biopsy, biopsy and/or molecular testing can be skipped. This can reduce the cost and patient discomfort associated with pre-surgical workup, especially when the results will not change management.

When assessing a patient with concern for thyroid malignancy, it is paramount to collect a complete personal and family history of malignancy. Twenty-five percent of medullary thyroid cancer is inherited; commonly due to multiple endocrine neoplasm syndromes 2A and 2B. Genetic counselling can be helpful with a strong family history of malignancies. Although there are no known hereditary syndromes associated with differentiated thyroid cancer, there is a higher risk among those with first-degree relatives who have a history of differentiated thyroid cancer.

20.5 Approach to Surveillance

The American Thyroid Association recommends that patients with thyroid nodules that do not meet biopsy criteria should undergo repeat ultrasound in 6–12 months if the ultrasound had highly suspicious features, 12–24 months if the ultrasound had intermediate features, more than 24 months if the nodule is greater than 1 cm and had very low suspicion features, and no repeat necessary if less than 1 cm and with very low suspicion features. If the nodule has progressed to meeting biopsy criteria, the patient should be referred to a surgeon for FNA. However, there is the caveat that these recommendations are based on low-quality or insufficient evidence. There is no consensus on how long stable thyroid nodules should be surveilled.

Patients with thyroid nodules meeting biopsy criteria should be referred to a surgeon. If the biopsy results are benign, the surgeon will determine the surveillance plan based on ultrasound features. The American Thyroid Association provides recommendations that can be found online and are listed as a suggested reading.

20.6 Rapidly Expanding Neck Mass

Any patient with a rapidly expanding neck mass should have an expedient workup as these often represent aggressive malignancies. Although surgery with curative intent is very much contingent on the stage of the malignancy at the time of diagnosis and often not possible, surgery is sometimes indicated for airway protection (tracheostomy) or palliation of compressive symptoms.

- Anaplastic thyroid carcinoma
  - Anaplastic thyroid carcinoma is an aggressive type of thyroid cancer accounting for 2% of thyroid cancers, with a poor prognosis as it often presents late and is locally invasive. Patients should be referred to a surgeon for evaluation, although surgical resection is not possible in many cases.
- Thyroid lymphoma
  - Thyroid lymphoma arises in the setting of previous autoimmune thyroiditis, leading to a rapidly expanding neck mass, B symptoms (fevers, night sweats, and weight loss), and lymphadenopathy of the neck. If there is suspicion for thyroid lymphoma based on the history and physical exam, the patient should undergo FNA or core needle biopsy with flow cytometry for definitive results and should be referred to a medical oncologist for management.
- Metastasis to the thyroid
  - Metastasis to the thyroid often presents similarly to a primary thyroid cancer and FNA is required for an accurate diagnosis. The role of surgical intervention is often limited only to palliation for aerodigestive compression or invasion. The most common primary cancers to metastasize to the thyroid are renal cell carcinoma and lung cancer.

20.7 Thyroiditis

Thyroiditis describes a group of conditions characterized by inflammation of the thyroid. Most are managed medically, but there are some instances where surgical referral is warranted.

- Subacute (de Quervain's) thyroiditis
  - De Quervain's thyroiditis is inflammation of the thyroid secondary to viral illness. Patients may present with a swollen, tender thyroid. Patients typically experience an acutely painful hyperthyroid state, followed by a euthyroid state, a hypothyroid state, and then resolution with return to euthyroid state. Patients do not need to be referred to a surgeon as the condition is self-limiting.
- Autoimmune (Hashimoto's) thyroiditis
  - Hashimoto's thyroiditis is an autoimmune condition leading to lymphocytic invasion of the thyroid with destruction of the thyroid architecture and resulting hypothyroidism. Patients will present with symptoms of hypothyroidism, including fatigue, weight gain, constipation, feeling chilled, dry skin, hair loss, and brain fog. Elevated thyroid peroxidase (TPO) antibodies support a diagnosis of Hashimoto's thyroiditis. Over time, the thyroid gland may become enlarged and lead to compressive symptoms of dysphagia, palpable enlargement, and a globus sensation. Patients may desire surgical excision for symptomatic relief, and as most are already on lifelong thyroid hormone replacement, this is not a major lifestyle adjustment.
- Riedel's thyroiditis
  - Riedel's thyroiditis is a progressive condition causing fibrosis of the thyroid gland often associated with other fibrosing pathologies. Historically, isthmectomy was performed to relieve tracheal compression; now, medical management with tamoxifen or steroids is more commonly pursued.
- Suppurative thyroiditis
  - Suppurative thyroiditis is an infection of the thyroid due to a bacterial or fungal infection; it is rather uncommon due to the highly vascular nature of the thyroid. Patients will present with a tender, swollen thyroid and often symptoms of systemic infection. Antibiotics are the mainstay treatment; however, an ultrasound should be performed to evaluate for abscesses. Any patient with a thyroid abscess should be expeditiously referred to a thyroid surgeon for incision and drainage.

20.8 Care of the Patient Following Thyroidectomy

- Following thyroid lobectomy, a TSH level should be measured in 2–3 weeks and levothyroxine prescribed if necessary.
- Following total thyroidectomy, patients will require daily levothyroxine, which may be titrated by an endocrinologist or primary care provider.
- Patients with confirmed thyroid cancer will be followed by their surgeon for a minimum of 5 years. The frequency of surveillance is influenced by the stage of the patient at the time of surgery and the results of dynamic surveillance (thyroglobulin levels and ultrasound).
- Patients complaining of hoarseness following neck surgery might have sustained a recurrent laryngeal nerve injury (temporary or permanent) and should return to their surgeon for laryngoscopy.
- Patients complaining of numbness or tingling of fingers, toes, or lips or muscle cramping should have calcium and magnesium checked. Postoperative hypocalcemia can result from devascularization of the parathyroid glands and may require temporary or lifelong calcium supplementation.

Presenting complaint	Recommended triage
Expanding neck hematoma following surgery Difficulty breathing Tetany following surgery	Patient should present to the emergency room
Hoarseness following surgery Numbness/tingling of extremities following surgery Rapidly growing neck mass (prior to surgery, without airway compromise) Suppurative thyroiditis with concern for abscess	Patient should be seen by surgeon urgently

(continued)

Presenting complaint	Recommended triage
New thyroid nodule with suspicious imaging findings Compressive symptoms due to thyroid nodule or goiter	Patient can be referred to surgeon according to typical referral scheduling
Newly diagnosed hyperthyroidism Difficult to manage hypothyroidism	Patient should be referred to endocrinology
Hypothyroidism Stable, asymptomatic thyroid nodule without suspicious ultrasound characteristics	Patient should continue under care of PCP

Workup and management prior to surgeon referral
All patients should have thyroid function tested and appropriate medical management initiated
Hypothyroidș—levothyroxine
Hyperthyroid—antithyroid medication and beta-blockers titrated to goal of normal heart rate
Patients with abnormal thyroid function should have autoantibodies tested
All patients should have basic labs tested, including creatinine to evaluate renal function and calcium to evaluate for concomitant hyperparathyroidism
Patients with concern for goiter or nodule should have a neck ultrasound
Patients with hyperthyroidism not clearly consistent with Graves' should have a thyroid scintigraphy scan
Patients with suspicious nodules should be referred to a surgeon PRIOR to biopsy

Suggested Readings

1. Wang TS, Lyden ML, Sosa JA. Thyroidectomy. UpToDate. 2023. https://www.uptodate.com/contents/thyroidectomy
2. Chen AY, Bernet VJ, Carty SE, et al. American thyroid association statement on optimal surgical management of goiter. Thyroid. 2014:181–9. https://doi.org/10.1089/thy.2013.0291.

3. Kravets I. Hyperthyroidism: Diagnosis and Treatment. Am Fam Physician. 2016;93(5):363–70. Available from: https://www.aafp.org/pubs/afp/issues/2016/0301/p363.html
4. Haugen BR, Alexander EK, Bible KC, et al. 2015 American Thyroid Association Management Guidelines for Adult Patients with Thyroid Nodules and Differentiated Thyroid Cancer: The American Thyroid Association Guidelines Task Force on Thyroid Nodules and Differentiated Thyroid Cancer. Thyroid. 2016;26(10):1–133. https://doi.org/10.1089/thy.2015.0020.

Parathyroid Disease 21

Nicholas A. Rawson, Katie Marrero,
Daniel Chase, and Uretz Oliphant

21.1 Presentation

Abnormal hypersecretion of parathyroid hormone (PTH) can result from several etiologies. The most common is due to primary hyperparathyroidism (HPT), that is, altered function of the gland itself. This can usually be traced back to a single adenoma, glandular hyperplasia, or in rare circumstances malignancy. Secondary HPT typically results from poor kidney function,

N. A. Rawson
Carle Health, Urbana, IL, USA

K. Marrero
Carle Health, Urbana, IL, USA

Carle Illinois College of Medicine, Urbana, IL, USA

Pennsylvania State University Milton S. Hershey Medical Center, Hershey, PA, USA

D. Chase
Carle Illinois College of Medicine, Urbana, IL, USA

Carle Hoopeston Regional Medical Center, Hoopeston, IL, USA

U. Oliphant (✉)
Carle Health, Urbana, IL, USA

University of Illinois College of Medicine at Chicago, Chicago, IL, USA
e-mail: Uretz.oliphant@carle.com

G. P. Kohn et al. (eds.), *The SAGES Manual of Surgical Referral for Primary and Emergency Care*,
https://doi.org/10.1007/978-3-031-92678-5_21

resulting in an inability to convert vitamin D into its active form. The lack of 1,25-cholecalciferol then prevents adequate intestinal absorption of calcium creating an environment where increased PTH levels will be required to maintain homeostasis. Additionally, high levels of serum phosphorus will stimulate the parathyroid glands to hypertrophy. Tertiary HPT occurs in those patients with secondary hyperparathyroidism who receive a kidney transplant. Despite the renal graft, the parathyroid gland will remain hyperfunctional, resulting in hypercalcemia.

Historically, the presentation of HPT was characterized by the classic "stones, groans, moans, and psychic overtones" of hypercalcemia and radiographic findings of osteitis fibrosa cystica (brown tumors) on long bones or erosive bone disease. In the modern Western world, this has been replaced by largely asymptomatic disease identified through hypercalcemia on routine laboratory evaluation. Subtle symptoms suggesting changes in mood, memory, energy levels, attention, bowel or bladder habits, appetite, and thirst can be found in even those who are previously thought to be asymptomatic. These can include fatigue, changes in attention, mood, or memory, changes in bowel or bladder habits, and polydipsia. In either symptomatic or asymptomatic disease, examination of the neck is usually normal. In the rare circumstance that a nodule is palpated, this should raise concern for either a thyroid nodule or a parathyroid neoplasm.

21.2 Diagnostics

A single episode of hypercalcemia alone is insufficient to make the diagnosis of HPT. Table 21.1 summarizes the workup that should be completed prior to referral to a surgeon. Measuring serum PTH levels and confirming the calcium elevation on a subsequent lab draw can confirm the diagnosis in many cases. An ionized calcium does not usually provide additional benefit in confirming the diagnosis and can be reasonably excluded in the initial workup. The overwhelming majority of patients with HPT will demonstrate PTH levels above the normal limit. However, approximately 20% of patients with HPT will have normal PTH

Table 21.1 Testing that should be completed prior to surgical referral

Should be completed prior to referral for all patients	Should be completed for asymptomatic patients
Serum calcium	Bone densitometry
Serum PTH	Renal ultrasound, radiography, or cross-sectional imaging
Serum vitamin D	Vertebral radiographs or cross-sectional imaging
24 h urine calcium	
Serum creatinine	

measurements. It is imperative to distinguish this group of patients with HPT from those with familial hypocalciuric hypercalcemia (FHH). A 24-h urine calcium, serum creatinine, and serum vitamin D can be helpful in delineating the underlying cause. Patients with FHH will have normal vitamin D levels, a 24-h urine calcium <200 mg, and a calcium/creatinine ratio of <0.01. Ca/Cr ratio can be calculated by (Serum Cr * 24 h Urine Ca) / (Serum Ca * 24 h Urine Ca). Low 24-h urine calcium and vitamin D deficiency is usually indicative of secondary HPT.

It is important to quantify how far over the upper limit of normal the serum calcium is elevated. The majority of asymptomatic patients will have mild disease that is <1.0 mg/dL over the upper limit of normal. Bone mineral density quantification is also useful in characterizing the severity of the disease.

Asymptomatic patients should be classified into those who have evidence of end-organ damage and who do not. End-organ damage should be assessed in all patients who do not meet immediate indications for parathyroidectomy (discussed in the next section). Important adjuncts include kidney imaging with ultrasound, X-ray, or CT to evaluate for nephrocalcinosis and nephrolithiasis as well as vertebral imaging with X-ray, CT, or MRI to assess for occult fracture.

Localization studies are helpful, but can generally be ordered by the surgeon once a decision for operative intervention is made. These studies include ultrasound, MRI, and nuclear medicine (Sestamibi) scans. Surgical decision-making regarding these studies is important as their use is controversial if bilateral neck exploration is planned. In the case of a palpable abnormality on a physical exam, we would still recommend sonographic evaluation concomitantly with surgical referral.

21.3 Indications for Surgical Referral

All symptomatic patients should undergo surgical evaluation as parathyroidectomy remains the mainstay of therapy. Medical management is possible in those patients who have contraindications to surgery, but this should not preclude evaluation by a surgeon. If there is any doubt as to whether the patient is symptomatic, consider surgical evaluation for final determination.

Asymptomatic patients are recommended surgery on the basis of *The Fifth International Workshop on the Evaluation and Management of Primary Hyperparathyroidism* guidelines:

1. Patients whose serum calcium is >1.0 g/dL above the upper limit of normal.
2. Bone densitometry measurements of ≤ -2.5 standard deviations below the mean as measured at the hip, lumbar spine, or distal radius.
3. Previous asymptomatic vertebral fracture.
4. Estimated glomerular filtration rate < 60 mL/min/1.73m^2.
5. 24 h urine Ca levels >250 mg/day in women and > 300 mg/day in men.
6. Nephrolithiasis or nephrocalcinosis on imaging.
7. <50 years old.

Some surgeons will also weigh the patient's access to medical and surgical care into the decision to operate. Patients who are not planned to undergo parathyroidectomy require close monitoring in order to avoid sequelae. If this is not possible, parathyroidectomy may remain the safest option for these patients.

If doubt remains at any step, surgical evaluation remains the safest approach to patients with HPT of any variety. Table 21.2

Table 21.2 Indications for the type of referral to be made

Emergency department referral	1. Airway compromise 2. Serum calcium >14 g/dL 3. Altered mental status 4. Cardiovascular symptoms such as EKG changes 5. Muscle weakness causing pulmonary compromise
Urgent surgical referral	1. Parathyroid carcinoma 2. Mass effect 3. Moderate hypercalcemia secondary to hyperparathyroidism (serum calcium 12–14 g/dL)
Routine surgical referral	1. Primary hyperparathyroidism 2. Tertiary hyperparathyroidism 3. Mild hypercalcemia secondary to hyperparathyroidism
No referral required	1. Vitamin D deficiency 2. Secondary hyperparathyroidism (can consider nephrology consultation) 3. Familial hypocalciuric hypercalcemia

summarizes the indications and type of referral that should be placed based on the patient's presentation.

21.4 Surveillance and Follow-Up

Patients who are not planned to undergo surgical intervention should be surveilled on either an annual or biannual basis for symptomatic disease, worsening of their hypercalcemia, or other indications for surgery as listed above. Serum calcium, glomerular filtration rate, and bone densitometry should be reviewed. Abdominal radiographs to rule out urolithiasis remain somewhat more controversial. These can certainly be ordered at the discretion of the primary care provider or if clinical concern arise. Surgical referral is indicated at the time that any of these complications arise.

Suggested Readings

1. Parathyroid Disorders | AAFP.
2. Workup and Indications for Surgery for Hyperparathyroidism (pennmedicine.org).
3. Primary hyperparathyroidism: Diagnosis, differential diagnosis, and evaluation – UpToDate.
4. Evaluation and Management of Primary Hyperparathyroidism: Summary Statement and Guidelines from the Fifth International Workshop – PubMed (nih.gov).

Severe Obesity 22

R. Wesley Vosburg

In 2013, the American Medical Association recognized obesity as a disease. Most healthcare providers are well aware of the multifactorial etiology, chronicity, and far-reaching impact on health that are associated with it. Meanwhile, about 70% of patients with this disease have reported that they perceived bias from physicians in the way they were treated during appointments (weight bias). These instances also took place at centers that were primarily focused on the disease of obesity. Some things that helped improve the patient's experience included the use of patient-first language. As an example: "the patient with obesity" rather than "the obese patient." Focusing on objective BMI and comorbid conditions rather than classification of patients as overweight, obese, or morbidly obese also helped. When thinking about weight loss surgery stating that "an operation may be the best option for you" rather than "you are a candidate for weight loss surgery" has also been found to be helpful. Even after attempts were made to decrease weight bias, providers often felt as though they did not have the resources available to fully support the treatment of patients with obesity. These include access to frequent follow-up, dietary and behavioral health support, exercise education and support groups.

R. W. Vosburg (✉)
HCA Grand Strand Medical Center, Myrtle Beach, SC, USA

G. P. Kohn et al. (eds.), *The SAGES Manual of Surgical Referral for Primary and Emergency Care*,
https://doi.org/10.1007/978-3-031-92678-5_22

Referral of a patient to a center that focuses on weight is one great option for primary care providers. Generally, patients with a BMI of 27 kg/m^2 or more with one obesity-related comorbidity or a BMI of 30 kg/m^2 or above are good candidates for referral. Patients in this group may benefit from a multidisciplinary evaluation and individualized treatment plan for their obesity. Registered dietitians, behavioral health providers, medical bariatricians, and antiobesity medications may all be helpful to them in combination with one another.

Metabolic and bariatric surgeons perform seven different procedures that are approved by the American Society of Metabolic and Bariatric Surgery. The two most commonly performed operations are sleeve gastrectomy and Roux-en-Y gastric bypass. Sleeve gastrectomy is the most commonly performed weight loss operation in the United States. Gastric bypass is the second most common. For every one patient who has a gastric bypass, three patients will have sleeve gastrectomy. Both operations are excellent in terms of weight loss and comorbidity improvement or resolution. They have been shown to be superior to maximal nonsurgical treatments for obesity. Patients can expect to lose and keep off about 20–40% of their starting weight with either procedure. Weight loss is the fastest in the first year following surgery. Long-term strategies are needed for maintenance of weight loss; they predominantly focus on dietary, exercise, and, occasionally, antiobesity medication therapy.

In 2022, the guidelines for selecting adult patients who would benefit from weight loss surgery were updated by the International Federation for the Surgery of Obesity and Metabolic Disorders (IFSO) and American Society of Metabolic and Bariatric Surgery (ASMBS). The following criteria are used as guidelines for offering surgery:

1. Anyone with a BMI of 35 kg/m^2 or greater.
2. Patients with a BMI of 30–34.9 kg/m^2 with an obesity related comorbidity*.

   *Common obesity-related comorbidities include hypertension, sleep apnea, and type 2 diabetes, among others.

Lower BMI cutoffs might be appropriate for patients in the Asian population as comorbidities are worse for those in that group at a lower BMI cutoff. It has therefore been suggested that patients in an Asian population be offered surgery at a lower weight loss range of 27.5 kg/m^2 or above. There are no absolute guidelines in terms of the upper limit for age. There is also no minimum weight requirement.

Recommendations were also made to offer metabolic and bariatric surgery to adolescents who are appropriately selected. These patients are best served by referral to a tertiary care center with ample resources appointed to weight management in this specific group of adolescents with obesity. Patients should have access to medical, behavioral health, and nutritional specialists. The center should be experienced with adolescent obesity treatment, and a pathway into an adult program should exist. Adolescence was defined by the group as aged 10–19 years old.

In this group of patients, surgery may be a good option for those with.

1. A BMI at or above 120% of the 95th percentile with an obesity-related comorbid condition.
2. A BMI at or above 140% of the 95th percentile.

Specific decision-making regarding the individual benefit to a patient, consent process, and optimal perioperative planning should take place within the tertiary center specialized in adolescent obesity surgery.

Emergency requiring ER presentation	No specific treatments for obesity mandates ER referral. This condition is best managed outpatient.
Requires referral to surgeon as an outpatient	Any patient with a BMI above 35 kg/m^2 or above 30 kg/m^2 with an obesity-related comorbidity should be referred to a bariatric surgeon for counseling about weight loss options
What to check before referring to a surgeon	No testing is needed prior to referral. Surgeons can see patients wherever they are on their weight loss journey. Surgeons work in a multidisciplinary group with behavioral health and dietitian providers to assess all patients

(continued)

What can be managed by a PCP	Patients with BMI of 27 kg/m^2 or higher should be screened for obesity related comorbidities at least annually: Accurate height and weight measurements at every visit Documentation of any weight management efforts in progress notes Blood pressure assessment, STOP BANG sleep apnea questionnaire with referral to sleep lab for any positive screens, annual hemoglobin A1c levels Common deficiencies should be assessed including: thiamine (B1), folate, B12, iron, vitamin d, thyroid-stimulating hormone (TSH)

Suggested Readings

1. Eisenberg D, Shikora SA, Aarts, et al. American Society for Metabolic and Bariatric Surgery (ASMBS) and International Federation for the Surgery of Obesity and Metabolic Disorders (IFSO): Indications for Metabolic and Bariatric Surgery. Surg Obes Relat Dis. 2022;18(12):1345–56. https://doi.org/10.1016/j.soard.2022.08.013. Epub 2022 Oct 21. PMID: 36280539.
2. Eisenberg D, Noria S, Grover B, Goodpaster K, Rogers AM. American Society for Metabolic and Bariatric Surgery Clinical Issues Committee. ASMBS position statement on weight bias and stigma. Surg Obes Relat Dis. 2019;15(6):814–21. https://doi.org/10.1016/j.soard.2019.04.031. Epub 2019 May 10. PMID: 31196777.

Pancreatitis

23

Joe Bean, Elisa C. Calabrese,
and Stefan Scholz

23.1 Initial Assessment

Pancreatitis can be delineated as acute or chronic. The hallmark of the clinical presentation of acute pancreatitis is most commonly constant, epigastric abdominal pain. Other symptoms can include nausea, vomiting, and fever [1]. A thorough history should be obtained to help distinguish the etiology, including alcohol consumption, biliary colic, trauma, recent instrumentation, toxin exposure, family history or personal history of pancreatitis, and medications. In adults, the most common etiologies are gallstone disease and alcohol abuse. The most common etiologies in adolescents are gallstones and in children trauma and systemic disease [2].

J. Bean
Department of Surgery, University of Pittsburgh, Pittsburgh, PA, USA

E. C. Calabrese
Department of Surgery, University of California San Francisco-East Bay, Oakland, CA, USA

Department of Surgery, University of Adelaide, The Queen Elizabeth Hospital, Adelaide, SA, Australia

S. Scholz (✉)
Department of Surgery, University of Pittsburgh, Pittsburgh, PA, USA

Division of General and Thoracic Pediatric Surgery, UPMC Children's Hospital of Pittsburgh, Pittsburgh, PA, USA
e-mail: stefan.scholz@chp.edu

G. P. Kohn et al. (eds.), *The SAGES Manual of Surgical Referral for Primary and Emergency Care*,
https://doi.org/10.1007/978-3-031-92678-5_23

The physical exam may demonstrate evidence of dehydration. The abdominal exam can vary between no abdominal tenderness or severe epigastric abdominal tenderness depending on the severity of the disease. Abdominal distention and rigidity can also be present in severe cases. Flank or periumbilical ecchymosis are rare findings that indicate retroperitoneal bleeding in severe, often necrotizing pancreatitis. The presence of jaundice may indicate choledocholithiasis or compression of the common bile duct from pancreatic edema [2].

In the ambulatory setting, patients should be sent to the emergency department if there is a high clinical suspicion of acute pancreatitis for close monitoring and prompt workup. Ultimately, diagnosis will be based on clinical symptoms, laboratory findings, and imaging findings as based on the Atlanta Classification [3] (Fig. 23.1).

Chronic pancreatitis can present as dull epigastric abdominal pain, often worse after meals, and can vary in pattern [1]. Other symptoms can include weight loss and diarrhea. Chronic pancreatitis can also be superimposed by episodes of acute pancreatitis. There are a wide range of presentations and some with no previous clinical manifestation of acute pancreatitis [4, 5]. Patients with elevated hemoglobin A1c, steatorrhea, or vitamin deficiency should prompt concern for endocrine or exocrine dysfunction, respectively. These symptoms are often found later in the disease process as about 90% of gland dysfunction needs to be present to manifest some of these symptoms [2]. Etiologies include idiopathic, alcohol abuse, genetic, autoimmune, recurrent severe acute pancreatitis, hypertriglyceridemia, anatomic abnormalities,

Abdominal pain consistent with acute pancreatitis
Serum lipase (or amylase) at least three times greater than the upper limit of normal
Characteristic findings of acute pancreatitis on contrast-enhanced computed tomography (CECT) or magnetic resonance imaging (MRI)

Fig. 23.1 Definition of the diagnosis of acute pancreatitis using the Atlanta Classification. Two of the three features must be present for diagnosis [4]

with alcohol abuse being the most common [4]. As with acute pancreatitis, a thorough history should be obtained.

23.2 Laboratory Testing

A laboratory workup should be obtained, including complete blood count (CBC), comprehensive metabolic panel (CMP), amylase, lipase, and lipid panel. An amylase and lipase level greater than three times the upper level of normal is suggestive of acute pancreatitis; however, it is not required to make the diagnosis. In patients who present later than 24–48 hours after symptoms, lipase is more sensitive as it has a longer half-life [2]. If lipase is normal, this does not rule out that an episode of pancreatitis occurred or that the patient is suffering from chronic pancreatitis, and the other methods of diagnosis discussed in the chapter should be used to help make the diagnosis. Elevated liver enzymes should raise suspicion for gallstone pancreatitis. These laboratory derangements should prompt right upper quadrant abdominal sonographic evaluation looking for cholelithiasis and/or choledocholithiasis. If there is concern for chronic pancreatitis secondary to autoimmune etiology, immunoglobulin G4 testing can be considered. If the patient has symptoms or labs concerning for hyperparathyroidism, such as hypercalcemia, then parathyroid hormone testing can be considered as a possible etiology.

23.3 Imaging

1. *Computed tomography (CT) of the abdomen/pelvis with intravenous (IV) contrast*

   This imaging modality can help characterize the severity of the disease and help confirm the diagnosis for both acute and chronic pancreatitis. This is indicated upon presentation when there is diagnostic uncertainty, for confirmation of severity, Ranson score > 3 or APACHE score > 8, during failure to respond to conservative treatment, or when there is clinical deterioration [2, 6]. It can also help identify peripancreatic fluid collections if the patient is presenting several days after their initial symptoms or after a trauma. This may need to be repeated MRI is an alternative to CT. The CT Severity Index Score, demonstrated in Fig. 23.2, can be used to grade the severity of acute pancreatitis and predict morbidity and mortality based on imaging findings [7]. Chronic pancreatitis can demonstrate duct dilation, calcifications, or atrophy of the pancreas.

2. *Right upper quadrant (RUQ) abdominal ultrasound*

   This imaging modality can be used to determine the presence of cholelithiasis. If there is suspicion for choledocholithiasis as well, then decision for further imaging with magnetic resonance imaging (MRI) versus endoscopic retrograde pancreatography (ERCP) can be obtained [2].

3. *Magnetic resonance cholangiopancreatography (MRCP)*

   Should be considered if CT results are negative with high clinical suspicion of pancreatitis and risk factors for chronic pancreatitis. This imaging modality will best identify ductal stricture in chronic pancreatitis. It should also be used when there is unexplained or recurrent pancreatitis to further delineate the pancreatic and biliary ductal anatomy [2].

FEATURE	*POINTS*
Pancreatic Inflammation	
Normal pancreas	0
Focal or diffuse pancreatic enlargement	1
Intrinsic pancreatic alterations with peripancreatic fat inflammatory changes	2
Single fluid collection or phlegmon	3
Two or more fluid collections or gas, in or adjacent to the pancreas	4
Pancreatic Necrosis	
None	0
≤30%	2
30%–50%	4
>50%	6

CTSI 0–3, mortality 3%, morbidity 8%; CTSI 4–6, mortality 6%, morbidity 35%; CTSI 7–10, mortality 17%, morbidity 92%.

Fig. 23.2 Computed Tomography Severity Index (CTSI) for acute pancreatitis [1, 2]

4. *Endoscopic ultrasound (EUS)*

   This imaging modality can be useful in chronic pancreatitis diagnosis if both CT imaging and MRCP are negative but continued high clinical suspicion remains. It can also be used when there is concern for choledocholithiasis, such as jaundice, persistent sepsis, severe pain, and elevated liver function tests in the setting of gallstone pancreatitis.

23.4 Referral to Surgery for Acute Pancreatitis

Acute pancreatitis should be managed medically with conservative measures, including fluid resuscitation, pain control, and early nutrition [2]. Acute pancreatitis can be divided into interstitial edematous pancreatitis or necrotizing pancreatitis based on imaging findings (Fig. 23.3). Fluid collections can also be discovered on imaging and are generally classified as acute, if less than 4 weeks from acute pancreatitis onset, or chronic, if present greater than 4 weeks from onset. They can also be simple or necrotizing in nature. A simple, acute collection is an acute peripancreatic fluid collection. A simple, chronic collection is a pancreatic

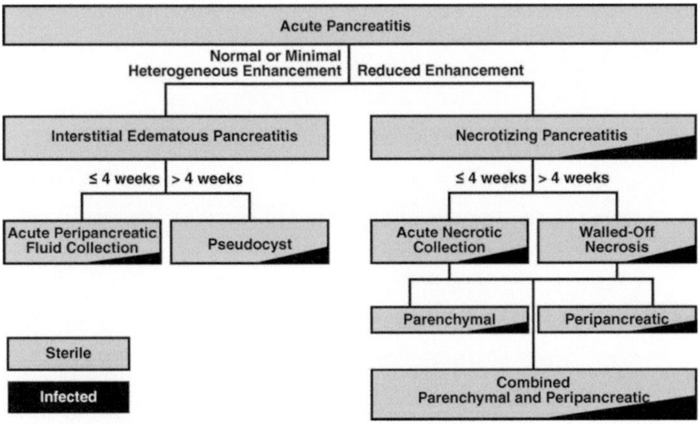

Fig. 23.3 Classification of acute pancreatitis based on Atlanta Classification with associated risk of infection at each stage [2, 8]

pseudocyst. A necrotic, acute collection is an acute necrotic collection. A necrotic, chronic collection is walled off necrosis [3].

Acute peripancreatic fluid collections have been reported in approximately 1/3 to ½ of acute pancreatitis cases. These fluid collections should not be intervened upon as most will resorb with time [3]. They can sometimes become infected, but the usual signs of infection are unreliable as they can be present in the natural course of pancreatitis. Concern for infection should be raised if there is gas within the fluid collection on imaging, rapid clinical decline, or lack of improvement after 10–14 days [2]. CT-guided fluid sampling can be performed if there is high clinical suspicion for infection. Percutaneous or endoscopic drainage and IV antibiotics are appropriate therapies for infected collections [2], and an operative intervention is not indicated.

Acute necrotizing collections occur in up to 20% of patients with acute pancreatitis and can be associated with a more complicated course. The risk of infection is directly related to the amount of necrosis [2]. If possible, an intervention should be postponed until the collection is chronic and walled off. Sterile necrotizing collections should be intervened upon when there is clinical decline despite maximal support, especially if there is suspicion of or confirmed infection. In these cases, the "step-up approach"

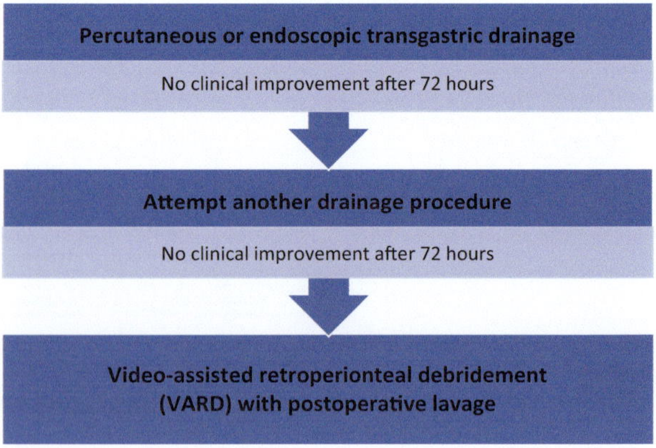

Fig. 23.4 Step-up approach [9, 10]

should be followed (Fig. 23.4) [9]. This approach is associated with significantly less morbidity and mortality than surgical open necrosectomy [9, 10]. Referral or consultation to a surgical provider should be initiated if initial endoscopic and percutaneous measures in the "step-up approach" fail and the patient continues to decline.

Pancreatic pseudocysts are simple, chronic collections that occur in approximately 10% of patients with peripancreatic fluid collection after acute pancreatitis [2]. They typically mature between 4 and 8 weeks following the inciting event. About 1/3 will spontaneously resolve in adults and even more in children [11]. Other etiologies include chronic pancreatitis, previous pancreatic operation, or previous trauma, which can impact the likelihood of spontaneous resolution [12]. Patients can present with early satiety, pain, nausea, vomiting, weight loss, or upper gastrointestinal bleeding. Diagnosis is confirmed by cross-sectional imaging. Referral for EUS with fine-needle aspiration (FNA) can be done if the diagnosis is unclear. Intervention is reserved for complicated pseudocysts (see Fig. 23.5). If the stomach and the duodenum are in proximity to the matured cyst wall (<1 cm), then endoscopic drainage approaches can be performed. Surgical referral should be sought when endoscopic treatment fails, the cyst recurs, or if endoscopic intervention is not possible due to the location of the cyst [2].

Gallstone pancreatitis has a 30% recurrence rate if left untreated [2]. Referral to a surgeon for cholecystectomy is advised and should ideally be performed within the same hospital admission prior to discharge. If the patient cannot have an operation safely performed during the same admission due to severe pancreatitis or logistical reasons, conservative management for at least 6 weeks is recommended before cholecystectomy [13]. If the patient is presenting with concomitant cholangitis or persistent choledocholithiasis seen on imaging, then ERCP should be performed. Choledocholithiasis can also be cleared during laparoscopic cholecystectomy with common bile duct exploration under one single anesthesia, a more cost-saving approach. In patients who are not safe surgical candidates, ERCP could only be performed under sedation including sphincterotomy to help prevent recurrent disease [2].

Complicated pancreatic pseudocysts (one criterion sufficient)

- Compression of large vessels (clinical symptoms or seen on CT scan)
- Gastric or duodenal outlet obstruction
- Stenosis of the common bile duct due to compression
- Infected pancreatic pseudocysts
- Haemorrhage into pancreatic pseudocyst
- Pancreatico-pleural fistula

Symptomatic pancreatic pseudocyst

- Satiety
- Nausea and vomiting
- Pain
- Upper gastrointestinal bleeding (10–20%)

Asymptomatic pancreatic pseudocyst:

- Pseudocysts >5 cm, unchanged in size and morphology for more than 6 weeks [2]
- Diameter >4 cm and extrapancreatic complications in patients with chronic alcoholic pancreatitis [40]
- Suspected malignancy: median 5-year survival rate after resection 56% [57]

Fig. 23.5 Indications for intervention of pancreatic pseudocyst [3, 12]

Surveillance for any of the above pathologies varies based on severity and symptoms. Patients should be seen promptly after discharge from the hospital by their general practitioner to manage symptoms and check for development of any of the above pathologies discussed. Recurrence rates for acute pancreatitis approximate 20% depending on the etiology and typically occur within the first few years from the initial occurrence [14]. It is helpful to ensure risk factors are mitigated, for example, cholecystectomy planned if appropriate, or cessation of alcohol. Repeat episodes of acute pancreatitis could lead to chronic pancreatitis. Following an episode of acute pancreatitis, indications for repeat imaging include change in clinical status 2–7 days after initial presentation, if CT severity score is 3–10 at presentation/grade 3, to determine response to treatment after surgery/interventional procedure, or before discharge in patients with severe acute pancreatitis [6].

Surveillance for peripancreatic fluid collections depends on the specific collection and on the intervention the patient undergoes.

23.5 Referral to Surgery for Chronic Pancreatitis

The mainstay of treatment for chronic pancreatitis is management of symptoms and removal of predisposing factors. This may include pancreatic enzyme replacement and glycemic control. If the patient continues to be symptomatic, then they should be evaluated for ductal obstruction or strictures with MRCP and be considered for endoscopic therapy with possible stenting.

Surgical therapy is considered for patients who have failed medical and endoscopic management and continue to have significant pain (Figs. 23.7 and 23.8) [4]. One surgical option is longitudinal/lateral pancreatico-jejunostomy, also known as the Puestow procedure, wherein the pancreatic duct is flayed open longitudinally and anastomosed via a Roux-en-Y jejuno-jejunostomy to allow for maximal pancreatic drainage. Pain relief is reported in up to 80% of patients [13, 14]. The Frey procedure is another option that can be seen as a modification of the Puestow procedure; in addition to a lateral Roux-en-Y pancreatico-jejunostomy, portions of the pancreatic head are resected to include the major and minor pancreatic ducts. The Beger procedure also involves resection of the pancreatic head, but different from the Frey procedure in resection of nearly the entirety of the pancreatic head while sparing the duodenum, common bile duct, and the stomach. Both procedures have similar rates of success (about 90% of patients are pain-free after 5 years), morbidity, and mortality. Distal pancreatectomy is considered in some patients with distal pancreatic disease and/or small duct diameter, but generally has lower rates of success, with about 60% long-term pain relief. The Whipple procedure, resection of the pancreatic head including the duodenum and the pylorus, was historically used for chronic pancreatitis with about 40% pain relief but carries higher morbidity/mortality that has shifted its indication mostly to pan-

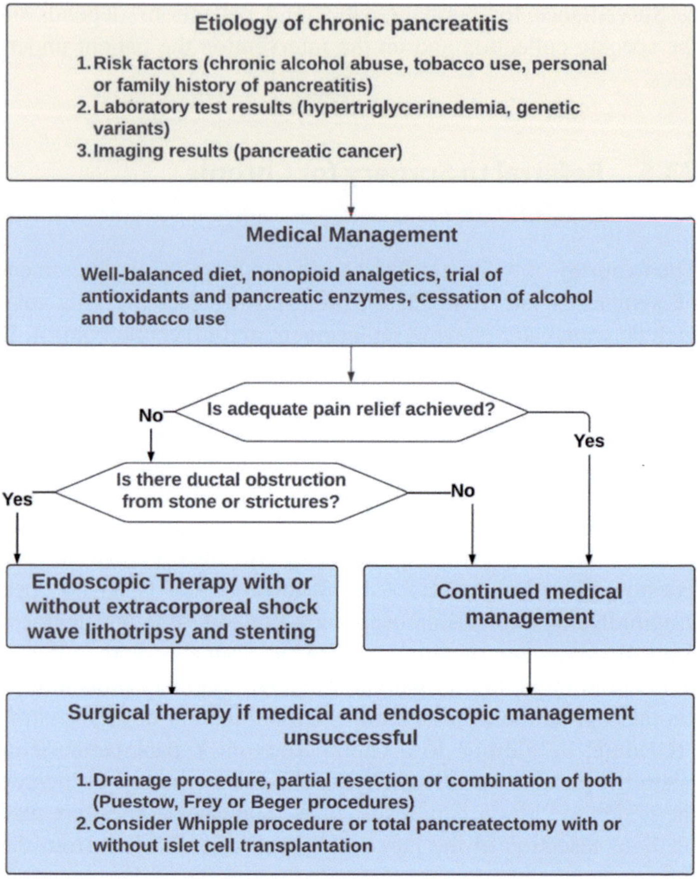

Fig. 23.6 Algorithm for the management of chronic pancreatitis. This algorithm has not been validated in randomized trials

Emergency requiring ER presentation	- Evidence of acute pancreatitis - Suspicion of acute pancreatitis or peripancreatic fluid collection with symptoms or clinical concerns such as fever, tachycardia, early satiety with inability to tolerate PO - Severe pain
What requires urgent surgical review	- Worsening clinical status despite conservative management - New peri-pancreatic fluid collection with clinical deterioration - Evidence of GI obstruction with inability to tolerate PO - Known peri-pancreatic fluid collection with evidence of superimposed infection or enlargement or clinical deterioration - Evidence of hemorrhage from fluid collection or gastrointestinal bleed
Non-urgent surgical review	- Non-resolving peri-pancreatic collection with sub-acute symptoms - Cases of acute severe pancreatitis that are high risk for developing complications - Clinically worsening chronic pancreatitis patients despite conservative management
Management by Primary Care Provider (PCP)	Chronic pancreatitis and its sequelae can generally be managed by PCP Post-hospitalization follow-up and lab work
Management by Gastroenterology/Interventional Radiology(dependent on resources at facility)	Gastroenterology can perform endoscopic necrosectomy or cyst-gastrostomy in the setting of complications related to acute pancreatitis – regardless surgery should be informed of the patient Gastroenterology may be more involved in progressive chronic pancreatitis for management and decision to refer to surgeon Interventional radiology can be helped when there are drainable fluid collections – regardless surgery should be informed of the patient

Fig. 23.7 Overview of surgical involvement and referral

Acute pancreatitis	Chronic pancreatitis
• CT abdomen/pelvis • RUQ U/S if concern for choledocholithiasis as etiology • MRCP in select cases with concern for choledocholithiasis or with concern for pancreatic or common bile duct obstruction or malformation/anomalies • Complete blood count, metabolic panel, lipase, INR/prothrombin time	• **MRCP** • Complete blood count, metabolic panel, INR/prothrombin time • Other labs may be appropriate depending on suspicion of etiology and deficiencies (see "Laboratory Testing")

Fig. 23.8 Overview of tests to obtain *prior* to referral to surgery

creatic cancer today [15, 16]. For extreme cases of chronic pancreatitis and pain, total pancreatectomy with possible islet cell transplantation can be considered (Fig. 23.6).

23.6 Resources for Readers

1. International Association of Pancreatology (IAP) Guidelines for Acute Pancreatitis
   https://pubmed.ncbi.nlm.nih.gov/24054878/
2. Classification of acute pancreatitis
   https://www.ncbi.nlm.nih.gov/pmc/articles/PMC5074676/
3. Step-up approach
   https://pubmed.ncbi.nlm.nih.gov/20410514/
4. Ashraf H, Colombo J, Marcucci V, et al. A Clinical Overview of Acute and Chronic Pancreatitis: The Medical and Surgical Management. Cureus. 2021;13(11): e19764.
   https://doi.org/10.7759/cureus.19764

References

1. Mederos MA, Reber HA, Girgis MD. Acute Pancreatitis: A Review. JAMA. 2021;325:382–390
2. Townsend CM, Daniel Beauchamp R, Mark Evers B, Mattox KL. Sabiston textbook of surgery: the biological basis of modern surgical practice. Elsevier health sciences. 2016.
3. Banks PA, Bollen TL, Dervenis C, et al. Classification of acute pancreatitis--2012: revision of the Atlanta classification and definitions by international consensus. Gut. 2013;62:102–11.
4. Singh VK, Yadav D, Garg PK. Diagnosis and Management of Chronic Pancreatitis: A Review. JAMA. 2019;322:2422–34
5. Catalano MF, Sahai A, Levy M, et al. EUS-based criteria for the diagnosis of chronic pancreatitis: the Rosemont classification. Gastrointest Endosc. 2009;69:1251–61
6. Busireddy KK, AlObaidy M, Ramalho M, et al. Pancreatitis-imaging approach. World J Gastrointest Pathophysiol. 2014;5:252–70.
7. Sahu B, Abbey P, Anand R, et al. Severity assessment of acute pancreatitis using CT severity index and modified CT severity index: Correlation with clinical outcomes and severity grading as per the Revised Atlanta Classification. Indian J Radiol Imaging. 2017;27:152–60.

8. Zhao K, Adam SZ, Keswani RN, Horowitz JM, Miller FH. Acute pancreatitis: revised Atlanta classification and the role of cross-sectional imaging. Am J Roentgenol. 2015;205(1):W32–41.
9. Besselink MGH, van Santvoort HC, Nieuwenhuijs VB, et al. Minimally invasive "step-up approach" versus maximal necrosectomy in patients with acute necrotising pancreatitis (PANTER trial): design and rationale of a randomised controlled multicenter trial [ISRCTN13975868]. BMC Surg. 2006;6:6.
10. van Santvoort HC, Besselink MG, Bakker OJ, et al. A step-up approach or open necrosectomy for necrotizing pancreatitis. N Engl J Med. 2010;362:1491–502
11. Pan G, Wan MH, Xie K-L, et al. Classification and Management of Pancreatic Pseudocysts. Medicine. 2015;94:e960.
12. Aghdassi AA, Mayerle J, Kraft M, et al. Pancreatic pseudocysts--when and how to treat? HPB. 2006;8:432–41.
13. Larson SD, Nealon WH, Evers BM. Management of gallstone pancreatitis. Adv Surg. 2006;40:265–284.
14. Wu BU, Conwell DL. Acute pancreatitis part II: approach to follow-up. Clin Gastroenterol Hepatol. 2010;8:417–22.
15. Bouwense SAW, Kempeneers MA, van Santvoort HC, Boermeester MA, van Goor H, Besselink MG. Surgery in Chronic Pancreatitis: Indication, Timing and Procedures. Visc Med. 2019;35(2):110–18. https://doi.org/10.1159/000499612.
16. Benjamin O, Lappin SL. Chronic Pancreatitis. [Updated 2022 Jun 21]. In: StatPearls [Internet]. Treasure Island (FL): StatPearls Publishing; 2024 Jan-.Available from: https://www.ncbi.nlm.nih.gov/books/NBK482325/.

Splenomegaly 24

Lindel Dewberry
and Mackenzie Donoho

24.1 Introduction

The spleen is part of the lymphatic system and functions to filter blood via the reticuloendothelial system and optimize immune cell function through the maturation of B and T lymphocytes. It is specifically important to the development of immunity against encapsulated bacteria. The spleen is located in the left upper quadrant within the peritoneal cavity and has ligamentous attachments to the kidney, diaphragm, colon, and stomach. The arterial blood supply includes the splenic artery that can have either a magistral or distributed branching pattern. The venous drainage is along the splenic vein, which then joins the mesenteric vein to confluence into the portal vein.

An enlarged spleen, referred to as splenomegaly, can occur for a variety of reasons. These can be organized into several categories, as defined by the American Academy of Family Physicians. This includes congestive, neoplastic, infectious, parasitic, autoimmune, hematologic, and infiltrative causes. Depending on the etiology, splenomegaly may be transient and self-resolving, or an

L. Dewberry (✉) · M. Donoho
University of Kentucky, Lexington, KY, USA
e-mail: Lindel.Dewberry@uky.edu

G. P. Kohn et al. (eds.), *The SAGES Manual of Surgical Referral for Primary and Emergency Care*,
https://doi.org/10.1007/978-3-031-92678-5_24

indication of a significant pathology that requires specialist evaluation and surgical removal.

Defining splenomegaly according to size requires an individualized approach as size varies according to age, sex, and body mass index. Splenomegaly is historically characterized by splenic length > 12 cm; however, the individual's characteristics should be considered rather than using a hard cutoff at 12 cm.

24.2 Initial Evaluation

24.2.1 History

Patients can present with a wide variety of symptoms depending on the etiology of splenomegaly. Most commonly, patients may report left upper quadrant pain that is referred to the left shoulder. Other symptoms include early satiety and upper abdominal distention. A thorough review of systems, medical history, and family history may elucidate a cause for the splenomegaly. A history of recent systemic illness, sick contacts, and travel should also be obtained (Table 24.1).

24.2.2 Exam

A normal spleen should not be palpable on exam. During the physical exam, the patient should be supine on the exam table. The examiner's hand should move caudal to cranial along the left abdomen with gentle deep palpation on inspiration to appreciate the tip of the spleen. The patient may also be rolled into the right lateral decubitus position with bent knees to aid in abdominal relaxation when trying to palpate the spleen. Percussion may help the examiner estimate splenic span, focusing along the mid-axillary line tracing from below the nipple to beyond the most inferior intercostal space. Tenderness on exam may indicate infection or infarction.

Consideration should also be given to patient habitus, and splenomegaly cannot be ruled out in certain cases where manual

Table 24.1 Causes, symptoms, and medical history associated with splenomegaly

Cause	Symptoms[a]	Medical history
Liver disease	Jaundice, ascites, upper gastrointestinal bleeding, encephalopathy	Alcohol abuse Hepatitis
Venous thrombosis	Abdominal distention, upper GI (variceal) bleeding	Malignancy Liver cirrhosis Hemolytic anemia
Underlying malignancy	Fatigue, weight loss, fevers, night sweats, petechiae	Prior malignancy
Infectious disease	Pharyngitis, systemic symptoms (fever, malaise)	Sick contacts Environmental exposure Recent travel
Autoimmune disease	Inflammatory joint pain, fatigue, rashes	Systemic lupus erythematosus Sarcoidosis
Infiltrative	Fatigue, bruising, shortness of breath, hepatomegaly, ataxia	Gaucher disease Niemann–pick Amyloidosis
Hematopoietic	Abdominal pain, fatigue, shortness of breath, bone pain, easy bruising or bleeding	Thalassemia Myelofibrosis Hereditary spherocytosis Hemolytic anemia

[a]It is important to note that some etiologies of splenomegaly may be asymptomatic, with splenomegaly being the first indication of disease. Absence of symptoms should not rule out pathologic causes and may require additional evaluation

examination of the spleen is not accessible. In these cases, and particularly when symptoms are present and other physical exam findings are identified, imaging may be appropriate.

A complete physical examination should be conducted to elucidate possible causes. This includes evaluation for lymphadenopathy, signs of anemia with bruising, cardiac exam, and respiratory exam to evaluate for possible pleural effusion. A thorough abdominal examination should be completed as well, looking for ascites or hepatomegaly.

24.3 Ancillary Studies

24.3.1 Laboratory Studies

The first lab test that should be performed is a complete blood count (CBC) with a peripheral blood smear (PBS). This testing can provide information on hematologic and lymphocytic causes of splenomegaly, as well as indicate overall splenic function. Care should be taken to examine each aspect of this testing, in the context of the specific patient presentation, and determine if further testing or specialist referral is appropriate (Table 24.2).

In cases of hemolysis causing splenomegaly, the CBC may show a normocytic anemia, with a decreased hemoglobin and mean corpuscular volume within normal limits. Reticulocytes may be elevated as well. Further testing to elucidate causes of hemolysis, particularly if autoimmune hemolysis is suspected, would include lactate dehydrogenase level, bilirubin level, and direct antiglobulin testing. Platelet count can also reveal hemolytic disease leading to splenomegaly, specifically immune thrombocytopenic purpura (ITP). In this scenario, platelet count may be decreased while hemoglobin remains within normal limits. Thalassemia, a collection of hereditary blood disorders, can present as a microcytic anemia.

Myeloproliferative disorders are a major cause of splenomegaly. There are multiple types of myeloproliferative disorders, and

Table 24.2 Evaluation and treatment prior to referral to surgeon

Lab testing	Imaging	Additional intervention
CBC, INR Infectious disease workup[a] CMP ESR, CRP	US of LUQ and liver with Doppler CT abdomen with IV contrast[b]	Referral to appropriate specialist based on laboratory and imaging workup. Patient should be seen by a hematologist prior to referral to surgeon in a patient with splenomegaly secondary to hemolytic anemia or thrombocytopenia.

[a]Including HIV, viral hepatitis, EBV, TB, histoplasmosis, and malaria
[b]Indicated for patients with refractory hemolytic disease or malignancy

they may present differently on laboratory testing depending on the specific cell line that is affected. Polycythemia vera can present with elevated red blood cells, white blood cells, and platelets. Malignancy, including chronic myelogenous leukemia, may present with elevated white blood cells without alterations in red blood cells or platelets. Later stages of disease, however, may show alterations in all cell lines. Rarer forms of myelogenous disease, like chronic eosinophilic leukemia, can present with alterations in specific white blood cells. A CBC with differential may be indicated in these cases where nonspecific CBC changes are noted in patients with history indicating potential malignancy.

One of the most common causes of splenomegaly is infectious mononucleosis. In these patients, CBC may reveal an elevated white blood cell count. A differential can further characterize this disease with elevated lymphocytes up to greater than 50% and the presence of atypical lymphocytes. Further evaluation includes EBV antigen and antibody testing.

The peripheral smear can provide insight into the morphology of cells, which can elucidate causes of splenomegaly that may be difficult to identify through CBC alone. Malignancy may present with immature white blood cells. Hallmarks of genetic conditions leading to splenomegaly can also be identified on peripheral smear, with the presence of spherocytes potentially indicating hereditary spherocytosis, and target cells associated with thalassemia. Heinz bodies are associated with multiple blood disorders that can present with splenomegaly, including thalassemia and hemolytic anemia. In splenic sequestration crisis, sickle cells may be seen on peripheral smear indicating the presence of homozygous disease.

The peripheral smear can also show signs of impaired splenic function. This includes red blood cells with Howell–Jolly bodies or membrane pitting. Parasitic organisms can also be identified on peripheral smear (e.g., *Erlichia, Bartonella, Babesia, Malaria*).

Additional laboratory evaluation may include liver function testing, with transaminase levels, bilirubin, and international normalized ratio. Infectious diseases are also a potential cause of splenomegaly and should be assessed when appropriate based on history and exam findings. This may include serologic testing for

HIV, HBV, and HCV, CMV, skin or blood testing for tuberculosis, and blood and sputum culture for histoplasmosis.

Rarer causes of splenomegaly, including infiltrative and autoimmune disease processes, may require additional specific testing. These cases warrant referral to appropriate specialists.

24.3.2 Imaging

Ultrasound is the preferred imaging modality as it accurately provides splenic measurements and avoids radiation. The spleen size is measured in an oblique craniocaudal direction. Surrounding organs should be evaluated during ultrasound as well if hepatic or other intra-abdominal pathologies are suspected. Vascular ultrasound may also be appropriate in cases where splenomegaly appears to be related to thrombosis (splenic or portal vein). US findings indicating urgent surgical evaluation would include free peritoneal fluid and heterogeneity and lucencies within the spleen as these would indicate splenic rupture.

CT and MRI also play a role in spleen imaging. If a focal lesion is noted on ultrasound, a CT or MRI may be obtained for further characterization. CT with intravenous contrast of the spleen allows for visualization of any associated thromboses (splenic or portal vein). Infarct would be suspected on contrast CT with areas of low attenuation. CT can also identify the presence of calcifications, typically present in granulomas, or older hematomas. These imaging modalities also aid in characterizing diseases related to splenomegaly.

If there is concern for ITP, imaging should also evaluate for any accessory splenic tissues that will have to be removed during splenectomy.

24.4 Management

An otherwise asymptomatic patient with incidentally discovered splenomegaly with a normal complete blood count and peripheral smear may be observed; the splenomegaly may be monitored with

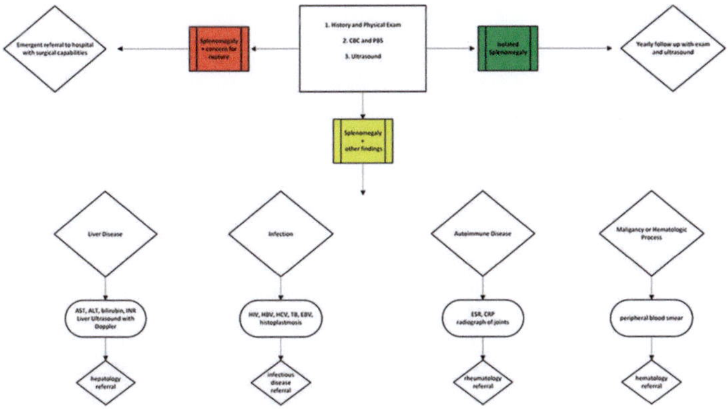

Fig. 24.1 Splenomegaly management flowchart

yearly exams and ultrasounds (Fig. 24.1). Patients with infectious etiology should be managed with appropriate antimicrobial or antiparasitic treatment.

24.4.1 Specialists

For patients with symptoms, an outpatient referral is appropriate if the patient is well appearing with normal vital signs. The first referral should be to a hematologist (Fig. 24.1 and Table 24.3). If a malignancy is suspected, a bone marrow or lymph node biopsy or testing of peripheral blood through flow cytometry rather than a splenic biopsy is recommended due to the risk of significant bleeding with splenic biopsy. If liver disease is suspected, a referral to a hepatologist should be placed (Fig. 24.1 and Table 24.3).

24.4.2 Surgical Indications

A referral to the general surgeon is usually placed by the hematologist for several reasons (Fig. 24.1).

Table 24.3 Splenomegaly management

Features requiring ER referral	Splenomegaly with concern for rupture Marked tenderness in the upper left quadrant on exam Peritoneal signs Unstable vital signs Tachycardia and hypotension.
Urgent surgical evaluation	Splenomegaly with concern for rupture and unstable vital signs
Nonurgent surgical evaluation	Hypersplenism with cytopenia Thrombocytopenia Hemolysis Evidence of inherited or autoimmune hemolytic anemia refractory to medical therapy Malignancy of the spleen
Features requiring specialty referral	Features of concurrent liver disease, refer to hepatology Evaluate with transaminases, INR, bilirubin Features of infectious disease Screen for HIV, hepatitis viruses, TB, EBV, histoplasmosis, malaria Referral to ID when refractory to initial medical management Features of autoimmune disease Initial laboratory testing includes ESR, CRP If joint involvement, XR may be appropriate Refer to rheumatology Features of malignancy or hematologic process Abnormality in CBC or PBS Additionally, may utilize LDH, haptoglobin, bilirubin Discrete mass on imaging Refer to hematology oncology for further workup
Features to be managed by PCP	Initial diagnostic workup can be managed by PCP including history, physical, CBC with PBS and US Isolated splenomegaly may be managed with yearly exam and US Recommendation to avoid abdominal injury in splenomegaly secondary to EBV

- Need for lymph node biopsy to establish diagnosis.
- Diagnostic splenectomy (last resort if all other testing is unrevealing).
- Therapeutic splenectomy if unresponsive to medical treatment (depending on the underlying cause) in cases of hypersplenism or sequestration events.

24.4.3 Emergent Indications

If the patient appears ill with abnormal vital signs, they should be evaluated urgently in an emergency department with inpatient admission (Fig. 24.1 and Table 24.3). Splenomegaly may rarely lead to splenic rupture that requires urgent surgical consultation.

24.4.4 Other Considerations

Avoidance of high-risk contact sports is recommended in patients with splenomegaly due to the risk of splenic rupture.

Suggested Reading

SplenoCalc

1. Expected spleen size. https://reference.medscape.com/calculator/384/expected-spleen-size. Accessed 18 Dec 2023.

Splenomegaly: Diagnosis and Management in Adults

2. Aldulaimi S, Mendez AM. Splenomegaly: diagnosis and management in adults. afp. 2021;104(2):271–6.

25 Small Bowel Obstruction

Brynley Dean and Jonathan Dort

25.1 Etiology

Small bowel obstruction (SBO) is the impediment of the passage of bowel contents, and its causes can be classified in terms of the relationship of the obstructing lesion to the intestinal wall: intraluminal, intramural, and extramural. Intraluminal causes include foreign bodies and gallstones. Intramural causes are tumors or Crohn's disease-associated inflammatory strictures. Extramural sources of obstruction include adhesions, hernias, carcinomatosis, and abscesses. By far the most common etiology of small bowel obstruction in the developed world is the presence of intra-abdominal adhesions related to prior abdominal surgery (up to 75% of SBOs). Other causes include hernias, malignancy, infectious or inflammatory sources, intussusception, and gallstone ileus. Determining the specific etiology of a small bowel obstruction is not critical in the initial stages of evaluation; it is more important to determine the patient's condition, the urgency of evaluation and treatment, and the necessity for and timing of appropriate surgical consultation.

B. Dean · J. Dort (✉)
Inova Fairfax Medical Campus, Falls Church, VA, USA
e-mail: Brynley.dean@inova.org; jonathan.dort@inova.org

G. P. Kohn et al. (eds.), *The SAGES Manual of Surgical Referral for Primary and Emergency Care*,
https://doi.org/10.1007/978-3-031-92678-5_25

25.2 Pertinent History and Physical Findings

A careful history to identify pertinent risk factors for small bowel obstruction is essential in diagnosing and determining possible etiologies of this disease. The examiner should inquire about previous abdominal or pelvic surgeries, including cesarean sections, known hernias, a history of inflammatory bowel disease or neoplasms, and previous abdominopelvic radiation exposure. A thorough medication review should also be completed to elucidate potential contributing factors to poor gut motility. Patients with SBO will typically describe the abrupt onset of colicky abdominal pain as the intestines contract against the obstructed segment. A more gradual onset of symptoms may be present in patients with partial SBO. Progression from this colicky pain to a more severe, localized, or constant pain may indicate progressive bowel ischemia or necrosis. Patients may experience significant nausea and vomiting, leading to a cessation of oral intake. Signs and symptoms of dehydration such as low urine output, dry mucous membranes, tachycardia with thready pulses, orthostatic hypotension, and loss of skin turgor may be present depending on the time since onset of obstruction. Vomitus is more likely to be feculent if the obstruction is prolonged or located more proximally. Obstipation and constipation are indicative of complete small bowel obstruction, although patients may initially report passage of diarrhea after symptom onset as the bowel distal to the obstruction continues to evacuate its contents. Abdominal distention is often reported in more distal obstructions but may not be as prominent in patients with more proximal or closed-loop obstructions.

Signs and symptoms of strangulated obstruction or intestinal ischemia include severe abdominal pain out of proportion to physical exam findings, and findings of developing sepsis such as tachycardia, tachypnea, fever, and acute mental status changes. Patients presenting with abdominal pain and any of these findings warrant immediate surgical consultation, prior to waiting for the results of laboratory or imaging studies to help identify the specific cause. These can be done simultaneously so as not to delay surgical planning. Physical findings of significant tenderness with palpation or abdominal rigidity are signs of peritonitis, and also warrant immediate surgical consultation, as they can indicate perforation, sepsis, or current or impending ischemia.

25.3 Differential Diagnosis

Other entities that can present similarly to SBO include constipation and Ogilvie's syndrome, both forms of large bowel obstruction, as well as postoperative ileus and gastroenteritis. While the presenting symptoms of these entities can mimic a small bowel obstruction, the primary treatment for all of them is nonsurgical.

A patient with constipation will often present with a chronic history of poor bowel function. An abdominal examination can show distention, and imaging may reveal diffuse colonic distention without a transition point. These findings can also be seen in Ogilvie's syndrome, which is colonic pseudo-obstruction without an identifiable structural source of obstruction. However, this entity is typically associated with medications or an underlying condition such as a neurologic, cardiac, renal, or pulmonary pathology.

Postoperative ileus refers to the disruption of coordinated motor activity throughout the bowel following a surgical procedure. Patients are at higher risk for developing prolonged postoperative ileus after prolonged or open procedures, surgery on the lower portion of the gastrointestinal tract, or procedures involving an infected field.

Gastroenteritis can present with pain, nausea, and emesis, similar to patients presenting with true bowel obstruction. Gastroenteritis can often present with diarrhea as well, but not always in the initial phase of the condition. Therefore, for all of these conditions, a thorough history and a high index of suspicion are required to help distinguish them from a true obstruction. Additionally, cross-sectional imaging can help identify a true transition point that is seen in small bowel obstruction but not for these other conditions. Patients with known diagnoses that can present as a small bowel obstruction, such as Crohn's disease or a malignancy, still require the same approach as all patients without these conditions.

25.4 Laboratory and Imaging Workup

Initial laboratory workup of small bowel obstruction should include a complete blood count (CBC), basic metabolic panel (BMP), and a lactic acid level. These tests do not play a role in the diagnosis of small bowel obstruction but are helpful to establish the degree of dehydration, guide fluid and electrolyte resuscitation, and assess for possible bowel ischemia or necrosis. CBC may demonstrate hemoconcentration, evidenced by elevated hemoglobin and hematocrit, due to the presence of dehydration. Leukocytosis and elevated bands or neutrophilia may indicate the presence of bowel compromise or perforation. A BMP may reveal electrolyte derangements, including hypokalemia, hypochloremia, and metabolic alkalosis, in the setting of prolonged emesis. An elevated BUN is indicative of dehydration. The presence of lactic acidosis is concerning for intestinal ischemia. However, a normal lactic acid level does not rule out the possibility of compromised bowel perfusion.

Various imaging modalities are useful in the diagnosis and treatment of small bowel obstruction. Abdominal X-ray (AXR) is cost-effective, portable, and can be used for serial examinations. In comparison to CT scan, abdominal X-ray has relatively lower radiation exposure but is less able to identify the level or cause of the small bowel obstruction. Signs of small bowel obstruction on abdominal X-ray include the presence of gastric dilation and gas or fluid-filled small bowel loops >3 cm. CT scans of the abdomen and pelvis with IV contrast are considered to be the gold standard in the imaging workup of a small bowel obstruction. They are generally more sensitive and specific than abdominal X-ray in determining the level of an obstruction. Dilated small bowel loops >3 cm with air-fluid levels are consistent with the diagnosis of small bowel obstruction. CT scans are generally very effective at establishing a transition point, with dilated small bowel loops proximal and decompressed small bowel loops and colon distal to the point of obstruction. Extrinsic sources of compression, such as an abscess or tumor, may also be more easily identified on CT scan. Small bowel volvulus or closed-loop obstruction can be identified with this modality as well. CT scans can also identify abdominal wall hernias, as well as the extent of bowel involvement and potentially the condition of the involved bowel.

CT scans with IV contrast are also more effective than abdominal X-rays in identifying early signs of bowel ischemia. Abdominal X-rays may demonstrate free air under the diaphragm late in the progression of bowel ischemia, after perforation has occurred. CT findings concerning for ischemia include bowel wall thickening, mesenteric venous congestion, mesenteric fluid and ascites, pneumatosis intestinalis, and portal venous gas.

Ultrasound can be a useful adjunct as well and has comparable accuracy to abdominal X-ray in diagnosing small bowel obstruction, but is highly operator dependent, and resolution can be adversely affected by air. MRI carries no radiation burden but is more expensive and lengthier than CT scan, and may not be as reliable in identifying the cause of obstruction.

25.5 Decision Tree

A patient presenting with symptoms of nausea, vomiting, abdominal pain, obstipation or constipation, and a physical exam with distention, tenderness, or signs of dehydration, should undergo a workup to identify the presence of a small bowel obstruction. This workup includes CBC, BMP, lactic acid, AXR or CT AP with IV but not oral contrast due to the concern over aspiration. While evidence exists that small bowel follow-through studies with gastrografin may be useful in the treatment of small bowel obstruction, these studies should not be attempted prior to surgical consultation. The hyperosmolarity of the water-soluble gastrografin contrast can help reduce wall edema and improve peristalsis. However, reports of gastrografin pneumonitis exist, even in amounts as low as 50 ml, and the outcome was fatal in nearly all of the reported events. Once the diagnosis of small bowel obstruction is established, an assessment of threatened bowel viability should be made. Any patient found to have free air, pneumatosis, peritoneal signs, signs of sepsis, an abdominal wall hernia that cannot be reduced, or an abdominal operation within the prior

4 weeks should receive immediate surgical consultation. Additionally, any patient found to have small bowel obstruction by imaging who presents with symptoms of constipation, nausea, or emesis should receive urgent surgical consultation. Although the majority of small bowel obstructions will resolve without surgical intervention, the final determination as to the need for surgical intervention should be made by the surgeon. Surgical consultation should thus not be delayed. Patients with an imaging study read as having a small bowel obstruction but who do not exhibit obstructive symptoms or have any of the above concerning features for bowel compromise may be admitted to a medical service. If a patient previously without any concerning features has a change in signs or symptoms or develops any indications of bowel compromise, surgical consultation should be obtained immediately.

Patients who present with symptoms and signs of small bowel obstruction in the setting of a previously known medical diagnosis can present a different set of challenges. Patients with Crohn's disease who present with obstructive symptoms can be managed with steroids and parenteral nutrition provided that they do not exhibit any of the signs or findings of compromised bowel. Patients who present with recurrent obstructions on medical therapy are candidates for surgical intervention. Those who initially respond to medical therapy but show a lack of progression or clinical deterioration should also be considered for surgical intervention. Patients with a known malignancy who present with obstruction will still have a benign etiology in up to a third of cases, but up to half of these patients will still require surgery. Although malignancy-related obstructions rarely lead to ischemia, these patients should still undergo the same decision algorithm for initiation of a surgical consultation. Patients with known carcinomatosis, palpable masses, or ascites, in the absence of an already determined advanced directive, warrant a longer nonoperative trial of treatment, but should still be offered surgical consultation based on the same criteria. A diagnosis of intussusception on imaging should always prompt a surgical consultation as nearly all intussusceptions in the adult population are associated with a specific structural finding, most commonly neoplasms. For patients presenting with a nonreducible hernia, surgical consultation should always be sought. On presenting physical exam, the hernia must be easily reducible, and no escalated efforts through additional pressure or use of relaxing medications should be used. Hernias that are easily reduced are not likely to be the source of a bowel obstruction. Abdominal wall hernias that do not easily reduce, especially when found in a patient with a potential bowel obstruction, already have the potential for bowel wall ischemia, and therefore require evaluation by a surgeon. These hernias may ultimately require surgical intervention or close nonoperative observation, but this decision should be made by the surgical team. The forced reduction of compromised bowel can lead to undiagnosed ischemia, perforation, sepsis, or death. Even a CT scan failing to show concerning findings of bowel incarcerated in a hernia should not negate the need for surgical consultation in these circumstances as the scan may be early in the process or the imaging may fail to show findings indicative of compromised bowel.

Regardless of the etiology of the SBO or timing of surgical consultation, immediate care of the patient should be initiated (Table 25.1). This includes IV placement with volume resuscitation, electrolyte replacement, and nasogastric tube decompression to reduce the risk of aspiration and improve patient symptoms. This course of treatment should also be initiated for conditions that mimic small bowel obstruction, such as Ogilvie's syndrome, gastroenteritis, and postoperative ileus. Due to emesis, dehydration, and diarrhea, these patients can also suffer electrolyte and acid–base disorders as well as volume contraction requiring fluid

Table 25.1 Checklist for workup and management of SBO prior to surgical consultation

Prior to surgery consultation	
Labwork	CBC, BMP, lactic acid
Imaging	CT abdomen/pelvis with IV contrast preferred AXR if CT unavailable
Management	Correct any existing electrolyte derangements Insert NGT and maintain to low continuous suction Place patient on aspiration precautions

resuscitation. Isotonic fluids such as normal saline or lactated Ringer's solution should be used. Based on laboratory findings, electrolytes should be replaced as necessary, and repeat lab evaluations should be instituted to determine the success of these interventions. These measures can and should be initiated prior to and during the workup to determine the diagnosis, and prior to or concomitant with surgical consultation. Additionally, any patient suspected of having a small bowel obstruction should be made NPO (nothing to eat) with consideration of parenteral nutritional supplementation if prolonged enteric obstruction is anticipated. Adequate pain control for the patient should be assured once a diagnosis and treatment plan are determined and executed. Serial abdominal exams are a critical portion of the evaluation of a patient with potential small bowel obstruction as these findings can change suddenly, and patients can deteriorate quickly. Patients who receive pain medication for their discomfort should have their medication titrated to provide the necessary analgesic effect without altering the patient's mental status and ability to verbalize symptoms and undergo a reliable physical exam. This requirement can be relaxed for patients where the decision for surgical intervention has already been made and no further serial evaluations by physical exam are deemed necessary. However, this should only be attempted where aspiration concerns are minimal, and personnel are present who have the expertise and resources to quickly secure the patient's airway.

The requirement for surgical evaluation does not change depending on the availability of that consultation. If surgical consultation is either unavailable or will be significantly delayed, plans should be expedited to transfer the patient to a facility where appropriate surgical consultation is readily available. In that situation, only those laboratory and imaging studies necessary to determine the need for surgical consultation should be done, and no unnecessary delays in transfer and definitive care should result from waiting for studies or treatments not immediately required for care prior to the transfer. Resuscitation efforts such as IV placement, IV fluid administration, basic labs necessary to aid in the decision for transfer, and placement of a nasogastric tube for stomach decompression and aspiration risk reduction, are all useful and necessary procedures that can and should be undertaken prior to transfer. Direct communication should be made between the referring physician and the receiving surgeon when possible. While it should not require discussion, insurance, financial, and practice politics should never be part of the consideration in the transfer of a patient for necessary care.

25.6 Summary

Small bowel obstruction remains a significant cause of emergency department visits and consultation to surgical services. The most common causes are adhesive disease from prior operations, incarcerated or strangulated abdominal wall hernia, and malignancy, as well as many other less prevalent causes. Although the majority of these patients can be managed successfully non-operatively, it is difficult to determine in advance which patients these will be. Therefore, it is important to maintain a high index of suspicion and to recognize the factors on presentation and findings that should warrant surgical consultation (Fig. 25.1). Patients with abdominal pain in association with significant tenderness or peritoneal signs, presence of a nonreducible hernia, fever, tachypnea, tachycardia, leukocytosis, or lactic acidosis should be seen urgently by a surgeon. Patients who present with abdominal pain, nausea, emesis, and obstipation should get a CBC, BMP, lactic acid level, and plain abdominal films with a CT scan of the abdomen and pelvis with IV contrast. Findings of free air, a transition point in the small bowel, pneumatosis, ascites, volvulus, a mesenteric swirl sign, or other signs of ischemia should prompt immediate surgical consultation. If the clinical picture is not clear or the referring physician is uncomfortable with the interpretation of the exam or findings, a surgical consultation is always appropriate. Finally, patients who present with no specific finding necessitating an immediate surgical consult but who have changes or worsening of their symptoms, physical exam, or adjunct laboratory or imaging findings, should always lead the referring physician to ask for surgical consultation. Patients who have been deemed to be safe to manage initially without that consultation must be

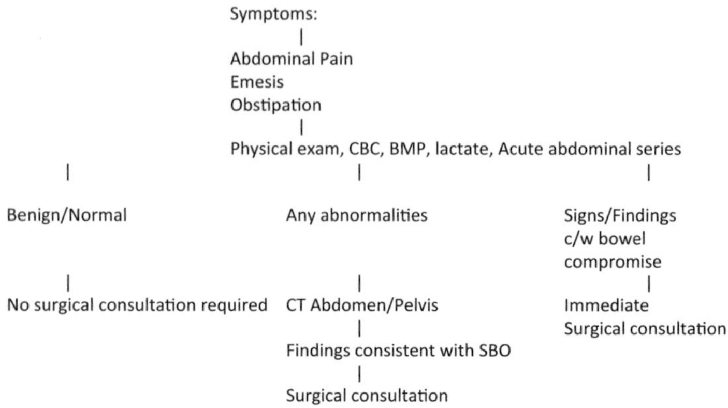

Fig. 25.1 Algorithm for determining the need for surgical consultation for an SBO

resuscitated appropriately and followed with exams and repeat imaging and lab testing aggressively. While patients who have worsening of their symptoms, clinical exams, or lab or X-ray findings should certainly necessitate surgical consultation, so should patients who fail to show progress or improvement. The survival likelihood of a patient with intestinal ischemia is strongly negatively correlated to the delay in diagnosis and subsequent definitive treatment of the condition. Therefore, if unavailable locally and deemed necessary, transfer to a facility where surgical consultation is available should never be delayed. When in doubt, the timely and collaborative discussion of a patient with potential small bowel obstruction with a surgeon is never the wrong move.

References

1. https://www.ncbi.nlm.nih.gov/books/NBK572336/
2. https://www.east.org/education-resources/practice-management-guidelines/details/smallbowel-obstruction-evaluation-and-management-of
3. https://www.uptodate.com/contents/etiologies-clinical-manifestations-and-diagnosis-of-mechanical-small-bowel-obstruction-in-adults?search=small%20bowel%20obstruction&source=search_result&selectedTitle=1~150&usage_type=default&display_rank=1

Appendicitis 26

Celeste Hollands

26.1 Background

Appendicitis is the leading reason for emergency surgery in adults and children in the United States. Surgery has long been the mainstay of therapy. Nonoperative treatment with antibiotics alone began to be used for select adult and pediatric patients with uncomplicated appendicitis about 10 years ago. The Covid-19 pandemic saw a rise in the use of this nonoperative therapy due to limitations of healthcare access during this time. Additional studies in adults and children have shown that nonoperative therapy in carefully selected patients results in fewer complications, better pain control, and decreased disability days over those patients treated with surgery as first-line therapy. These results should be balanced with the findings that patients treated nonoperatively have a 30–50% risk of needing an appendectomy within 5 years. The decision for operative versus nonoperative therapy is best made during a shared decision-making conversation between the surgeon and the patient. All patients diagnosed with acute appendicitis whether uncomplicated or complicated require emergent surgical evaluation.

C. Hollands (✉)
Texas Tech University Health Sciences Center, Amarillo, USA

G. P. Kohn et al. (eds.), *The SAGES Manual of Surgical Referral for Primary and Emergency Care*,
https://doi.org/10.1007/978-3-031-92678-5_26

26.2 Definitions

Acute appendicitis: Acute, severe inflammation of the appendix. Acute appendicitis may be uncomplicated or complicated.

Simple or uncomplicated appendicitis: Early or suppurative phases of inflammation when appendix has not perforated. No phlegmon or abscess on imaging.

Perforated or complicated appendicitis: Progression of inflammation resulting in perforation of the appendix. Patients present with evidence of diffuse peritonitis with or without evidence of sepsis or with advanced localized disease with evidence of phlegmon or abscess on imaging.

Chronic appendicitis: Less severe inflammation that is recurrent and self-limited. Briefly, chronic appendicitis usually presents as recurrent abdominal pain that does not progress to acute appendicitis. These patients generally present with symptoms that prompt an evaluation for acute appendicitis and there may be recurrent episodes. Patients with this history may benefit from referral to a surgeon to evaluate their chronic abdominal pain for possible chronic appendicitis. Diagnostic laparoscopy and appendectomy can be diagnostic and therapeutic for these patients.

26.3 Clinical Presentation

26.3.1 History

A complete history should be taken from all patients, particularly focusing on the abdominal pain and associated symptoms. It is important to ask the patient if they have been diagnosed with or treated for appendicitis previously. Menstrual and urinary histories are also important.

Patients with acute uncomplicated appendicitis typically present with abdominal pain present for 12–24 hours that begins in the periumbilical location and radiates into the right lower quadrant.

The pain worsens with ambulation, sudden movement, or jarring. The pain will likely only be lessened with the administration of pain medication. Associated symptoms may include nausea, vomiting, fever, and anorexia. Pregnant patients may have pain localized higher on the right side depending on the trimester of presentation since the appendix may become displaced upward by the fetus. Patients with complicated appendicitis are more likely to present with fever and vomiting and diffuse abdominal pain.

Pediatric patients may not accurately describe the pain or associated symptoms and also may not have anorexia. One tip is to ask the patient to point with one finger where the pain is. Most patients with appendicitis can pinpoint a single spot, not outline a general area.

26.3.2 Physical Exam

All patients should be assessed with attention to general appearance, vital signs, and volume status. A complete physical exam with focused abdominal exam should be performed. The focused abdominal exam consists of visual assessment with particular attention to surgical scars or distention. Auscultation in all four quadrants with gentle pressure can aid in assessing bowel sounds, significant tenderness, and guarding (both voluntary and involuntary). Palpation in all four quadrants starting in the left lower quadrant and moving counterclockwise to the right lower quadrant should be performed, noting any tenderness.

Patients with uncomplicated appendicitis will likely have normal vital signs and focal rebound tenderness in the right lower quadrant. Adjuncts to test for rebound tenderness include obturator sign (pain on internal rotation of the thigh), Rovsing's sign (pain in right lower quadrant when palpating or percussing left lower quadrant), and psoas sign (pain with passive extension of right leg posteriorly by the examiner while the patient is lying on their left side). Pregnant patients may have tenderness higher than McBurney's point in the right lower quadrant. Patients with perforated appendicitis may have generalized or localized peritonitis and may have a palpable mass in the right lower quadrant.

Pediatric patients who are initially examined for rebound by the traditional method of depressing the abdomen and quickly releasing will likely not be amenable to any further examinations or interventions. A better way to examine pediatric patients is by percussion only, starting in the left lower quadrant and progressing counterclockwise to the right lower quadrant. If percussion tenderness exists, the patient most likely has peritoneal irritation. If percussion tenderness does not exist, then proceed with palpation in the same counterclockwise fashion.

Genitourinary examination may be needed to rule out pelvic inflammatory disease and scrotal pathology in patients with confusing or atypical presentations.

26.4 Labs (Table 26.1)

Chemistry panel: Basic electrolytes, glucose, liver function tests, amylase, lipase on all patients

hCG: Obtain on all patients who anatomically and physiologically could be pregnant. Some hospitals have a lower age limit

Table 26.1 Diagnostic tests

Labs	Prior to surgical evaluation	After discussion with surgery
	Complete blood count (CBC) with differential	
	Basic electrolytes, glucose, liver function tests, amylase, lipase	
	Beta-Human Chorionic Gonadotropin (bHCG)	
	Urinalysis (UA) with microscopy	
	C-Reactive Protein (CRP)	
Imaging		
		Ultrasound-focused RLQ (male and female) Ultrasound pelvic (female reproductive organs)
		CT scan with IV and/or oral contrast
		MRI with oral contrast

(9–10 years of age), an upper age limit (55 years of age), and exclusions (hysterectomy, postmenopausal).

CRP: This can be a helpful adjunct, especially in children

UA with microscopy: Obtain on all patients

In pediatric patients, consideration should be given to starting an IV at the time labs are drawn.

26.5 Imaging (Table 26.1)

Focused right lower quadrant ultrasound (US) is often the first study that should be performed to identify signs of acute appendicitis. Consideration should be given to doing a complete abdominal ultrasound in patients who are not able to clearly communicate the exact location of their pain or in pregnant patients whose appendix may be displaced upward.

Computed tomography scan (CT) with intravenous contrast of abdomen and pelvis in nonpregnant patients can be used if the clinical diagnosis cannot be made with history, physical, labs, and ultrasound results. Radiology protocols differ as to whether to add oral contrast, and this should be discussed with surgery and radiology prior to obtaining. Facilities with an available surgeon to care for a patient with appendicitis should give consideration to discussing the utility of obtaining a CT scan with the evaluating surgeon so as to avoid unnecessary radiation exposure. Facilities that would have to transfer the patient to another facility in order to obtain surgical care should obtain a CT scan as described if it will not delay disposition and if it will negate the need for transfer if the patient does not have appendicitis. If the patient will be transferred to another facility for surgical evaluation regardless of the CT scan results, then it should be deferred to the accepting facility to decide about obtaining this study.

Magnetic resonance imaging (MRI) of the abdomen and pelvis with oral contrast avoids radiation to the fetus and mother in pregnant patients and is widely being used as the study of choice for this patient population. This study should be ordered only after discussion with surgery, radiology, and obstetrics unless an institutional protocol or policy exists to follow. Gadolinium is not given as it is known to cross the placenta. MRI is also being used in some hospitals for pediatric patients who need additional workup to aid in making the diagnosis after labs and ultrasound have returned equivocal results. This is done to avoid increased radiation exposure in childhood. It can also be useful in ruling out other causes of abdominal pain in children. MRI will take longer than a CT scan, and thus it is important to note that the child will need to be able to lie still in order to obtain quality images. Younger patients may require sedation to be able to lie still for this long and then the risks and benefits of sedation versus radiation from a CT scan need to be carefully considered and discussed.

26.6 Diagnosis

The diagnosis of acute appendicitis can likely be made using the history, physical exam, and laboratory results. Some studies report a higher negative appendectomy rate when imaging is not incorporated in the diagnostic workup. Routine imaging may not be standard globally. The Prospective Observational Study on Acute Appendicitis Worldwide (POSAW) of 4282 patients in 116 worldwide surgical departments from 44 countries reported imaging played a cardinal role in the diagnosis of acute appendicitis. Reliable imaging in patients with clinical suspicion of appendicitis reduced the rate of negative appendectomy by almost 15%.

For some patients, the diagnostic test results or the clinical presentation may not be straightforward. Several scores have been developed and validated to aid in making the diagnosis of acute appendicitis. The Alvarado score, pediatric appendicitis score, and appendicitis inflammatory response score have all been reported and evaluated in the literature. Several articles include associated algorithms based on the index of suspicion to help guide safe patient disposition from the initial point of healthcare access and evaluation.

The appendicitis inflammatory response (AIR) score is accurate at excluding appendicitis in those deemed low risk and more accurate at predicting appendicitis than the Alvarado score in those deemed high risk. The pediatric appendicitis score (PAS) has also been found to be more predictive than the Alvarado score. The usefulness of all of these scoring systems is most sensibly used to determine which patients need immediate imaging and which are safe to be discharged with precautions. Online calculators are available to calculate these scores AIR: https://www.mdcalc.com/calc/3984/appendicitis-inflammatory-response-air-score and PAS: https://www.mdcalc.com/calc/3926/pediatric-appendicitis-score-pas.

Patients with AIR scores ≤4 and PAS scores <4 are low risk for acute appendicitis and may be safely observed as an outpatient for worsening symptoms. Patients with AIR scores of 5–8 and PAS scores 4–7 are considered intermediate risk for acute appendicitis and require additional evaluation by US and consideration for surgical evaluation depending on the results of the US or clinical judgment of the evaluating provider. Patients with AIR scores ≥9 and PAS scores ≥8 are high risk for acute appendicitis and require surgical emergent surgical evaluation.

26.7 Referral (Table 26.2)

All patients diagnosed with acute appendicitis should be referred for urgent surgical evaluation. In most communities, this will be best done in the hospital emergency room (ER). Some communities may have the ability to perform point-of-care labs and imaging in the outpatient setting (office or urgent care) and diagnose acute appendicitis allowing for either emergent outpatient evalua-

Table 26.2 Referrals

	Referral type	Emergent	Elective
Diagnosis			
		Acute uncomplicated or complicated appendicitis	
			Chronic appendicitis

tion by the surgeon or direct admission to the hospital for surgical evaluation and treatment. It is important that emergent surgical evaluation is achieved by whatever mechanism expedites this process in the individual community.

26.8 Surveillance/Reassessment

Those who are low risk for appendicitis do not need immediate imaging and can be reassessed the following day in the outpatient setting with instructions to return for reassessment sooner if pain worsens or associated symptoms develop. Those who are intermediate and high risk should have immediate imaging and surgical consultation as discussed above.

Several articles include clinical guidelines or pathways that are reasonable to follow. The SAGES appendicitis guideline supports that workup and management remain nuanced, and thus each facility may have slightly different approaches to the diagnostic workup and the surgeon and patient choice of management for acute appendicitis.

All patients with acute appendicitis should be monitored and reassessed for pain control, signs of sepsis, and hydration status throughout their course of treatment.

26.9 Treatment

Patients with significant pain should be treated with pain medication most appropriate for their general medical condition and level of pain. This will not interfere with the ability to obtain an adequate abdominal exam for peritonitis and should not be withheld pending the surgical team's bedside evaluation of the patient.

Isotonic intravenous fluids should be started immediately if the patient is dehydrated, with consideration given to administering a 20 cc/kg bolus prior to starting the maintenance rate. If the patient does not appear dehydrated, then maintenance intravenous fluids should be started once the diagnosis of acute appendicitis is made.

The decision to administer antibiotics as well as the choice of antibiotics is best made in collaboration with the evaluating surgeon. Uncomplicated appendicitis is a localized infection, and, if the operative approach to treatment is planned, then a single dose of antibiotics within one hour of incision is adequate surgical prophylaxis. Patients who have decided with their surgeon to be treated with antibiotics only should be given intravenous broad-spectrum antibiotics once this decision has been made. Complicated appendicitis presents a risk of sepsis, and broad-spectrum intravenous antibiotics should be given as soon as that diagnosis is suspected.

26.10 Special Considerations

26.10.1 Pregnant Patients

Pregnant patients may have pain and tenderness localized higher on the right side depending on the trimester of presentation since the appendix may become displaced upward by the fetus. For diagnostic imaging, MRI with oral contrast avoids radiation to the fetus and mother in pregnant patients and is widely being used as the study of choice. This study should be ordered only after discussion with the surgeon, radiologist, and obstetrics unless an institutional protocol or policy exists to follow. Gadolinium is not given as it is known to cross the placenta.

26.10.2 Pediatric Patients

Pediatric patients may not accurately describe the pain or associated symptoms and also may not have anorexia. One tip is to ask the patient to point with one finger where the pain is. Most patients with appendicitis can pinpoint a single spot, not outline a general area. Pediatric patients who are initially examined for rebound by the traditional method of depressing the abdomen and quickly releasing will likely not be amenable to any further examinations or interventions. A better way to examine pediatric patients is by percussion only, starting in the left lower quadrant and progressing counterclockwise to the right lower quadrant. If percussion tenderness exists, the patient most likely has peritoneal irritation. If percussion tenderness does not exist, then proceed with palpation in the same counterclockwise fashion. In addition, consideration should be given to starting an IV at the time labs are drawn. Finally, for diagnostic imaging, if an US is not diagnostic, MRI is often recommended instead of CT scan if available.

26.10.3 Patients Previously Treated with Antibiotics Alone for Uncomplicated Appendicitis

Patients diagnosed with acute appendicitis should be asked if they have previously been diagnosed with and treated for acute appendicitis. Patients who have previously been treated for acute appendicitis on the nonoperative pathway would likely not be offered nonoperative treatment a second time.

Suggested Reading

1. Salminen P, Paaianen H, Rautio T, et al. Antibiotic therapy vs appendectomy for treatment of uncomplicated acute appendicitis: the APPAC Randomized Clinical Trial. JAMA. 2015;313:2340–8. https://doi.org/10.1001/jama.2015.6154.
2. Minneci PC, Mahida JB, Lodwick DL, et al. Effectiveness of patient choice in nonoperative vs surgical management of pediatric uncomplicated acute appendicitis. JAMA Surg. 2016;151(5):408–15. https://doi.org/10.1001/jamasurg.2015.6154.
3. Minneci PC, Hade HM, Lawrence AE, et al. Association of nonoperative management using antibiotic therapy vs laparoscopic appendectomy with treatment success and disability days in children with uncomplicated appendicitis. JAMA. 2020;324:581–93. https://doi.org/10.1001/jama.2020.10888.

4. Lamm R, Kumar SS, Collings AT, et al. Diagnosis and treatment of appendicitis: systematic review and meta-analysis. https://Sages.org/publications/guidelines/diagnosis-and-treatment-of-appendicitis-sr-and-meta
5. Kollár D, McCartan DP, Bourke M, Cross KS, Dowdall J. Predicting acute appendicitis? A comparison of the Alvarado score, the Appendicitis Inflammatory Response score and clinical assessment [published correction appears in World J Surg. 2015;39(1):112]. World J Surg. 2015;39(1):104–9.

Supraumbilical Lumps and Bulges (Epigastric Hernias and Diastasis Recti)

27

Vahagn C. Nikolian and Vamsi V. Alli

27.1 Introduction

Abnormalities of the upper abdominal wall can present in a variety of ways. Commonly, these are related to either primary ventral hernias or rectus diastasis. These can also be related to prior operations, resulting in iatrogenic injuries manifest as bulges, weakness, or asymmetry. This chapter will focus on the evaluation and diagnostic workup for common upper abdominal wall bulges that may warrant surgical referral.

27.2 Initial Evaluation

Presentation of abdominal wall bulges is varied and can range from asymptomatic incidental findings to patients who have severe symptoms. For patients presenting with localized symptoms or concerns, a thorough history should be obtained focused on pain or discomfort, physical disability attributable to the bulge,

V. C. Nikolian
Oregon Health & Science University, Portland, OR, USA

V. V. Alli (✉)
Penn State Milton S. Hershey Medical Center, Hershey, PA, USA
e-mail: valli@pennstatehealth.psu.edu

G. P. Kohn et al. (eds.), *The SAGES Manual of Surgical Referral for Primary and Emergency Care*,
https://doi.org/10.1007/978-3-031-92678-5_27

and whether gastrointestinal symptoms are associated with the discomfort. Questions about core instability should supplement examination. Patients should be asked about pain scores while resting, with light activity, and with more strenuous activity. A review of medical history should include an assessment of obesity, prior pregnancies, smoking status, diabetes status, and collagen vascular diseases. A surgical history should be obtained, with a review of the surgical approaches used (e.g., laparotomy vs. laparoscopic surgery). A review of patient surgical history should specifically focus on if any prior hernia repair has been performed, the approach to the operation (e.g., open vs. minimally invasive), and if a mesh prosthesis was placed.

27.3 Physical Exam

Physical exam is critical for patients presenting with abdominal bulges and contour irregularities. An exam of the abdominal wall while standing can be helpful and generally will allow for obvious asymmetry to be noted. Patients should also be assessed with dynamic engagement of the abdominal wall—either by observing the patient transition from a seated position to a supine position or having patients perform a straight leg raise while in a supine position. These simple maneuvers may highlight bulges, prominences, asymmetry, and further assess abdominal wall functional limitations. Skin quality is an important factor for planning repair of a hernia but is seldom a concurrent issue in rectus diastasis. Skin integrity should be documented, specifically taking note of any overlying ulcerations, discoloration, and nonhealing wounds, which should prompt a more expedited workup or referral.

In patients with no significant surgical history, rectus diastasis will often present as a symmetric bulging when the core is engaged. This occurs because the rectus muscles have a space between them through which the midline tissues bulge upon tightening. It most commonly occurs in infants, who are likely to outgrow the problem, and postpartum women who developed it in pregnancy. The bulge is most commonly in the central, upper abdomen though it can extend from the xiphoid process to the pubis. On palpation, no obvious fascial defects should be identified and pain to palpation is considered atypical. However, small epigastric hernias can occasionally be palpated in the diastasis, especially in children. Quantification of the inter-rectus width and the dimensions of the bulge should be recorded.

If a fascial defect is palpated, then the diagnosis is likely a hernia. Hernia assessment should include whether the bulge is reducible or incarcerated. Chronic incarceration is common and does not warrant emergency consultation unless there are any concerns for an acute complication or intestinal strangulation. Identification of surgical scars can be helpful, but it should be noted that surgical scars may not align well with fascial defects, particularly for patients with obesity or those who have had significant fluctuations in their weight. Bulges or hernias adjacent to incisional scars should be considered incisional hernias until proven otherwise.

27.4 Diagnostic Imaging and Clinical Decision-Making

Diagnostic workup of abdominal wall abnormalities is focused on imaging studies (Table 27.1). As understanding of abdominal wall anatomy has improved and contemporary techniques for repair have expanded, reliance on surgical planning with dedicated imaging has increased. Due to the cost and potential for unnecessary testing, imaging is not mandatory for surgical referral, despite the potential for facilitating efficient patient care. We describe strategies for diagnostic workup and referral for common clinical scenarios in the following.

Table 27.1 Prereferral imaging

	Workup prior to surgical referral
Diastasis	None
Hernia <4 cm	Optional ultrasound with Valsalva
Hernia >4 cm	Noncontrast CT abdomen and pelvis

27.4.1 Rectus Diastasis

In general, rectus diastasis is a benign condition and can be safely observed by the primary care physician without imaging. However, should the findings be uncertain, ultrasound is useful in pediatric patients, but a noncontrast CT of the abdomen and pelvis can be used to verify the diagnosis, though it may be best deferred until after a surgical consultation. Some patients benefit from a trial of physical therapy. If the patient is presenting with primarily cosmetic concerns, referral to cosmetic surgical specialists can be considered. In patients under observation, development of a separate bulge within the symmetric midline diastatic bulge should prompt concern for the development of a primary ventral hernia through attenuated midline fascia and trigger referral to a general surgeon. Additionally, if the bulge is associated with functional limitations, or gastrointestinal symptoms analogous to hernia symptoms, referral to general surgeons is warranted.

27.4.2 Primary Ventral Hernias

Primary ventral hernias with obvious fascial defects or incarcerated bulges can be managed with or without imaging. This is often at the discretion of the surgeon, and a variety of factors will contribute to decision-making. For patients presenting with smaller defects (<4 cm), imaging in advance of referral is not necessary. A US with and without Valsalva may impart information related to the hernia in specific cases, such as when trying to characterize contents of an incarcerated hernia. General surgeons are well-versed in managing these problems and can address them with a variety of techniques. For larger hernia defects (>4 cm), cross-sectional imaging in the form of a noncontrast CT of the abdomen and pelvis is often desired and can provide important information for directing management.

27.4.3 Incisional Hernias

The presence of a bulge adjacent to a prior surgical scar likely indicates the presence of an incisional hernia, which may prompt evaluation by a surgeon. Similar to primary hernias, hernias that are larger than approximately 4 centimeters or hernias arising within a larger incision should be further characterized through a noncontrast CT of the abdomen and pelvis. It is important to recognize that radiology impressions do not always convey the necessary level of detail or full clinical picture needed to assess for the appropriate method of reconstruction. It is imperative to clinically correlate imaging to the patient's history and concerns and have a low threshold for further surgical evaluation.

27.4.4 Complicated Hernias

Patient may present with complex problems related to their hernias, warranting expedited surgical referral. Chronic incarceration can be associated with pain or gastrointestinal symptoms, including early satiety, constipation, and less focal, vague abdominal pain. This is to be distinguished from acute incarceration, which is a surgical emergency and may lead to bowel obstruction or strangulation. Additional complications such as compromised overlying skin and soft tissue, fistula formation, mass effect on limbs, and limitations on mobility as a result of hernias can have a profound impact on patients and their quality of life and health. In the event of acute incarceration, overlying skin changes, skin breakdown, or the presence/emergence of a fistula, potential presentation to an emergency department and acute surgical management is warranted (Table 27.2).

Table 27.2 Red flags that would prompt emergency department evaluation of a hernia

Urgent referral signs and symptoms
Localized severe pain
Acute incarceration
Bowel obstruction
Overlying skin changes: warmth, erythema, skin breakdown
Fistula formation or drainage from bulge

27.5 Adjuncts to Surgical Referral

Surgical evaluation for patients with hernias can take time, leading patients to seek advice on interim management. As such, it is important to recognize supportive strategies to managing these patients and preparing them for their consultation.

27.5.1 Exercise Programs

It is common for patients to be advised to refrain from strenuous exercise, weight lifting, or core exercises because of the presence of hernias. However, there is no data to suggest that these activities are associated with progression in hernia disease or acute complications. In general, it is recommended that patients work to maintain an active lifestyle and exercise as tolerated. Core exercises should not be discouraged as core deconditioning can contribute to further dysfunction. Collaborating with physical and occupational therapists can help patients further improve their overall abdominal core health, though there are no significant studies to recommend exercise as a means of preventing or treating abdominal wall defects.

27.5.2 Preoperative Optimization

In advance of meeting with a surgical specialist, patients should be informed about the importance of prehabilitation for surgical outcomes. Surgeons will often work to optimize patient nutritional status and exercise tolerance in advance of surgery, with data suggesting improved short- and long-term outcomes. In particular for patients undergoing major abdominal wall interventions, it is worthwhile to optimize management of diabetes, target weight loss for patients with morbid obesity (BMI > 35 kg/m^2), and encourage smoking cessation in advance of surgery.

27.5.3 Binders and Other Supportive Garments

Many patients will desire support of their hernias with belts, bands, and other garments. These are low-risk and low-cost interventions that may allow patients to perform more activities and may reduce the strain on accessory muscles. Binders can be used as needed by patients.

27.6 Conclusion

Upper abdominal wall bulges and diastasis are common problems. Diagnosis of these issues is primarily accomplished with physical examination and correlating to symptomatology. Imaging is often guided by the size of the defect and the patient's symptoms. Surgical management of these problems continues to evolve as our understanding of these issues improves. A multidisciplinary approach for the management of these problems is in the best interest of patients.

Suggested Reading

1. Hernández-Granados P, Henriksen NA, Berrevoet F, Cuccurullo D, López-Cano M, Nienhuijs S, Ross D, Montgomery A. European hernia society guidelines on management of rectus diastasis. Br J Surg. 2021;108(10):1189–91. https://doi.org/10.1093/bjs/znab128. PMID: 34595502; PMCID: PMC10364860.
2. Henriksen NA, Kaufmann R, Simons MP, Berrevoet F, East B, Fischer J, Hope W, Klassen D, Lorenz R, Renard Y, Garcia Urena MA, Montgomery A; on behalf of the European Hernia Society and the Americas Hernia Society. EHS and AHS guidelines for treatment of primary ventral hernias in rare locations or special circumstances. BJS Open. 2020;4(2):342–353. https://doi.org/10.1002/bjs5.50252. Epub 2020 Jan 9. PMID: 32207571; PMCID: PMC7093793.
3. Beck WC, Holzman MD, Sharp KW, Nealon WH, Dupont WD, Poulose BK. Comparative effectiveness of dynamic abdominal sonography for hernia vs computed tomography in the diagnosis of incisional hernia. J Am Coll Surg. 2013;216(3):447–53; quiz 510–1. https://doi.org/10.1016/j.jamcollsurg.2012.11.012. Epub 2013 Jan 26.
4. Joslyn NA, Esmonde NO, Martindale RG, Hansen J, Khansa I, Janis JE. Evidence-based strategies for the prehabilitation of the abdominal wall reconstruction patient. Plast Reconstr Surg. 2018;142(3 Suppl):21S–9S. https://doi.org/10.1097/PRS.0000000000004835.
5. Martindale RG, Deveney CW. Preoperative risk reduction: strategies to optimize outcomes. Surg Clin North Am. 2013;93(5):1041–55. https://doi.org/10.1016/j.suc.2013.06.015. Epub 2013 Aug 6.

28 Incisional Hernias

Sergio Mazzola Poli de Figueiredo,
Aldo Fafaj, and Charlotte Horne

28.1 Introduction

Incisional hernias represent one of the most common pathologies requiring referral for surgical evaluation. Up to 41% of patients undergoing abdominal operation will develop an incisional hernia. Although watchful waiting is a reasonable option in patients with incisional hernias, particularly in high-risk and complex patients, most patients ultimately end up undergoing hernia repair as it is associated with significant improvement in quality of life and functional status.

Patients with incisional hernias present with a wide spectrum and severity of symptoms. Regardless of symptoms, it is ideal to refer patients with incisional hernias for surgical evaluation for elective ventral hernia repair as emergent hernia repair is associated with significantly higher morbidity and mortality. However, it is common to encounter patients with significantly symptomatic

S. M. P. de Figueiredo
University of North Carolina, Chapel Hill, NC, USA

A. Fafaj
The University of Tennessee Health Sciences Center, Knoxville, TN, USA

C. Horne (✉)
Mayo Clinic, Rochester, MN, USA

G. P. Kohn et al. (eds.), *The SAGES Manual of Surgical Referral for Primary and Emergency Care*,
https://doi.org/10.1007/978-3-031-92678-5_28

hernias in the emergency room, especially those with bowel incarceration, obstruction, or strangulation at the hernia site that often mandate emergency surgery.

28.2 Clinical History and Physical Exam

Incisional hernias can be defined as a hernia located at a previous surgical site or incision, which may occur in various locations of the abdominal wall depending on the index surgical procedure. Although there is a wide spectrum of symptoms related to incisional hernias, most commonly patients will notice a bulge associated with either pain or discomfort; however, up to 25% of patients might be asymptomatic.

A thorough history is critical to determine a patient's baseline comorbidities that may impact decision-making when assessing patients with an incisional hernia. It is essential to identify important risk factors for complications, such as smoking, diabetes, obesity, immunosuppression, previous abdominal wall infection, and history of prior hernia repairs. It is important to inquire about previous episodes of incarceration requiring manual reduction, worsening pain at the hernia site, or obstructive symptoms such as nausea, vomiting, constipation, and overlying skin changes as they would require urgent surgical consultation. It is also essential to instruct the patient to obtain all operative records of prior operations before consultation with a surgeon, especially prior hernia repair operations, as this may determine appropriate options for repairs and mechanisms of recurrence.

The next step when evaluating a patient with incisional hernias is a thorough physical exam noting all previous incisions, hernia location, size, accompanying overlying skin concerns, and additional features within the abdominal wall such as stomas and other devices implanted within the abdominal wall. It is imperative to note if the exam is associated with pain and if the hernia contents are reducible. Findings during the history and physical examination help delineate appropriate imaging required for further workup and determine appropriate timing of surgical referral.

Table 28.1 summarizes appropriate preoperative imaging requirements and emergency of referral based on presenting symptoms.

Emergent referral to the emergency department is necessary if new overlying skin changes are noted at the site of the hernia or if a patient has clinical signs and symptoms of a current bowel obstruction. These symptoms include nausea, vomiting, and new-onset tenderness at the location of the hernia. Additionally, if a patient is having obstructive symptoms and the hernia cannot be reduced, the patient should be directed to the emergency department. Urgent surgical intervention is necessary in patients with hernias that report intermittent obstructive episodes that are managed at home, hernias that are rapidly enlarging, or hernias that are causing a significant amount of pain, even if the patient does not have any concomitant obstructive symptoms.

It is recommended that all patients with a clinically diagnosed incisional hernia should be referred and evaluated by a surgeon, ideally in an elective setting. A watchful waiting approach is not recommended in patients with an incisional hernia, and while not all hernias require urgent intervention, the patient should be

Table 28.1 Appropriate management based on clinical presentation of patients with hernia disease

Hernia symptoms	Imaging required	Appropriate treatment
Obstructive symptoms	CT abdomen and pelvis	Refer to the emergency department
Overlying skin changes	CT abdomen and pelvis	Refer to the emergency department
Draining ascites		Refer to the emergency department
Rapidly enlarging hernia	CT abdomen and pelvis	Urgent surgical evaluation
New or worsening pain	CT abdomen and pelvis	Urgent surgical evaluation
New umbilical bulge	Imaging not routinely required	Elective surgical evaluation
New incisional bulge	CT abdomen and pelvis	Elective surgical evaluation

referred to a surgeon to thoroughly discuss the risks, benefits, and alternatives to surgical intervention. In regard to preoperative optimization, patients who are currently smoking should be encouraged to enroll in smoking cessation programs and appropriate referrals for smoking cessation specialists should be considered. Diabetic patients should also be referred to their primary care physicians or endocrinologists to ensure optimal glycemic control to minimize perioperative complications. Obesity is also a significant risk factor for postoperative complications in patients undergoing hernia repair, and all obese patients, especially with body mass index (BMI) greater than 35 kg/mg^2, should attempt medical weight loss through weight loss specialists either with medical, pharmacological, or surgical weight loss. Patients currently on immunosuppression could also benefit from medication optimization as some immunosuppressive agents such as steroids and sirolimus have been shown to significantly impact wound morbidity. Patients with extensive pulmonary and cardiac history should also be evaluated by their respective subspecialty physicians, given that undergoing incisional hernia repair may impact respiratory function and require additional preoperative testing or perioperative management of medication.

Most patients undergoing hernia repairs will require temporary cessation of most anticoagulants perioperatively. The decision to resume anticoagulation following hernia repair highly depends on surgical technique and intraoperative findings. The management of perioperative anticoagulants is highly individualized, and the risks of holding anticoagulation should be balanced with the risks of postoperative bleeding.

All patients with acutely symptomatic hernias in the emergency department warrant emergent surgical consultation, especially in the setting of obstructive symptoms, incarceration, or associated skin changes. For these patients, often there is no time to undergo preoperative optimization, and the priority should be to resolve the surgical emergency.

28.3 Laboratory and Imaging Workup

Although incisional hernias can be diagnosed clinically, preoperative imaging is an essential component of incisional hernia repair. We recommend that all patients who are symptomatic and are potential surgical candidates or those who are interested in surgical options undergo further imaging to characterize the incisional hernia. We prefer to obtain a computed tomography (CT) of the abdomen and pelvis without any oral or intravenous contrast. Although most commonly a noncontrast CT is sufficient, oral contrast can be considered in the presence of gastrointestinal symptoms and intravenous contrast can help evaluate soft tissue abnormalities and perfusion to the hernia contents, usually in the emergency settings. Additional imaging modalities that can be used include magnetic resonance imaging (MRI) and ultrasound (US).

Several laboratory tests can be helpful when evaluating patients with hernias. In the emergency department and for patients with significantly symptomatic hernias, a complete set of labs should be obtained with attention noted to markers such as white blood cell count and serum lactate, which could indicate concomitant bowel compromise mandating emergent repair. In the elective setting, obtaining hemoglobin A1C can be a valuable tool to evaluate longer-term glycemic control. Nutritional markers such as albumin and prealbumin can also be beneficial to diagnose malnutrition, especially in the setting of weight loss, which can have significant effects on perioperative outcomes. Preoperative lab studies in general are guided by the patient's comorbidities to ensure the patient is fully optimized prior to undergoing elective surgery.

28.4 Conclusion

All patients with incisional hernias should be referred to a general surgeon for hernia repair consideration. Appropriate history and physical, with detailed prior operative notes, can be of immense value during surgical evaluation. Additional referrals placed before surgical consultation can help expedite patient's preoperative optimization and maximize the chances of the best outcome possible without significant delay. Finally, all patients with acutely symptomatic hernias who present in the emergency department require an emergent surgical consultation.

Suggested Reading

1. Sanders DL, Pawlak MM, Simons MP, et al. Midline incisional hernia guidelines: the European Hernia Society [published correction appears in Br J Surg. 2023 Oct 26]. Br J Surg. 2023;110(12):1732–68. https://doi.org/10.1093/bjs/znad284.
2. Liang MK, Holihan JL, Itani K, et al. Ventral hernia management: expert consensus guided by systematic review. Ann Surg. 2017;265(1):80–9. https://doi.org/10.1097/SLA.0000000000001701.
3. Schlosser KA, Renshaw SM, Tamer RM, Strassels SA, Poulose BK. Ventral hernia repair: an increasing burden affecting abdominal core health. Hernia. 2023;27(2):415–21. https://doi.org/10.1007/s10029-022-02707-6.
4. Wolf LL, Ejiofor JI, Wang Y, et al. Management of reducible ventral hernias: clinical outcomes and cost-effectiveness of repair at diagnosis versus watchful waiting. Ann Surg. 2019;269(2):358–66. https://doi.org/10.1097/SLA.0000000000002507.

Umbilical Hernias 29

Martin Walsh and Bethany J. Slater

29.1 Adult Patients

29.1.1 Introduction

Umbilical hernias are a common surgical condition, occurring in 10–30% of adults. They are a subclassification of ventral hernias and involve a protrusion of abdominal contents through a defect in the umbilical ring. While some umbilical hernias are congenital, most umbilical hernias in adults are acquired secondary to increased intra-abdominal pressure and/or weakening of the umbilical ring and fascia from prior abdominal surgery, obesity, pregnancy, or ascites. Umbilical hernias often contain mesenteric fat, omentum, or bowel, and can become incarcerated or strangulated. An incarcerated hernia becomes stuck in the defect and cannot be reduced, while a strangulated hernia is an incarcerated hernia that results in compromised blood supply and threatened bowel integrity. While incarcerated or strangulated hernias require

M. Walsh
Department of Surgery, Advocate Lutheran General Hospital, Park Ridge, IL, USA

B. J. Slater (✉)
University of Chicago, Chicago, IL, USA

G. P. Kohn et al. (eds.), *The SAGES Manual of Surgical Referral for Primary and Emergency Care*,
https://doi.org/10.1007/978-3-031-92678-5_29

urgent or emergent referral, reducible hernias warrant more elective surgical evaluation or may not require surgical referral altogether. This chapter aims to better elucidate the optimal workup and referral strategy for umbilical hernias in adults.

29.1.2 Presentation and Initial Evaluation

Adult patients presenting with umbilical hernias can elicit a wide range of symptoms. Patients typically present in the primary care office setting with complaints of an umbilical protrusion that enlarges with actions that increase intra-abdominal pressure. A thorough history should be taken to identify risk factors, medical comorbidities, contributory history (prior abdominal surgery, prior umbilical hernia repair, etc.), and assess the duration and progression of symptoms, with emphasis on prior episodes of pain, obstruction, or incarceration. On exam, the physician should note the size of the hernia defect, the condition of the overlying skin, and determination of a reducible versus irreducible hernia. If a patient with an irreducible hernia presents with obstructive symptoms (nausea, emesis, abdominal distention) or peritoneal signs (diffuse abdominal tenderness to palpation, rebound tenderness, guarding, fever, leukocytosis), they should be referred to the emergency room for prompt evaluation for surgical evaluation.

Imaging is not routinely indicated for reducible umbilical hernias. However, imaging can be useful in certain situation including strangulation, incarceration, or complicated hernia. Urgent assessment can include an upright abdominal X-ray for free air or obstruction. Additionally, an abdominal CT with oral and intravenous contrast can provide further detail. In the absence of symptoms/signs of incarceration, imaging should be deferred pending surgical evaluation as few require it (Table 29.1).

29.1.3 Indications for Surgical Referral

Guidelines from SAGES and the European Hernia Society have been published on indications for operative management of umbilical hernias, and these can serve as a basis for guiding appropriate referral and management. In general, guidelines suggest repair for symptomatic umbilical hernias, hernias with defects >2 cm, previously incarcerated hernias that have been successfully reduced, or actively incarcerated or strangulated hernias (with or without evidence of bowel obstruction). For patients with larger (>2 cm defect size) reducible hernias without pain or other symptoms, surgical referral is warranted but can be done on a routine basis (2–8 weeks). More urgent referral (within 2 weeks) may be considered for patients with any pain symptoms (regardless of hernia size) or incarcerated hernias successfully reduced by the referring clinician (given the high risk of recurrence). Emergent surgical evaluation is warranted for persistently incarcerated umbilical hernias, strangulated hernias, or any hernia type with associated peritoneal signs.

For patients with small (<1 cm defects), easily reducible hernias without additional symptoms, surgical referral can likely be delayed with continued monitoring for worsening of symptoms and/or progression in size. Routine referral can also be considered for patients who would prefer to discuss surgical options with a specialist (Table 29.1).

Table 29.1 Overview for surgical referral indications

	Emergent evaluation	Elective referral	Referral deferred
Adult	Irreducibility Strangulation Obstructive symptoms Peritoneal signs	Symptomatic hernias >2 cm defects Ascites	Asymptomatic <1 cm Pregnancy (referral after delivery)
Pediatric	Incarceration Strangulation Obstructive symptoms Peritoneal signs	Any size (>4-5y) High-risk features[a]	Reducible (<4y)

[a]Large defect (>3.5 cm), proboscis, extreme prematurity (28wks), connective tissue disorders, pulmonary conditions, and neurologic conditions

29.1.4 Surgeon Selection

Most umbilical hernias can be repaired by any available board-certified general surgeon. For very large (>10 cm), recurrent, or otherwise complex umbilical hernias, referral to a fellowship-trained hernia specialist can be considered given they have focused, advanced training in complex abdominal wall reconstructions with access to more minimally invasive techniques. Referral to a surgeon with the appropriate expertise and resources for the complexity of the case helps ensure optimal outcomes after umbilical hernia repair.

29.1.5 Patient Optimization and Symptomatic Control

While patients await surgical evaluation and repair, there are optimization measures and conservative options to consider. Smoking cessation should be encouraged to reduce pulmonary risks with anesthesia. Weight loss for obese patients prior to elective repair may reduce operative risks and improve outcomes. Nutritional optimization is also important. Abdominal binders can provide external support and symptom relief for large umbilical hernias causing pain. Over-the-counter pain medications like acetaminophen or nonsteroidal anti-inflammatories can help manage intermittent discomfort or pain associated with the hernia. Regardless of the hernia specifics and patient characteristics, optimizing modifiable risk factors preoperatively and providing symptomatic relief are important while patients await surgical evaluation (Table 29.2).

29.1.6 Special Consideration for High-Risk Surgical Patients

29.1.6.1 Pregnancy

In pregnancy, umbilical hernias occur commonly in the third trimester with uterine growth. In these patients, repair is delayed until approximately 6 weeks after delivery in the absence of incar-

Table 29.2 Primary care considerations

	Workup prior to referral	Management if deferred referral	Referral considerations
Adult	History/ physical	Patient education Smoking cessation Symptom control Medical optimization Lifestyle modification[a]	Tertiary center referral if ascites or large hernia
Pediatric	History/ physical	Parent education Close monitoring Return precautions	Pediatric surgeon preferred

[a]Weight loss, constipation prevention, nutritional optimization, and limiting straining

ceration or strangulation. This approach has been shown to be safe, decreasing utilization costs and reducing recurrence rates. While awaiting repair, these patients can undergo lifestyle modifications by limiting heavy lifting/straining, applying an abdominal binder, and treating constipation. Patients with evidence of incarceration or strangulation undergo emergent treatment using established precautions for pregnancy.

29.1.6.2 Ascites

In patients with cirrhosis complicated by ascites, umbilical hernias have a reported incidence of 20% given increased abdominal pressure and abdominal wall weakness. In these patients, there is a considerably increased risk of strangulation/incarceration if pursuing conservative management (5% vs 0.5–1% for non-cirrhotic patients). In these patients, mesh placement is standard over primary suture repair and both open and laparoscopic repair are safe. Additionally, optimization of the patient's ascites and underlying disease is paramount and may require nutritional optimization, diuresis, paracentesis, transjugular intrahepatic portosystemic shunts (TIPS), and/or temporary peritoneal dialysis catheters. Referral to a specialized hernia center and multidisciplinary approaches with medical specialists is recommended when available due to the increased risk of postoperative complications (Table 29.2).

29.1.7 Postoperative Considerations

Most patients undergoing elective repair are discharged the same day. A multimodal pain regimen limiting narcotics as able adequately treats expected pain from the surgical incision. While complications such as minor bleeding and mild pain can occur, early recurrence, evidence of bowel injury (with peritonitis, obstruction), and surgical site infection warrant prompt evaluation of the treating surgeon for possible urgent intervention. Patients with mesh placement have a risk of complications from the prosthetic, including infection, seroma, and chronic pain, but a lower risk of recurrent hernias.

29.1.8 Conclusion

Umbilical hernias in adults are a common surgical problem that primary care and emergency providers will encounter. Large, symptomatic, incarcerated, and strangulated umbilical hernias warrant urgent surgical evaluation for repair. Smaller, asymptomatic hernias can be repaired on an elective basis or deferred with close monitoring. With appropriate diagnosis, referral practices, and good preoperative optimization, outcomes after umbilical hernia repair are generally excellent.

29.2 Pediatric Patients

29.2.1 Introduction

Umbilical hernias are a common surgical condition in pediatric patients. However, the management in this population is notably different than in adults. Diagnosed in 10–30% of infants and 10% of patients at age 3, the majority (80–90%) of these hernias spontaneously resolve by age 4 or 5. Thus, after acute complications such as incarceration or strangulation are ruled out, most can be successfully managed with watchful waiting and reassurance—

with only refractory, symptomatic, or growing hernias needing referral for surgical evaluation (Table 29.1).

29.2.2 Presentation and Initial Evaluation

In a pediatric primary care and emergency medicine setting, evaluation should emphasize identifying symptomatic, irreducible umbilical hernias. Given pediatric patients are often unable to elicit symptoms, careful and thorough evaluation must be pursued. Reducible hernias in pediatric patients usually present as a soft, reducible mass at the umbilicus that is nontender and typically increases with crying, coughing, or straining. Notably, while constipation with straining can cause a hernia to become more apparent, umbilical hernias do not cause constipation in the absence of incarceration or strangulation. While pediatric umbilical hernias are statistically less likely to be incarcerated/strangulated compared to adults (0–1% for children compared to 4–30% for adults), symptoms of irreducibility, obstructive symptoms (emesis, obstipation), increased fussiness (especially upon umbilical palpation), and/or colicky abdominal pain should raise clinical suspicion. Later signs of strangulation can include dusky/purple discoloration at the hernia site, fever (or hypothermia), or shock (secondary to intra-abdominal sepsis from necrotic bowel). Any child exhibiting these concerning symptoms/signs warrants prompt referral/transfer to the emergency department and prompt surgical evaluation for consideration of immediate surgical intervention. While awaiting surgical evaluation, emergent workup can be pursued with plain film abdominal radiographs. In select cases, ultrasound and/or CT imaging with PO and IV contrast may be needed to understand the clinical picture.

For reducible hernias without concerning symptoms, emergency department referral and imaging are unnecessary. However, if the diagnosis is unclear, abdominal ultrasound can help distinguish between other umbilical etiologies such as urachal cysts, lipomas, hemangiomas, and umbilical granulomas (Table 29.1).

29.2.3 Delayed Referral for Asymptomatic Hernias

In 2019, the American Academy of Pediatrics (AAP) released guidelines recommending against routine surgical referral for asymptomatic umbilical hernias in children younger than 4–5 years old. This is based on the high observed percentage of spontaneous closure by age 5 (80–90%). Additionally, specific risks inherent to the umbilical hernia repair process (anesthesia complications, infection, pain, bleeding, recurrence) can be avoided. The low incidence of strangulation/incarceration and high likelihood of spontaneous closure also support a watchful waiting approach. Discussion with the parents regarding natural history of hernias, high success rate of spontaneous closure, and an emphasis on the low complication rate is paramount. Then, the hernia can be safely monitored on a routine outpatient basis for resolution or need for surgical referral (Tables 29.1 and 29.2).

29.2.4 Indications for Possible Early Referral

29.2.4.1 Large Hernia Size or Proboscis

Evidence suggests an association between increasing hernia size with decreased spontaneous closure rates. Closure rates are 50–60% for 2.5–3.5 cm and 10–30% for >3.5 fascial defects. Some patients will also develop proboscoid hernias where the umbilical skin over stretches leading to the tissue hanging over the diaper when upright or developing skin ulceration. While spontaneous closure is still possible for these larger hernias, earlier referral is reasonable if parents desire shared decision-making discussions around early repair.

29.2.4.2 Extreme Prematurity

Earlier referral (at 1–2 years of age) can be considered for infants of extreme prematurity (<28 weeks) with any size hernia due to decreased spontaneous closure rates.

29.2.4.3 Connective Tissue Disorders

For patients with connective tissue disorders, like Ehlers–Danlos syndrome or Marfan syndrome, earlier referral may be warranted given lower rates of spontaneous closure and possible increased complication rates.

29.2.4.4 Conditions That Increase Intra-abdominal Pressure

Patients with bronchopulmonary dysplasia, cystic fibrosis, or pulmonary hypertension can experience increased intra-abdominal pressure. Additionally, children with ascites or patients on peritoneal dialysis would also be considered candidates for early surgical referral. Limited evidence suggests these conditions may impart an increased incarceration risk in children warranting earlier intervention.

29.2.4.5 Abdominal Wall Defects

Patients with previously diagnosed abdominal wall defects, such as omphalocele or gastroschisis, are associated with decreased rates of spontaneous closure, though some may still close without repair.

29.2.4.6 Neurological Conditions

For patients with specific neurologic conditions that either impair their ability to reliably express or experience symptoms of incarceration/strangulation (such as cerebral palsy, spina bifida, Down syndrome, autism spectrum disorders) or predispose them to increased intra-abdominal pressure (hydrocephalus with concomitant ventriculoperitoneal shunt, seizure disorders), earlier referral is warranted to avoid complications and reliably identify symptoms for emergent intervention.

29.2.4.7 Family History

If a child has a sibling with an umbilical hernia complicated by incarceration, limited data suggests it may impart an increased risk of similar complications. Thus, earlier referral and discussion regarding risks/benefits may be warranted.

29.2.5 Postoperative Considerations

Laparoscopic repair is rarely performed for pediatric umbilical hernias unless there is a concomitant pathology such as urachal remnant or cyst requiring laparoscopic exploration. Open repair is the standard repair approach using an infra- or supra-umbilical incision. Most repairs for asymptomatic umbilical hernias are done on an elective, outpatient basis with same-day discharge. Typically, the surgery is well tolerated with mild postoperative pain (controlled well with Tylenol and/or ibuprofen). The child can return to his/her usual diet after surgery. Typically, the only restrictions are aggressive play or heavy lifting for limited periods of time based on surgeon preference. From a primary care perspective, it is important to monitor for more concerning postoperative complications such as wound dehiscence, hernia recurrence, and severe abdominal pain. These would warrant prompt notification of the treating surgeon for emergent evaluation.

29.2.6 Conclusion

Umbilical hernias are a common pediatric surgical problem that pediatricians and emergency providers will encounter. As in the adult population, careful evaluation is required to identify patients requiring surgical referral and determine the appropriate timing of referral based on the clinical presentation. Unlike in adults, surgical referral in pediatric patients can often be safely deferred until age 4–5 years old unless more concerning factors coexist. With this approach of watchful waiting, pediatric patients can receive optimal care while decreasing the risk of undergoing potentially unnecessary and risky surgical procedures.

Suggested Reading

1. Heniford BT. SAGES guidelines for laparoscopic ventral hernia repair. Surg Endosc. 2016;30(8):3161–2. https://doi.org/10.1007/s00464-016-5073-9. Epub 2016 Jul 15. PMID: 27422242.

2. Henriksen NA, Montgomery A, Kaufmann R, Berrevoet F, East B, Fischer J, Hope W, Klassen D, Lorenz R, Renard Y, Garcia Urena MA, Simons MP; European and Americas Hernia Societies (EHS and AHS). Guidelines for treatment of umbilical and epigastric hernias from the European Hernia Society and Americas Hernia Society. Br J Surg. 2020;107(3):171–90. https://doi.org/10.1002/bjs.11489. Epub 2020 Jan 9. PMID: 31916607.
3. He K, Hills-Dunlap JL, Kashtan MA, Riley H, Sawaya DE, Rangel SJ. Frequency of potentially avoidable surgical referrals for asymptomatic umbilical hernias in children. J Pediatr Surg. 2022;57(5):855–9. https://doi.org/10.1016/j.jss.2022.04.022.

Pediatric Inguinal Hernias

30

Kylie M. Callier, Joy Ayemoba, and Bethany J. Slater

30.1 Introduction

Inguinal hernia repair is one of the most common operations performed by pediatric surgeons. Reported incidences of inguinal hernias in children range from 1 to 5% and occur most commonly within the first year of life. They are more common in males, and there is a slight predominance of right-sided hernias. Bilateral hernias are present about 10% of the time. Risk factors for inguinal hernias include prematurity, history of a hydrocele or undescended testis, positive family history, connective tissue diseases, or any disease causing increased intra-abdominal pressure. The majority of pediatric inguinal hernias are congenital, resulting from the failure of the processus vaginalis to close during fetal or newborn development that creates a communication between the scrotum/labia and the peritoneal cavity. If large enough, abdominal contents, commonly bowel or an ovary, may herniate, resulting in an indirect inguinal hernia. Direct inguinal hernias are caused by a weakness in abdominal wall musculature and protrude through the wall of the inguinal canal. While common in

K. M. Callier (✉) · J. Ayemoba · B. J. Slater
University of Chicago, Comer Children's Hospital, Chicago, IL, USA
e-mail: kylie.callier@uchicagomedicine.org;
joy.ayemoba@uchicagomedicine.org

G. P. Kohn et al. (eds.), *The SAGES Manual of Surgical Referral for Primary and Emergency Care*,
https://doi.org/10.1007/978-3-031-92678-5_30

adults, children rarely present with a direct inguinal hernia. Unless otherwise indicated in this chapter, "inguinal hernia" refers to an indirect inguinal hernia.

The diagnosis of an inguinal hernia can usually be made based on the history and physical exam alone. Although the presentation may vary, all pediatric inguinal hernias require operative treatment. It is important to be aware of the wide range of patient presentations and apply a systematic approach to the assessment and management of pediatric hernias in order to prevent severe and potentially life-threatening complications.

30.2 Presentation

Inguinal hernias typically present as an intermittent bulge in the groin, scrotum, or labia. Most hernias are asymptomatic or minimally symptomatic, but often appear during times of distress (crying, straining, or activities causing increased intra-abdominal pressure), leading parents of infants and younger children to feel that the hernia is the cause of these symptoms. Older children may complain of vague "pain" or "discomfort" during exercise. In addition to a careful history of symptoms, a detailed medical history should be obtained, including history of prematurity, history of hydrocele or undescended testis, history of any diseases associated with increased intra-abdominal pressure, prior groin surgery, and family history of hernias.

Symptomatic hernias may present with incarceration (difficult or unable to reduce) or strangulation (loss of blood supply). Entrapment of bowel in an incarcerated hernia results in signs of bowel obstruction, such as abdominal distention, vomiting, and/or obstipation. The reported incidence of incarceration in the pediatric population ranges from 5 to 18% and may be as high as 30% in premature infants. If the hernia is not reduced, the blood supply to the incarcerated organ may be compromised to the point of infarction (strangulated hernia). Patients presenting with an incarcerated hernia who have a prolonged history of a bulge, erythema, severe pain, or systemic symptoms such as fever, tachycardia, or leukocytosis should be promptly evaluated by a pediatric surgeon for emergency surgery. Box 30.1 lists the signs and symptoms that should raise concern for incarceration or strangulation.

Box 30.1 (a) Incarcerated hernias may present with symptoms of bowel obstruction and these patients may benefit from nasogastric tube placement and decompression. (b) Severe or systemic signs or symptoms should raise concern for strangulation and emergent surgery is indicated

(a) Symptoms of *obstruction*
- Vomiting
- Obstipation
- Abdominal distension and/or pain

(b) Signs/symptoms of *strangulation*
- Severe abdominal or groin pain
- Skin erythema overlying hernia
- Peritonitis
- Tachycardia
- Fever
- Leukocytosis

30.3 Differential Diagnoses

30.3.1 Hydrocele

Hydroceles are common in pediatric patients and are often associated with the presence of an inguinal hernia. Hydroceles are also caused by the failure of the processus vaginalis to close during development and are classified as noncommunicating and communicating. These may be difficult to differentiate on exam, and communicating hydroceles are frequently confused with inguinal hernias based on similar presentations and symptoms reported by patients or families. However, a careful history and physical will often reveal the diagnosis.

Complete closure of the proximal portion of the processus leaving fluid surrounding the testicle results in a noncommunicating hydrocele. Noncommunicating hydroceles are common in newborn males and typically resolve within the first year of life. A communicating hydrocele results when the processus vaginalis persists but is narrow enough to only allow the passage of fluid into the inguinal canal. The free flow of fluid leads to swelling that often fluctuates daily, increasing in size during the day when the child is upright and decreasing overnight. Patients may also report a progressive increase in size. Alternatively, hydroceles may present acutely either secondary to an acute testicular process such as torsion or following a respiratory or diarrheal illness in which coughing or straining has forced fluid through an undetected patent processus vaginalis.

Hydroceles can usually be distinguished from inguinal hernias by physical exam. Hydroceles typically present as nontender swelling of the scrotum that surrounds the testicle and transilluminates. However, transillumination does not guarantee the diagnosis as gas-filled bowel may also transilluminate. For this reason, aspiration should never be attempted for diagnosis. It is possible for a hydrocele to present as a bulge in the upper scrotum or inguinal canal. This is a hydrocele of the cord that forms when the proximal and distal portions of the processus vaginalis close, but there is enough remaining processus in the canal to form a fluid collection.

Patients with communicating hydroceles are at risk for complications if bowel traverses the canal, and thus are treated in the same fashion as inguinal hernias with elective repair. Surgical treatment of noncommunicating hydroceles is reserved for those that persist or occur after 1–2 years of age or in cases where a hernia or communicating hydrocele cannot be ruled out (e.g., neonates).

30.3.2 Undescended Testis

Inability to palpate the testis in the scrotum suggests an undescended or retractile testis. The child may or may not also have a hernia. Occasionally an elevated testicle can be mistaken for a hernia, especially if the testis is in the inguinal canal. Identification of the testis is important as the need for a concomitant orchidopexy may impact the timing and surgical approach.

30.3.3 Inguinal Adenopathy

Inguinal lymph nodes may look similar to a hernia. A detailed history and physical exam can usually differentiate between the two, but ultrasound may be helpful if the diagnosis remains unclear. Alternatively, an ovary within an inguinal hernia sac or a testis in the canal may be confused with a lymph node.

30.4 Assessment

30.4.1 Physical Exam

To examine for an inguinal hernia, the patient should be undressed and placed supine. First, observe for an obvious mass or asymmetry of the groins. Both testes should be palpated to rule out an undescended testis. Use a finger to hold the testis within the scrotum while examining for a hernia to differentiate a retractile testis from a true inguinal bulge. Standing on the contralateral side and palpating along the inguinal canal at the external inguinal ring can reveal a smooth mass extending from the ring lateral to the pubic tubercle. You may feel loops of intestine or an ovary within the hernia sac. Both groins should be examined in all patients being evaluated for an inguinal hernia. If no mass is identified, maneuvers that increase intra-abdominal pressure may reveal the bulge such as crying, coughing, or a Valsalva maneuver. Older children may be asked to stand or jump.

If a mass is still not identified, an attempt should be made to palpate the spermatic cord. A thickened spermatic cord compared to the contralateral side, called the "silk glove sign," is indicative of the presence of a hernia sac. This is performed by using an index finger to gently pin the spermatic cord against the pubic tubercle and lightly rubbing over the cord from side to side. While this maneuver can be difficult and its accuracy is debated, an obviously positive exam can be useful in supporting the diagnosis of an inguinal hernia.

If no hernia is able to be identified on physical exam, this does not necessarily rule out the presence of an inguinal hernia. Hernias that come and go may not be easily found on examination if nothing is in the hernia sac. It may be helpful to ask parents to take a picture of the bulge or swelling when it is noticed at home. Many surgeons will proceed with an inguinal hernia repair on history alone if the story is compelling and there is an absence of findings to suggest an alternate diagnosis.

Most hernias are easily reducible. Those that are difficult or unable to be reduced are "incarcerated" hernias. If there is vascular compromise of the entrapped contents, it is a "strangulated" hernia. A tender, firm mass in the scrotum or groin should raise suspicion for incarceration or strangulation (Fig. 30.1).

30.4.2 Reduction

Attempts at reducing an inguinal hernia should be made in all patients presenting without obvious signs of shock or peritonitis. The child should lie supine and be as calm as possible. Pain medication and/or sedation may be appropriate if available and placing the patient in Trendelenburg position (feet elevated) may assist in reduction. General anesthesia is not recommended as there is a potential for gangrenous bowel to be reduced into the abdomen and go unrecognized.

Knowledge of inguinal anatomy is very helpful when attempting manual reduction. Figure 30.1 is a simplified diagram of normal inguinal anatomy to keep in mind when examining and reducing inguinal hernias. An important consideration when attempting reduction is that the inguinal canal in younger children is oriented more vertically than when they are older, and the inguinal rings are essentially overlapping. This creates an angle in the hernia sac as it exits the inguinal canal. Pushing the hernia sac toward the abdomen can cause the sac to overlap on itself or slide

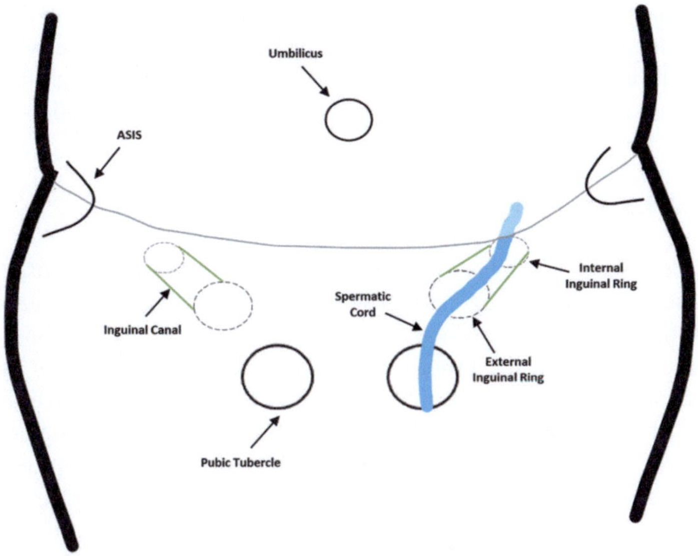

Fig. 30.1 Inguinal canal anatomy and landmarks. The inguinal canal begins at the internal inguinal ring and extends inferiorly and medially, ending at the external inguinal ring. The inguinal canal is much shorter in children than in adults and the internal and external inguinal rings essentially overlap in young children. Indirect inguinal hernias pass through the inguinal canal, following the path of the spermatic cord in males and the round ligament in females

over the external ring instead of reducing through the canal into the abdomen. This may be avoided by sweeping your fingers from the ipsilateral anterior superior iliac crest down along the inguinal canal. Then, with the same hand, grasping the apex of the hernia within the scrotum or labia and applying constant gentle traction to align the long axis of the hernia sac with that of the inguinal canal. Next, using the index finger and thumb of the other hand, apply pressure on either side of the hernia neck at the level of the internal ring. The goal of this technique is to straighten the canal and keep the external and internal inguinal rings open. Continue to apply pressure on either side of the inguinal canal with your index finger and thumb and, with the hand that is holding the apex of the hernia sac, slowly walk your fingers up the groin toward the inguinal ring applying steady, firm pressure. This may take several minutes. You may feel bowel or gas as it passes through the ring into the abdomen and, if successful, the hernia will disappear.

30.4.3 Imaging

The history and physical exam are the foundation of diagnosis, and very rarely is any kind of imaging indicated. There is a small subset of patients in which imaging may be helpful, such as those with a lump in the groin with unclear etiology. However, it is imperative to recognize that the diagnosis of an inguinal hernia can be made by history and physical exam alone in the vast majority of patients. Ordering of imaging studies may delay rather than expedite the diagnosis.

Plain Abdominal Radiograph An abdominal radiograph may reveal dilated bowel loops, suggesting a bowel obstruction or air in a hernia sac. This may be helpful in differentiating between an incarcerated inguinal hernias and testicular pathologies in a patient with acute scrotal swelling and pain.

Ultrasound When a patient's history or physical exam suggests a diagnosis other than an inguinal hernia or hydrocele, an ultrasound may be useful in identifying other diagnoses that mimic these conditions, such as an inguinal lymph node or testicular torsion. An ultrasound can identify the presence of fluid or bowel within a hernia sac but may not be sensitive enough to differentiate between a hernia or hydrocele, making it less useful when these are suspected.

30.5 Special Considerations

30.5.1 Patients <1 Year of Age

Inguinal hernias most commonly present within the first year of life and peak within the first few months. As mentioned above, it is not uncommon for parents to perceive the bulge is causing that patient pain. A detailed history often reveals that the bulge appears *after* crying or straining and disappears when the baby is sleeping. Not only are inguinal hernias much more common in infants than older children, but the incidence of incarceration is also much higher than the rest of the pediatric population. Over 50% of incarcerations will occur within the first six months of life. This risk gradually decreases after 1 year of age. Additionally, there is a concern that caregivers of these preverbal children may not recognize alarming signs or symptoms in a timely manner. It is imperative that families of infants waiting for elective hernia repair be counseled on the signs and symptoms that should prompt medical evaluation. However, it is also important to discuss that a crying or irritable infant without any other symptoms should be cared for in the normal fashion (feeding, diaper change, nap, etc.) and does not usually require immediate surgery.

As obliteration of the processus vaginalis occurs during the eighth month of pregnancy, it is not surprising that premature infants have the highest incidence of inguinal hernias. This risk correlates with the severity of prematurity. Premature infants also have a higher rate of incarceration and are more likely to have bilateral hernias.

There are several distinct challenges in the management of inguinal hernias in infants and neonates. The optimal timing of repair, particularly in preterm infants, remains controversial. There is significant variability in practice among pediatric surgeons. Given the increased risk of incarceration, many surgeons argue that repair should occur prior to hospital discharge in premature infants. Reasons for delaying repair include technical challenges, comorbid conditions, and risks associated with anesthesia such as postoperative apnea and/or ventilator dependence. Generally, the younger the patient's gestational and post-conceptual ages, the greater the risk for postoperative apnea. Other risk factors include a history of apnea or bradycardia, chronic lung disease, and anemia. Regional techniques such as spinal, epidural, or caudal anesthesia may be utilized to avoid this risk; however, it is not always available, and if additional sedation is needed at any time, the benefit is lost. Ultimately, providers must balance the risk of incarceration with the risks of postoperative respiratory complications.

General anesthesia has been shown to be very safe in healthy full-term infants, but concerns have been raised about the effect of general anesthesia on the developing brain and may affect decisions in management. This topic is actively debated, and there is currently no conclusive evidence to suggest that exposure to anesthetic for a relatively short duration adversely affects neurodevelopmental outcomes in healthy infants and children.

30.5.2 Adolescents

Although swelling may not be noticed for years, hernias in childhood are still almost always developmental defects due to a patent processus vaginalis and have been present since birth. While still extremely rare, acquired direct inguinal hernias are more likely to occur in adolescents compared to infants. Incarceration of an inguinal hernia is relatively rare after 5 years of age.

30.5.3 Predisposing Conditions

Inguinal hernias may be associated with underlying congenital or medical conditions, particularly those that may prevent the closure of the processus vaginalis or cause increased intraabdominal pressure. Excess fluid in the peritoneal cavity in patients with a ventriculoperitoneal shunt or on long-term peritoneal dialysis increases the incidence of hernias in this population. Both omphalocele and gastroschisis have also been shown to increase the odds of inguinal hernias, likely due to increased abdominal wall pressure preventing the closure of the processus vaginalis. Patients with inherited connective tissue disorders, such as Ehlers–Danlos and Marfan syndromes, have higher incidences of inguinal hernias and recurrence rates after operative repair. There is also an increased incidence of inguinal hernias in children with cystic fibrosis, which may be attributed to chronic cough and/or constipation.

30.6 Management

Initial management of inguinal hernias that can be performed by primary or emergency care providers while awaiting surgical evaluation is summarized in Table 30.1. Importantly, these should not delay surgical referral. Inguinal hernias do not resolve spontaneously, and operative treatment is recommended for all infants or children because of the risk of incarceration and its associated morbidity and mortality. Incarcerated and/or strangulated hernias can result in severe complications depending on which structure(s) is involved in the hernia sac, including bowel obstruction, necrosis, and/or perforation and testicular/ovarian necrosis or atrophy, and can be fatal.

Table 30.1 Management strategies that may be initiated by the primary or emergency care physician following diagnosis of inguinal hernia in a pediatric patient. Generally involves SUPPORTIVE care measures. Diagnostic studies are rarely indicated and not necessary prior to surgical referral

Management of inguinal hernias prior to surgical evaluation[a]
Asymptomatic/easily reducible hernia
No further diagnostic workup necessary
Counsel parents on symptoms that should prompt medical evaluation
Suspected incarcerated hernia
No further diagnostic workup necessary
Attempt manual reduction
Consider nasogastric decompression if obstructive symptoms present
Suspected strangulated hernia
Do not attempt reduction
If in outpatient setting, direct patient to the emergency room
Initiate intravenous fluids and broad-spectrum antibiotics
Consider nasogastric decompression if obstructive symptoms present
Obtain labs if able (complete blood count, coagulation profile, lactic acid, metabolic panel including electrolytes, blood urea nitrogen, creatinine, and bicarbonate)
May help guide resuscitation but should not delay surgical management

[a]All pediatric patients with inguinal hernia(s) should be referred to general or pediatric surgery. For suspected incarceration or strangulation, initial management should not delay surgical consultation and evaluation

Prompt referral to a pediatric surgeon or high-volume general surgeon who performs pediatric inguinal hernia repairs should occur following the diagnosis of an inguinal hernia in all pediatric patients. The urgency of evaluation and/or repair varies depending on patient characteristics, presentation, and physical exam findings. Figure 30.2 provides a general framework for the multidisciplinary evaluation and management of inguinal hernias.

Asymptomatic and/or easily reducible inguinal hernias do not require emergent intervention. Patients should be referred to pediatric or general surgery where they will be seen in clinic and scheduled for an elective operation. The timing of elective surgery varies among surgeons, and the actual risk of incarceration following the diagnosis of an inguinal hernia is unclear. In general, operative repair is performed within 1 month of the diagnosis, but may be recommended sooner, especially in patients known to be at higher risk for incarceration.

Patients have no activity restrictions while awaiting repair. Parents may be counseled on how to apply gentle pressure to reduce the bulge but there is no medical reason for regular reduction of the hernia. Patients will receive detailed instructions and have the opportunity to ask any questions regarding surgery at their outpatient surgical visit. Except for maintaining nothing by mouth status, there are no special preoperative steps or tests required for an elective hernia repair. Preoperative bloodwork is not needed unless otherwise indicated by a patient's comorbidities. For most patients, surgery can be performed safely in the ambulatory setting under general anesthesia. Full-term infants and children usually do not require overnight inpatient monitoring and go home the same day as surgery. Admission to the hospital for monitoring is suggested in high-risk patients including infants <50 weeks post-conceptual age.

In patients presenting with a suspected incarcerated hernia, manual reduction should be attempted. Most incarcerated hernias can be manually reduced using the techniques described previously in this chapter. Successful reduction will result in immediate relief of discomfort, resolution of any obstruction, and prevent strangulation. As with all pediatric inguinal hernias, a referral should be made to pediatric surgery. If the reduction is performed

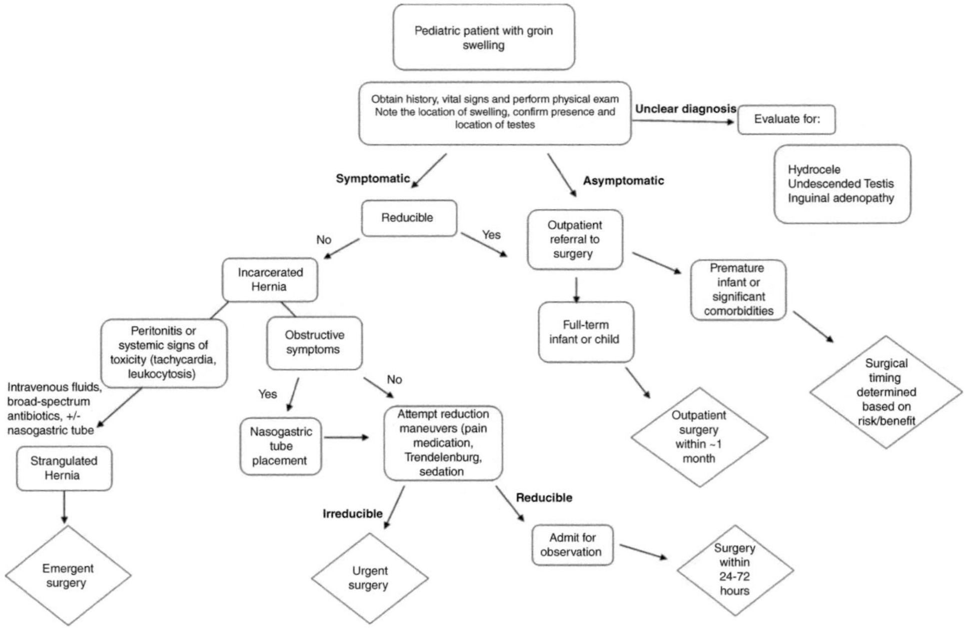

Fig. 30.2 Evaluation and management of inguinal hernia based on patient presentation

in the emergency room, children are often observed in the hospital for 24 hours, especially after a difficult reduction. Recurrent incarceration is common and definitive repair is usually scheduled within 24–72 hours of reduction to allow any edema to resolve. Unsuccessful reduction should prompt urgent evaluation by a pediatric surgeon.

If strangulation is suspected, successful manual reduction is likely impossible and should not be attempted. These patients should be directed to an emergency room, and emergent surgical exploration is indicated to assess the viability of the involved structures. Intravenous fluids and broad-spectrum antibiotics should be initiated. A nasogastric tube may be placed if signs of obstruction are present.

30.7 Surgical Approach

The key tenet of inguinal hernia repair in pediatric patients is performing a high ligation of the hernia sac at the level of the internal ring. In pediatric patients, the inguinal floor rarely requires repair and mesh is not routinely used. Elective inguinal hernia repair can be performed using an open or laparoscopic technique. The decision for either approach may be based on operative time, anesthesia, analgesia, and surgeon experience.

Open hernia repair has been the long-standing traditional approach in children. Laparoscopic repair boasts several advantages over open techniques in adults and has been commonly performed for many years but has only recently become an alternative for children. Many pediatric surgeons considered it unnecessary as the cited advantages of laparoscopy in adults (smaller incisions, ease of repair, less pain) are already features of the open technique in pediatric patients. Open repair is generally faster and might be preferred when the risks of prolonged general anesthesia are significant. An open approach also allows for the utilization of a regional anesthesia as opposed to general anesthesia.

Laparoscopic repair is being increasingly performed by experienced pediatric surgeons, and several variations of the technique have been developed. Laparoscopic approaches allow for visualization of both inguinal canals, which is advantageous in detecting contralateral inguinal hernias; there may be a prolonged learning curve for surgeons with less experience with laparoscopy, and initial studies suggested an increased hernia recurrence rate, but more recent studies have not supported this finding.

Incarcerated or strangulated inguinal hernias are commonly approached using an open technique, but laparoscopy has in certain situations. It can be used initially to reduce and visualize the hernia contents, visualize contents that spontaneously reduced before adequate inspection, or re-evaluate reduced contents after repair of the hernia defect.

Routine contralateral exploration is a widely debated topic. Given the lack of high-quality data, no firm recommendations can be made. Families are counseled preoperatively on the risk of developing a contralateral hernia with the potential for incarceration, and the potential need for additional surgery if only unilateral repair is performed.

30.8 Postoperative Care

Most pediatric patients do extremely well and recover quickly after surgical repair of their inguinal hernia. Some postoperative pain is to be expected and is typically mitigated with over-the-counter analgesics and should resolve in the first few days. Swelling in the groin or scrotal areas can occur after surgery and improves over time. Children will return to normal activity much sooner than adult patients. Most surgeons will allow normal activity when able with some restrictions on contact sports, strenuous activity, and heavy lifting. It is generally not necessary to limit the activities of infants and young children after undergoing inguinal hernia repair. There is no specialized wound care required after surgery. A postoperative appointment may be scheduled to assess wound healing.

30.9 Complications

Surgical complications from an inguinal hernia repair are very rare. Although the incidences are extremely low, complications may result from injury to surrounding structures during the operation. Injury to the testicular vessels can lead to testicular atrophy. A herniated ovary or fallopian tube is also susceptible to vascular compromise. A vas deferens injury may lead to the formation of spermatic antibodies causing infertility. Operative mortality is now rarely seen and is most often related to comorbidities such as prematurity and/or underlying lung or cardiac disease.

Hernia recurrence is possible, and certain patients are at higher risk. The reported recurrence rates in pediatric patients range from 1 to 5%. Patients with a history of incarceration or strangulation, connective tissue disorder, or conditions that increase intra-abdominal pressure are at an increased risk for recurrence. Additionally, an unrecognized tear in the hernia sac, failure to repair an enlarged inguinal ring, or damage to the inguinal floor at the time of operative repair are all associated with recurrence. Some studies have reported higher recurrence rates after laparoscopic repair; however, this may be related to surgeon experience, and there is now a growing body of evidence that the laparoscopic approach is at least as effective as open repair.

Recent studies demonstrate that surgical subspecialty training can lead to improved outcomes in pediatric patients. Fellowship-trained pediatric surgeons have the lowest rate of hernia recurrences. Higher recurrence rates of inguinal hernias have been associated with lower surgeon case volume, particularly when the repair is performed by a general surgeon. However, access to a pediatric surgeon may be challenging depending on location, and general surgeons who perform a reasonable amount of pediatric hernia repairs can achieve similar outcomes.

Suggested Readings

1. Glick PL, Boulanger SC. Chapter 76 - Inguinal hernias and hydroceles. In: Coran AG, editor. Pediatric surgery (Seventh Edition). Mosby; 2012. p. 985–1001.
2. Hirschl R, et al., editors. Inguinal Hernia. In: Pediatric Surgery NaT, American Pediatric Surgical Association, 2020. Pediatric Surgery Library, www.pedsurglibrary.com/apsa/view/Pediatric-Surgery-NaT/829066/all/Inguinal_Hernia.
3. Khan FA, Jancelewicz T, Kieran K, Islam S; Committee on Fetus and Newborn; Section on Surgery; Section on Urology. Assessment and Management of Inguinal Hernias in Children. Pediatrics. 2023;152(1):e2023062510.
4. Speck K, Smith AK. Pediatric laparoscopic inguinal hernia repair: a review of techniques. Soc Am Gastroenterol Endosc Surg. 2015;2:60–7.

Adult Inguinal Hernias

31

Hamza Nasir Chatha, Joshua L. Lyons, and Mazen R. Al-Mansour

31.1 Introduction

An inguinal hernia is a groin bulge that usually presents when an organ (e.g., intestines, bladder) or pre-peritoneal fat protrudes through a groin fascial defect. Generally, groin hernias can be divided into three categories based on their location: indirect inguinal, direct inguinal, or femoral hernias. Patients most commonly present with an inguinal hernia that can either be symptomatic or asymptomatic. Based on each patient's presentation, treatment can range from clinical observation to operative repair.

Inguinal hernias are the most common hernia type accounting for 75% of all abdominal wall hernias. The overall lifetime risk is 27% in men compared to 3% in women. 95% of patients presenting to primary care physicians are male. On the other hand, femoral hernias are more common in women, but women with a clinical groin hernia are still 5 times more likely to have an inguinal hernia than a femoral hernia.

H. N. Chatha · J. L. Lyons
University Hospitals, Cleveland, OH, USA

M. R. Al-Mansour (✉)
University of Florida, Gainesville, FL, USA
e-mail: mazen.al-mansour@surgery.ufl.edu

G. P. Kohn et al. (eds.), *The SAGES Manual of Surgical Referral for Primary and Emergency Care*,
https://doi.org/10.1007/978-3-031-92678-5_31

31.2 Etiology and Important Anatomical Landmarks

Generally, inguinal hernias present with a groin bulge above the inguinal ligament and femoral hernia below the inguinal ligament, but this subtlety is difficult to appreciate on a clinical exam because the inguinal ligament is difficult to visualize except in very thin patients (Fig. 31.1). Direct and indirect inguinal hernias differ in the location of the fascial defect. Clinical exam is not reliable in distinguishing direct from indirect hernias. However, the distinction between direct and indirect hernias is of little clinical significance since the approach of management and workup is the same. Oftentimes, a femoral hernia can be palpated inferior and lateral to the pubic tubercle, which can serve as an aid during the clinical exam.

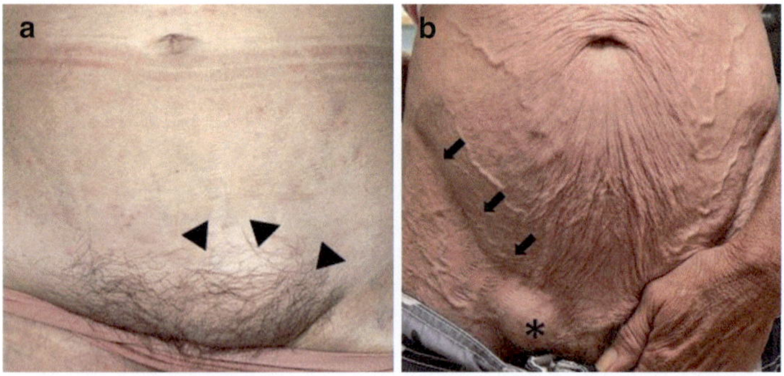

Fig. 31.1 (**a**) Female with left inguinal hernia (arrow heads). (**b**) Female with right femoral hernia (asterisk); arrows show visible inguinal ligament

31.3 Clinical Presentation

Inguinal hernias usually present with a bulge in the groin that can be reduced with manual pressure (often by the patient) or when the patient lies down. In men, large inguinal hernias can extend into the scrotum. Large inguinoscrotal hernias can often become irreducible. Some patients report hearing a gurgling noise in the bulge or upon attempting to reduce the bulge. Most inguinal hernias cause mild to moderate discomfort and a sensation of pressure that can be aggravated with activity, coughing, or sneezing. Severe pain is uncommon. The pain can be characterized as a dull aching, heavy, dragging, or burning sensation. Activities that increase intra-abdominal pressure such as straining, coughing, prolonged standing, and heavy lifting can exacerbate the pain or the size of the hernia. Many patients report worsening of their symptoms at the end of the day and improvement of the symptoms when they wake up from sleep. Pain can also radiate down to the scrotum or down the thigh.

Sometimes inguinal hernias can present with complications of acute incarceration or strangulation. These complications are uncommon, with a lifetime incidence of approximately 1%. Acute incarceration refers to an acutely irreducible hernia, one that cannot be pushed in, associated with pain or bowel obstruction (severe abdominal and/or groin pain, abdominal distension, nausea, vomiting, and failure to pass flatus/stool). This can progress to strangulation, which is indicative of bowel ischemia often manifesting with overlying erythema or skin discoloration of the groin bulge, signs of sepsis, fever, and chills. The abdomen or the groin bulge may be exquisitely tender. Acute incarceration and strangulation are more likely to occur with femoral hernias (Fig. 31.2). Acute incarceration and strangulation are surgical emergencies, and patients should be referred to the emergency department without delay. A chronically incarcerated (nonreducible) hernia without severe pain is not an emergency and can be addressed on an elective basis.

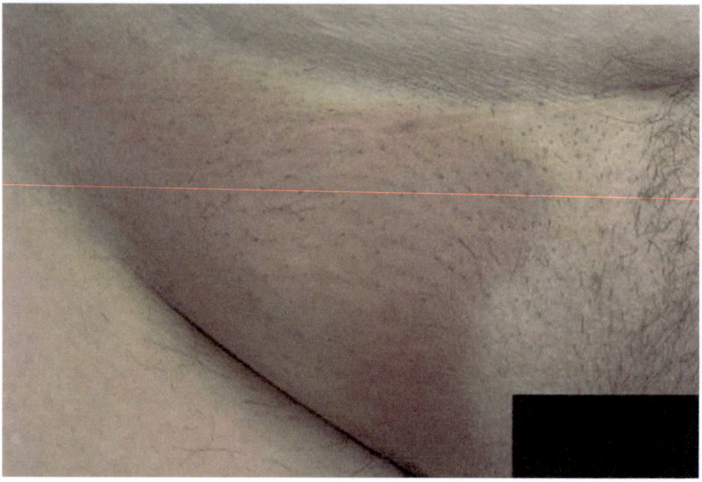

Fig. 31.2 Skin discoloration in a female patient with a strangulated femoral hernia

31.4 Clinical Workup

A proper detailed history and physical exam are necessary for the diagnosis and evaluation of an inguinal hernia. A detailed history should note the exacerbating and relieving factors and outline the symptoms of the patient. This should be followed by a thorough physical exam. The patient should be examined in a standing position with proper exposure. Standing allows a small hernia to become appreciable. Examining the patient in the supine position is important if assessing the reducibility of the bulge, which is more helpful for moderate- and large-size groin bulges. The groin area should be inspected for any visible bulges or asymmetry in the groin and scrotum. Any bulge or swelling should be noted at rest. If no obvious bulge is noted, asking the patient to perform the Valsalva maneuver or coughing may help demonstrate the bulge. Next, the groin and scrotum should be palpated to feel any masses or bulges. It is important to compare the examination of one side with the other for contrast and symmetry. Smaller hernias can present intermittently and sometimes may not be appreciable on clinical exams. If the patient reports a bulge but no bulge is detectable on exam after coughing/Valsalva, a repeat examination on a different day might be needed. A reducible groin bulge or a groin bulge with bowel sounds upon attempted reduction is diagnostic of a hernia.

When a patient presents with an inguinoscrotal bulge, the differential diagnosis includes an inguinal hernia and hydrocele. These can often be differentiated on clinical exam. Unlike a hydrocele, an inguinal hernia can be reducible, and the testicle can be palpated separate from the bulge. Gurgling (bowel) sounds can be heard during the attempted reduction of a hernia. A hydrocele, which represents fluid surrounding the testicle, makes it such that the testicle cannot be palpated on exam. Additionally, a transillumination test by shining a bright light behind the scrotum and appreciating the light shining through the fluid-filled scrotum is diagnostic of a hydrocele. If the clinical exam is not conclusive, a scrotal ultrasound is highly accurate in differentiating a hernia from a hydrocele. This distinction is important because hernias are often treated by general surgeons, while hydroceles are generally treated by urologists.

A positive history consistent with an inguinal hernia and a negative physical exam can warrant further investigation using radiological imaging. While the presence of bowel or bladder in the inguinal canal is diagnostic of a hernia, a downside of imaging is that it results in a significant false-positive rate when a fat-containing inguinal hernia is seen. This may simply represent normal fat in the spermatic cord. Therefore, we recommend that imaging only be used when the patient reports a bulge. If the patient reports groin pain without a bulge, the finding of "fat-containing inguinal hernia" should be interpreted with caution, and a search for an alternative diagnosis is warranted. Radiological modalities of choice can include computed tomography (CT), magnetic resonance imaging (MRI), and ultrasonography (USG). Dynamic groin ultrasound (performed in standing and supine positions with and without Valsalva) is our initial test of choice. A downside of ultrasound is that it is operator dependent and its accuracy depends upon the expertise of the examiner. Overall, radiological imaging has a sensitivity of 80–95% and a specificity of 65–95% in detecting hernias. MRI can be used to differentiate between musculoskeletal injuries and inguinal hernias when the chief complaint is groin pain without a bulge.

31.5 Treatment

Management of inguinal hernias is primarily dictated by the symptoms. Patients who present with minimal symptoms can be safely treated with watchful waiting. Multiple prospective trials have shown that watchful waiting for asymptomatic or minimally symptomatic inguinal hernias is associated with less than 1% risk of emergency surgery for acute incarceration or strangulation over 10 years. This is significant because in light of the risk of postop complications (particularly chronic post-herniorrhaphy groin pain and recurrence), providers and patients should understand that watchful waiting is safe and acceptable. However, these trials have also shown that nearly 70% of patients initially treated with watchful waiting crossed over to surgery over time due to symptom progression. Because femoral hernias have a high rate of acute incarceration and strangulation, watchful waiting is inappropriate for femoral hernias. Because femoral hernias are more common in females and differentiating femoral and inguinal hernias on the clinical exam is difficult, watchful waiting for groin hernias is not recommended in females and surgical repair should generally be offered.

Elective surgical repair should be offered for patients with significant symptoms and those with minimal symptoms who desire surgical repair. Minimally symptomatic chronic incarceration is not, in itself, an indication for surgery. Inguinal hernia repair can be performed either as an open (tissue or mesh-based) procedure or via a minimally invasive (laparoscopic or robotic) surgery. Patient factors play an important role in deciding the surgical approach such as overall health, comorbidities, and recurrent or bilateral hernia. The surgical approach also depends on the surgeon's practice and experience level. Patients presenting with signs of bowel obstruction or signs of strangulation require immediate surgery.

31.6 When to Refer

Male patients with an asymptomatic or minimally symptomatic inguinal hernia can be followed with watchful waiting in the primary care setting. Patients with a symptomatic inguinal hernia and those wishing to undergo surgical repair should be referred to a general surgeon on an elective basis. If the history and physical exam are equivocal, we suggest repeating the exam at a different time and/or proceeding with an imaging study (e.g., dynamic groin ultrasound, CT, or MRI) prior to referral to a surgeon. If an inguinal hernia diagnosis cannot be ruled out, then referral to a general surgeon is appropriate. All females with groin hernias should be referred to a general surgeon due to femoral hernias being quite difficult to rule out clinically and the high risk of acute incarceration or strangulation. If the patient presents with signs and symptoms of acute incarceration, bowel obstruction, or strangulation, the patient should be referred immediately to an emergency room. Figure 31.3 summarizes the clinical approach to groin bugle.

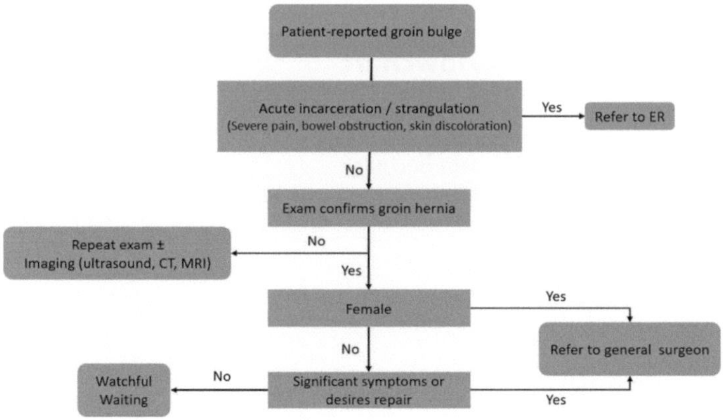

Fig. 31.3 Clinical approach to groin bulge

31.7 Groin Bulge After Hernia Repair

A groin bulge that develops after groin hernia repair is most likely to be a seroma or a recurrent hernia. Seromas represent the buildup of serous fluid at the site of surgery. Seromas are extremely common and tend to appear within 1–2 weeks of surgery. Seromas tend to be well-demarcated, firm, mobile, and nonreducible. Small- and moderate-sized seromas frequently resolve spontaneously over several months. Wearing compression garments may help in the resolution. Even a large seroma can shrink or resolve spontaneously over several months. Our approach is to follow moderate to large seromas with watchful waiting for 6–12 months postoperatively before any intervention. At that time if the seromas persist, surgical excision or drainage can be considered.

Inguinal hernia recurrence tends to present as a bulge at or near the site of a prior repair. Inguinal hernia recurrence after operative repair is seen in approximately 3% of patients. Most recurrences occur within the first 15 months of the repair. The clinical presentation, workup, and indication of surgery of a recurrent inguinal hernia are similar to that of an initial hernia.

31.8 Summary Flowchart

This flowchart summarizes the important checkpoints in workup and management of groin hernias.

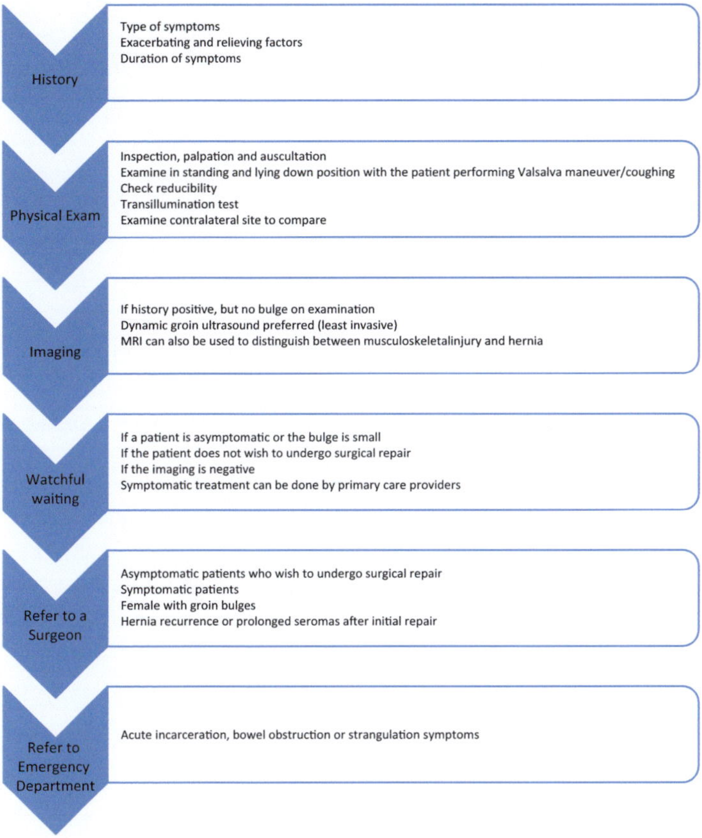

Suggested Readings

1. https://www.aafp.org/pubs/afp/issues/2020/1015/p487.html
2. https://doi.org/10.1159/000487278
3. https://link.springer.com/article/10.1007/s10029-017-1668-x

Femoral Bulge

32

Yashasvini Sampathkumar, Jalpa Patel,
and Nisha Narula

32.1 Presentation and Workup of Femoral Bulge

32.1.1 History

Despite the relatively small anatomic region, there are multiple diagnoses on the differential to consider when a patient presents with a femoral bulge or mass (Table 32.1). A full workup begins with a thorough history and careful physical exam. Some key aspects to consider when taking a history include the patient's age, baseline comorbidities, functional status, history of trauma/radiation/interventions to the groin, medical/surgical history, and family history (Table 32.2).

As we age, the femoral ring continues to expand, which makes femoral hernias more common in older patients. Malignancy is more common in older patients and those with a known cancer history or immunosuppression. A history of vascular disease makes femoral aneurysm higher on the differential. A personal history of heavy lifting, cough, straining, or other reasons for increased intra-abdominal pressure may make hernia more likely.

Y. Sampathkumar · J. Patel · N. Narula (✉)
Department of Surgery, Rutgers New Jersey Medical School,
Newark, NJ, USA

G. P. Kohn et al. (eds.), *The SAGES Manual of Surgical Referral for Primary and Emergency Care*,
https://doi.org/10.1007/978-3-031-92678-5_32

Table 32.1 Take-home points

What constitutes an emergency requiring emergency room presentation?	*Strangulated femoral hernia (signs include bulge that cannot be reduced, pain, skin changes, inability to eat or drink)* Expanding hematoma or pulsatile mass Loss of distal pulses, numbness of leg
What requires urgent surgical review?	The same clinical presentations requiring emergency room presentation would require emergent/urgent surgical evaluation upon arrival. Strangulated femoral hernia (signs include bulge that cannot be reduced, pain, skin changes, inability to eat or drink) Expanding hematoma or pulsatile mass. Loss of distal pulses, numbness of leg
What requires nonurgent surgical review?	Femoral hernia Lymphadenopathy Superficial skin pathology when infected, especially if concern for abscess Femoral artery aneurysm or pseudoaneurysm Benign or malignant mass
What features can be managed by primary care provider (as long as primary care provider is comfortable; also reasonable to refer)**?**	Superficial skin pathology DVT
What can be referred to nonsurgeon?	Superficial skin pathology—some can be referred to dermatology DVT—some may require referral to hematology, e.g., for workup of hypercoagulability disorder

Females have a higher rate than males of femoral hernia. A rapidly enlarging mass may be more concerning for malignancy or lymphadenopathy. Associated infectious symptoms would put abscess higher on the differential.

Table 32.2 Prior to surgical referral

Pathology	Tests to *consider ordering (in many instances of femoral bulge, no further testing beyond history and physical may be necessary prior to referral to a surgeon; testing may be warranted to help determine which specialty of surgeon to refer to when the diagnosis is unclear)*
Hernia	None; U/S or CT if diagnosis in doubt
Lymphadenopathy	CT if diagnosis in doubt
Superficial skin pathology	None
Vascular pathology	Duplex U/S or CTA
Benign and malignant soft tissue mass	CT or MRI

When obtaining a history about the bulge, it is important to clarify the duration of time the bulge has been present, precipitating factors, and other symptoms such as associated pain over the site or pain that radiates down the leg, fevers, chills, changes in weight, changes in diet tolerance, and obstructive symptoms (nausea, emesis, change in bowel habits, or inability to pass flatus or stool).

32.1.2 Physical Exam

A complete physical examination is one of the most critical tools in the evaluation of a femoral bulge. Some areas to focus attention on include checking for lymphadenopathy in all areas: cervical, supraclavicular, axillary, and bilateral groin nodal basins. The examiner should assess for hernias, including but not limited to ventral and umbilical hernias, incisional hernias if prior surgery has occurred, and groin hernias, which include inguinal and femoral hernias. In addition, a vascular exam should be carried out, namely assessing for abdominal aortic aneurysm and palpable pulses/bruits in the lower extremities. Attention should then be turned to careful examination of the bulge. Anatomic landmarks should be utilized. A femoral bulge refers to one that is located below the inguinal ligament. Starting with inspection of the femoral region, the examiner should look for skin changes such as ecchymosis, evidence of injury (e.g., puncture marks or skin lesions), and the presence of sanguineous or purulent drainage. These findings would be suggestive of infection. The examiner should have the patient both lie supine as well as stand up to help identify a bulge and if there are changes with movement and position. If a mass or bulge is not immediately detected, having the patient perform a Valsalva maneuver or cough can help with identification. Additionally, re-examining the patient after having them ambulate or stand for a period of time may reveal a bulge that was previously hidden. These all suggest femoral hernia. When encountered with an asymptomatic or painless bulge and a reported history consistent with a hernia, the examiner may attempt to manually reduce the bulge. This can be accomplished by laying the patient supine. One hand is placed at the proximal portion of the hernia at the fascial defect, and the second hand is placed at the distal portion of the hernia and provides steady, gentle pressure to guide the contents of the hernia back through the fascial defect and into the abdomen. Successful reduction of the contents and palpation of the defect confirms the diagnosis of a reducible femoral hernia. Sometimes a hernia cannot be reduced. If the patient endorses significant pain at the hernia site especially with an acute onset of a bulge or has signs of strangulation (e.g., skin changes over the site, a painful, hard mass on exam, nausea, vomiting, inability to pass flatus or bowel movements), then the bulge should not be reduced, and the patient should be referred to an emergency department for urgent evaluation by a minimally invasive or general surgeon. Findings of a pulsatile mass associated with a bruit on auscultation would be concerning for vascular pathology such as an aneurysm or pseudoaneurysm, which may or may not be associated with an overlying hematoma. A mass that does not change with Valsava, cough, or positioning, or one that is more solid and immobile is more concerning for a tumor, either benign or malignant, or lymphadenopathy.

Sometimes a patient has noticed a bulge, but it cannot be easily identified or further evaluated on exam. This is more common in obese patients or those who cannot participate in physical exam maneuvers. Imaging studies are not always needed for the evaluation of a femoral bulge but are more important in these clinical scenarios to aid in making the diagnosis.

32.1.3 Laboratory Evaluation

A complete blood count (CBC) with manual differential is crucial to obtain as part of the initial workup of a femoral bulge, with the white blood cell (WBC) count being the single most important lab value. High white blood cell counts can point to diagnoses of abscess or lymphoma, whereas low WBC counts (leukopenia) may prompt a further workup for conditions causing immunosuppression. HIV status is important to know particularly when lymphadenopathy, abscess, or malignancy is high on the differential, and if a patient has known HIV, a CD4 count and viral load should be obtained. A low red blood cell count (anemia) or low platelet count (thrombocytopenia) can also be helpful in evaluating for coagulopathies and to assess whether the patient is at higher risk of bleeding should a surgical intervention be warranted further down the line.

32.1.4 Imaging Studies

Not all femoral bulges need imaging for further workup, and oftentimes this is best determined by a surgeon. When considered, imaging studies such as ultrasonography (U/S), computed tomography (CT), and magnetic resonance imaging (MRI) are those that would be useful adjuncts in the diagnostic evaluation of a femoral bulge when unclear of physical exam. Ultrasound is most useful when the concern is for a vascular abnormality but also useful for hernias and lymphadenopathy. It is an affordable and expeditious test that can be used to help narrow down the diagnosis. Despite some important limitations, U/S has been proven to have a high degree of sensitivity and specificity in the detection of femoral hernias. The sensitivity of the ultrasound examination can be enhanced by having the patient perform a Valsalva maneuver, thus allowing the examiner to visualize pre-peritoneal fat or intra-abdominal viscera. Duplex ultrasonography is used to evaluate for vascular pathology as it utilizes Doppler to demonstrate flow through the vessels and can reveal the presence of aneurysms, pseudoaneurysms, false lumens, or thrombi. It is also useful in assessing for abscesses. Ultrasound, like physical examination, may yield fewer results in obese patients, and there is a high degree of variability depending on the skill of the ultrasonographer.

A CT scan is a very useful study to help further elucidate the anatomy and diagnosis and is most helpful when the diagnosis is in doubt. In addition to providing a higher quality image than an ultrasound, a CT scan is also significantly less operator-dependent compared to ultrasonography. While a noncontrast CT scan should be sufficient to identify pathology such as a hernia, lipoma, lymphadenopathy, or superficial skin mass, CT with IV contrast or CT angiography should be used when evaluating for vascular pathology such as an aneurysm/pseudoaneurysm, arteriovenous fistula, or varicosity, as long as renal function is adequate. If concerned for a bowel-containing hernia, then oral contrast can be given to better visualize the hernia contents and assess for an obstruction. Another advantage of CT is that it can often be quickly obtained at most centers at all hours and provides additional information that an ultrasound cannot provide. In practice at most institutions in the adult patient, a CT scan is often the imaging study that gives the most information. Notably, a CT scan can find no hernia when one is present as the patient is lying supine; therefore, when clinical suspicion of a femoral hernia exists, a negative CT scan cannot definitively rule out a hernia.

In the event that U/S and CT scan are both nondiagnostic, MRI of the groin can be considered. MRI offers greater tissue specificity, which can help when characterizing the origin of the bulge if thought to be soft tissue in origin or due to lymphadenopathy as well as during assessment for nerve compression. The disadvantages, however, are the increased length of exam, increased sensitivity to motion artifact, and greater associated cost of exam. It is typically not used as a first-line test.

32.2 Differential Diagnosis: Detailed Findings to Look for on Workup

32.2.1 Femoral Hernia

Femoral hernias usually present as a bulge below the inguinal ligament. They have a higher incidence in women than men but are a relatively uncommon type of hernia. However, the finding and diagnosis of a femoral hernia represent a condition that requires consultation by a surgeon and subsequent repair as they have a significant risk of incarceration. While a femoral hernia can certainly present as groin pain or bulge, it is important to note that groin hernias are not always symptomatic. One-third of patients report no symptoms. Typically, the hernias only become extremely painful and tender once they are incarcerated or strangulated. In addition to a painful femoral bulge, incarcerated bowel-containing femoral hernias would also be associated with obstructive symptoms such as nausea, vomiting, abdominal pain, and failure to pass flatus or bowel movements. Strangulation, which refers to vascular compromise to the hernia contents, results due to obstruction of arterial blood flow and is seen more commonly in femoral hernias versus inguinal hernias due to the smaller neck of the hernia. Pain related to a femoral hernia may occasionally present as chronic pelvic pain in some patients. Of note, femoral hernias can occur concomitantly in patients with inguinal hernias, so it is always important to perform a close physical exam and assess for the presence of multiple masses both above and below the inguinal ligament. The presence of a reducible mass on physical exam is suspicious enough for a hernia and can merit referral to a surgeon. No further imaging is needed beforehand. If the diagnosis is uncertain (e.g., physical exam is unreliable), then depending on the suspected diagnosis, an ultrasound and/or CT scan can be obtained beforehand to help confirm the diagnosis prior to referral to a surgeon to determine which specialty to refer to. However, in most cases, the referral to a surgeon can be made and the specific imaging test, if needed, can be determined at that time. If obtained, ultrasonography would demonstrate a mass lesion inferior to the inguinal ligament and medial to the femoral vein that protrudes with a Valsalva maneuver. On CT scans, the most sensitive and specific finding for femoral hernias is compression of the femoral vein, which may also lead to a secondary finding of dilation of the distal femoral vein and its collaterals. If a femoral hernia is not operated on, no specific surveillance is required, but patients should be counseled that if they develop pain/tenderness at the hernia, skin changes, inability to eat, or other concerning findings for strangulation, they need to go to the emergency room.

32.2.2 Femoral Lymphadenopathy

Lymphadenopathy of the groin can present as a soft, palpable, nonreducible mass. The history should be reviewed to assess for B symptoms, history of radiation exposure, and family history of malignancy. Additional lymph node basins should also be examined to differentiate between a generalized and localized process. Localized femoral lymphadenopathy may represent a benign pathology, metastatic disease, or a lymphoma and should be promptly further evaluated to form a final diagnosis. Ultrasound, CT, or MRI is particularly useful here. Typically, a biopsy in the form of a fine needle aspirate, core needle biopsy, or incisional or excisional biopsy may be required after evaluation by a surgeon. Lymphadenopathy requires further workup, and surveillance alone without a diagnosis would not be appropriate.

32.2.3 Superficial Skin Pathology

Skin pathology can be seen extending beyond the borders of the femoral canal and also involving the upper thigh or lower abdomen. In the case of an abscess or infected epidermal inclusion cyst, skin changes such as superficial tenderness, erythema, fluctuance, a central punctum, and purulent drainage can be observed. In patients with hidradenitis suppurativa, the presentation may vary from an isolated abscess to abscesses associated with deep scarring and sinus tracts. Folliculitis appears as multiple small, inflamed pustules and papules in a hair-bearing region. For a diagnosed superficial skin pathology, after treatment, clinical surveillance is likely enough; no further workup would be needed unless further clinical problems arise for the patient.

32.2.4 Vascular Pathology

Femoral artery aneurysms can present as pulsatile masses in the groin. The majority are asymptomatic on presentation, but some patients may have pain due to nerve compression. If there is a suspicion of a femoral artery aneurysm, then a full vascular pulse exam should be carried out as concomitant aneurysms are not uncommon. Duplex ultrasonography and CT angiography can be used as adjuncts to help confirm the diagnosis and aid in the identification of concomitant aneurysms. Femoral artery pseudoaneurysms are more common than true aneurysms, and they are associated with a history of percutaneous instrumentation, penetrating trauma to the lower extremities, or, in rare cases, from treatment of slipped capital femoral epiphysis. Pseudoaneurysms present as painful, pulsatile masses with associated bruits. They can be distinguished from true aneurysms based on history and imaging. In cases where there is an acquired arteriovenous fistula, there will be a continuous bruit and the patient may start having new-onset or worsening symptoms of lower extremity claudication or edema. Pseudoaneurysms may also be associated with a hematoma, which can be distinguished on ultrasonography. In regards to venous pathology, a deep vein thrombosis (DVT) in the femoral vein can also cause pain and swelling of the groin. Typically, these will cause swelling of the entire lower extremity. Femoral DVTs should be suspected in patients who recently underwent surgery, are bed-bound, have a history of cancer, coagulopathy, or trauma to the leg. Saphena varix, which is due to valvular incompetence, can also result in a reducible mass at the groin that swells with standing or Valsalva and reduces with lying flat. Duplex ultrasonography can be utilized to help delineate these vascular pathologies. Specific treatments depend on the vascular pathology identified. For those that do not require intervention, duplex ultrasound or CTA may be indicated but frequency depends on the specific diagnosis and will be best determined by a vascular surgeon.

32.2.5 Benign and Malignant Femoral Masses

Soft tissue tumors may occasionally present in the groin or thigh as a femoral bulge. The most common is a lipoma. Lipomas are benign fatty tumors that can present as symptomatic or asymptomatic masses. They are mobile, soft, and well circumscribed. Rarely they may undergo malignant transformation or present as a liposarcoma, a type of soft tissue sarcoma. Femoral bulges may also be the first sign of malignancy in some patients by presenting with a firm or soft nodular mass in the area representing lymphadenopathy related to metastatic disease, primary lymphoma, or malignant soft tissue disease such as sarcoma. Workup includes imaging and referral to a surgeon for possible biopsy. Either CT or MRI is appropriate but can be done after referral to a surgeon. After treatment, no surveillance of a benign mass is typically required. For a malignant mass, further surveillance may include clinical exam, CT, and/or MRI but will depend on the specific final pathology.

32.3 Conclusion: When to Refer to a Surgeon

Most femoral bulges should be referred to a surgeon given the above differential diagnosis (Table 32.1). Ideally, this occurs after the appropriate workup is completed, but given that many of the diagnoses require expeditious evaluation and treatment, it is better to refer first, especially if a complete workup with imaging will delay evaluation by a surgeon (Table 32.2). If the concern is for a femoral hernia, the patient should be referred to a general or minimally invasive surgeon for elective repair even if they are asymptomatic. This is due to the increased risk of incarceration and strangulation that exists with femoral hernias; it is higher than with inguinal hernias. Patients with lipomas and abscesses can also be referred to a general surgeon for excision or drainage, respectively. In the case of femoral lymphadenopathy or a soft tissue mass concerning for malignancy, referral to a general surgeon or surgical oncologist is warranted. Finally, if the bulge appears to be due to a vascular pathology, then referral should be made to a vascular surgeon. Children with findings of a femoral bulge or mass should be referred to a pediatric surgeon for further evaluation, though some general surgeons take care of pediatric patients.

Suggested Readings

1. International guidelines for groin hernia management. Hernia. 2018;22(1):1–165. https://doi.org/10.1007/s10029-017-1668-x.
2. Arenal JJ, Rodríguez-Vielba P, Gallo E, Tinoco C. Hernias of the abdominal wall in patients over the age of 70 years. Eur J Surg. 2002;168(8–9):460–3. https://doi.org/10.1080/110241502321116451.
3. Aurshina A, Ascher E, Hingorani A, Salles-Cunha SX, Marks N, Iadgarova E. Clinical role of the "venous" ultrasound to identify lower extremity pathology. Ann Vasc Surg. 2017;38:274–8. https://doi.org/10.1016/j.avsg.2016.05.113.
4. Bradley M, Morgan D, Pentlow B, Roe A. The groin hernia—an ultrasound diagnosis? Ann R Coll Surg Engl. 2003;85(3):178–80. https://doi.org/10.1308/003588403321661334.

Rectal Prolapse

33

Aditi Mishra, Nicholas Bartschat,
and Imran Hassan

33.1 Introduction

Rectal prolapse or rectal procidentia is the full thickness prolapse of the rectum, in which all layers of the rectal wall pass externally out through the anal canal beyond the internal and external sphincter complex. [1, 2] When this happens, it may spontaneously reduce or stay prolapsed and require manual reduction. In rare situations, it may not be reducible due to tissue edema and become ischemic.

This is an uncommon condition estimated to occur in less than 0.5% of the population, with a 9:1 female predominance [3]. While occasionally seen in younger patients, the incidence increases with age, with the peak incidence being in the seventh and eighth decades of life. Associated risk factors in younger patients include psychiatric conditions, developmental disorders, and substance abuse. Multiparity has not been found to be a risk factor.

A. Mishra · N. Bartschat · I. Hassan (✉)
Department of Surgery, University of Iowa, Iowa City, IA, USA

G. P. Kohn et al. (eds.), *The SAGES Manual of Surgical Referral for Primary and Emergency Care*,
https://doi.org/10.1007/978-3-031-92678-5_33

33.2 Presentation

The diagnosis of rectal prolapse can be made based on history and physical examination [4]. Patients generally report a prolapsing sensation or feel actual tissue coming out when they are having a bowel movement. In more advanced cases, they may report this happening without having a bowel movement or when they are standing up or walking. In taking a history, it is important to differentiate if the patient is experiencing an actual prolapse coming out of the rectum or bulging into the vagina, which would be more consistent with a rectocele.

Patients with full-thickness rectal prolapse will describe how they sense or feel tissue prolapsing out from the anus and whether it spontaneously reduces or stays out and has to be manually pushed back in. Associated symptoms include a pelvic fullness and tenesmus. Most patients also report rectal bleeding from ulceration or irritation of the rectal mucosa. If the rectum stays prolapsed, patients will report pain, mucous discharge, and fecal soilage. Fecal incontinence is generally present and can range from minimal soiling to gross loss of feces.

On physical exam, the classic finding is that of the rectum protruding from the anus with concentric folds visible (Fig. 33.1). The length of prolapse tissue can vary from 1 to 2 inches to several inches and is covered by healthy-appearing rectal mucosa. In patients with chronic prolapse, the tissue may appear excoriated or ulcerated from external trauma (Fig. 33.2).

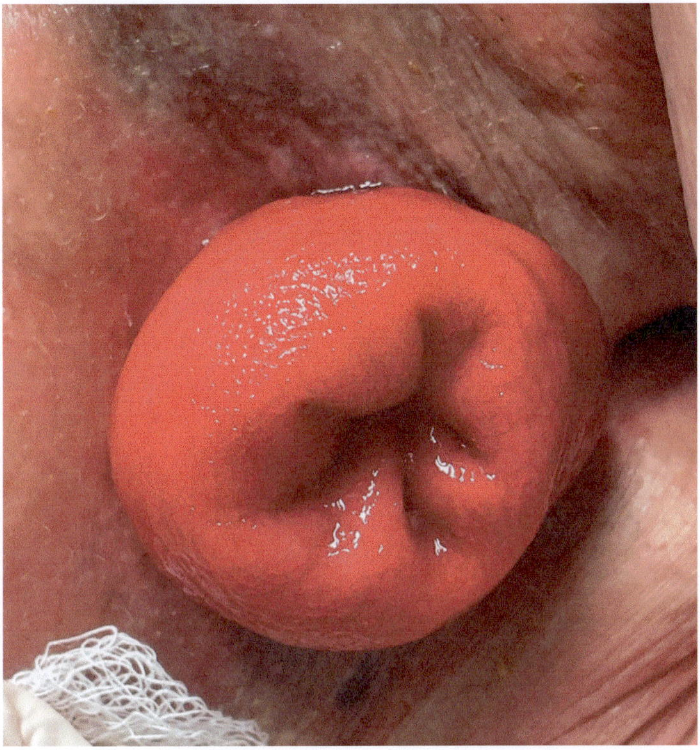

Fig. 33.1 Rectal prolapse

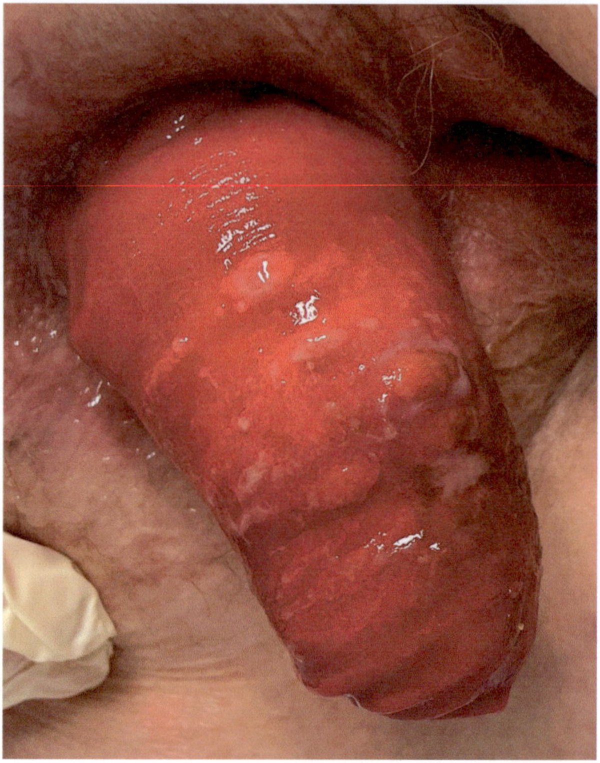

Fig. 33.2 Chronic rectal prolapse

33.3 Differential Diagnosis

Rectal prolapse should be distinguished from other anorectal pathologies such as a thrombosed external hemorrhoid, prolapsed internal hemorrhoids, or a rectal mass such as a prolapsed rectal polyp [5].

Prolapsed internal hemorrhoids represent mucosal prolapse, in which the muscular wall of the rectum remains in place. This can be differentiated from rectal prolapse by the fact that the tissue prolapses in columns corresponding to the anatomic hemorrhoidal columns, (Fig. 33.3) with grooves visible between the columns of tissue, compared to concentric folds that are seen in rectal prolapse. Prolapsed hemorrhoids may be spontaneously reducible or be strangulated and not be reducible.

Thrombosed external hemorrhoids usually present acutely but can be confused with rectal prolapse if they appear circumferential. However, external hemorrhoids are covered by skin and usually are exquisitely tender to touch (Fig. 33.4). A rectal mass such as a pedunculated rectal polyp may prolapse out of the rectum intermittently. These lesions will also be covered by rectal mucosa but will be seen coming through the anus and will not have the concentric appearance of a prolapse (Fig. 33.5).

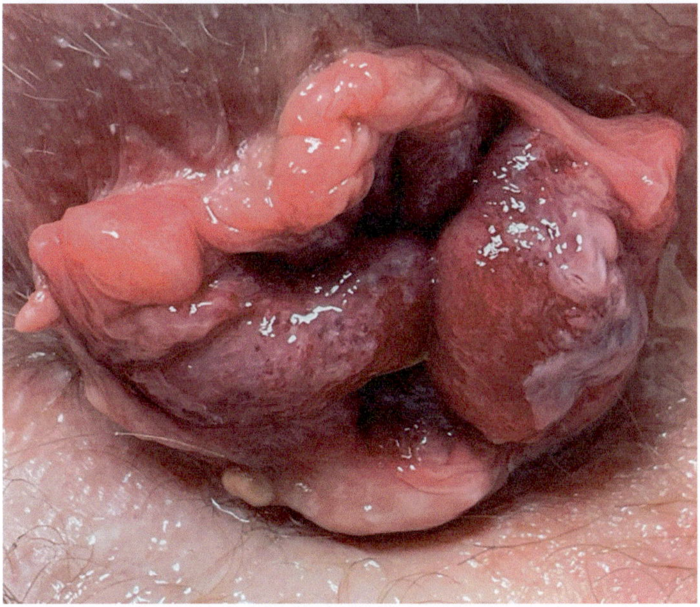

Fig. 33.3 Prolapsed internal hemorrhoid

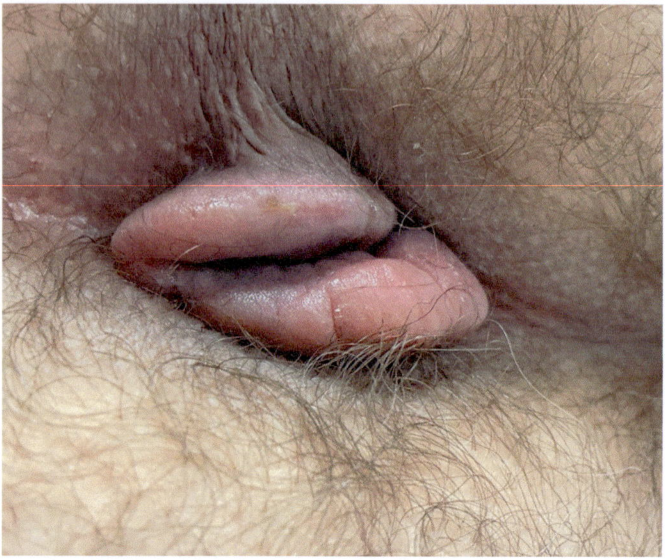

Fig. 33.4 Thombosed external hemorrhoid

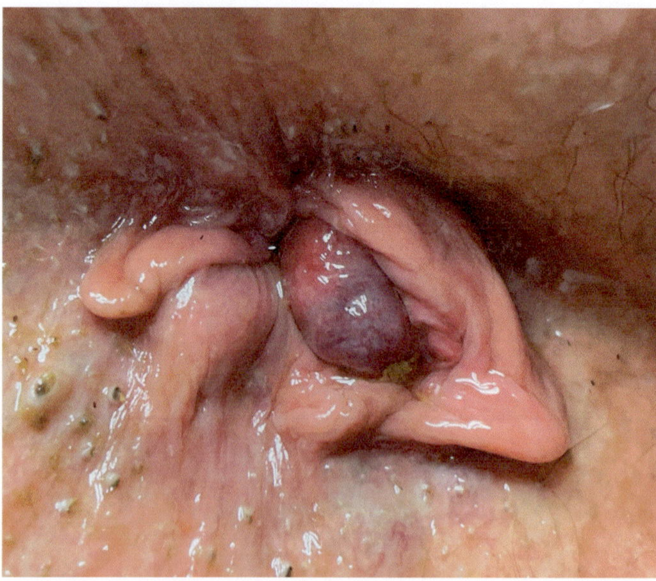

Fig. 33.5 Prolapsed polyp

33.4 Diagnosis

The diagnosis of a rectal prolapse can usually be made in the office based on the reported history and physical exam [4]. When examining the patient in the lateral decubitus position, if the patient is asked to bear down or Valsalva, the prolapse can be reproduced and visualized. In addition to identifying the rectal prolapse on physical exam, a digital rectal exam should be done to assess for any masses and assess sphincter tone. In patients with long-standing rectal prolapse, the anal sphincter complex is chronically stretched and appears patulous or with a diminished tone. Occasionally, an early prolapse will not be completely circumferential, but can be distinguished from hemorrhoids based on the lack of groves between columns of the prolapsing tissue [1]. In situations in which patients are unable to reproduce the prolapse on exam in the lateral decubitus position, they can be asked to sit on the commode and strain to reproduce the prolapse. In the current times of smartphones, a number of patients will present with a photograph on the phone to help in the diagnosis.

33.5 Management

In most patients presenting with rectal prolapse, the prolapsing tissue is reducible, and once a diagnosis is made, they can be referred to a surgical specialist for further workup and discussion for treatment (Table 33.1). In a small subset of patients, the prolapse is not reducible as the rectal mucosa becomes edematous and congested and cannot reduce itself leading to continued patient discomfort and pain. This represents an emergency and requires immediate referral; however, temporizing measures such as covering the prolapse with sugar to draw out the tissue fluids and decrease the congestion in order to allow the prolapse to reduce can be very effective. In extreme situations, the prolapsed tissue can become ischemic, and the tissue will appear dark and dusky with an ischemic appearance. This represents a surgical emergency and warrants prompt surgical referral and evaluation.

Table 33.1 Guidelines for referral

When the rectal prolapse is not reducible or there are signs of ischemia, an immediate surgical evaluation is needed
If the rectal prolapse is reducible, an elective outpatient referral can be made
In patients without symptoms or who do not want to have surgery, rectal prolapse can be managed nonoperatively

References and Suggested Reading

1. Cannon JA. Evaluation, diagnosis, and medical management of rectal prolapse. Clin Colon Rectal Surg. 2017;30(1):16–21. https://doi.org/10.1055/s-0036-1593431.
2. Oruc M, Erol T. Current diagnostic tools and treatment modalities for rectal prolapse. World J Clin Cases. 2023;11(16):3680–93. https://doi.org/10.12998/wjcc.v11.i16.3680.
3. Lohsiriwat V. Anorectal emergencies. World J Gastroenterol. 2016;22(26):5867–78. https://doi.org/10.3748/wjg.v22.i26.5867.
4. Bordeianou L, Paquette I, Johnson E, et al. Clinical practice guidelines for the treatment of rectal prolapse. Dis Colon Rectum. 2017;60(11):1121–31. https://doi.org/10.1097/DCR.0000000000000889.
5. Kwakye G, Maguire LH. Anorectal physiology testing for prolapse-what tests are necessary? Clin Colon Rectal Surg. 2021;34(1):15–21. https://doi.org/10.1055/s-0040-1714246.

34 Hemorrhoids

Pramod Nepal and Andreas M. Kaiser

34.1 Introduction

In all regions of the world, symptomatic hemorrhoids are a major health problem. In the United States, hemorrhoids have a prevalence rate of 4.4%, with a peak age between 45 and 65 years, of which one-third will seek medical treatment. However, patients and some nonspecialist physicians tend to attribute any anorectal symptoms to hemorrhoids without due symptom analysis and physical assessment. Understanding the anatomy of the anorectal region and of hemorrhoids is essential to choose the appropriate management. "Hemorrhoidal cushions," located in the right anterior, right posterior, and left lateral position, are a normal component of the anal anatomy and contribute to the physiological continence mechanism. In contrast, hemorrhoids represent a pathological engorgement of the submucosal vascular plexus—comparable to varicose veins. They develop as a result of disintegration of connective tissues, venous dilation, and local inflammatory

P. Nepal
Beth Israel Deaconess Medical Center, Harvard Medical School, Boston, MA, USA

A. M. Kaiser (✉)
City of Hope National Medical Center, Duarte, CA, USA
e-mail: akaiser@coh.org

G. P. Kohn et al. (eds.), *The SAGES Manual of Surgical Referral for Primary and Emergency Care*,
https://doi.org/10.1007/978-3-031-92678-5_34

reaction. Apart from a likely constitutional predisposition and age, extrinsic factors such as low-fiber dietary intake, chronic constipation, excessive straining, prolonged sitting, and pregnancy may contribute to the onset of hemorrhoidal pathology.

34.2 Classification

In classifying hemorrhoids, the most important distinction to be made is separating internal hemorrhoids from external hemorrhoids. Internal hemorrhoids originate from the vascular plexus proximal to the dentate line, are covered with a glossy transitional and columnar mucosa, and have comparably little pain innervation. The grading system only applies to internal hemorrhoids. However, a great number of patients present with a picture of mixed hemorrhoids, that is, a combination of internal and external components, which are best treated for whatever component predominates.

External "hemorrhoids" or anal skin tags are located distal to the dentate line, are covered by squamous, that is, skin-type epithelium, and have a very dense pain innervation.

Recognition and application of this distinction avoid many misdiagnoses, set the basis for the majority of clinical differential diagnoses, and clarify the pathways of decision-making.

The second most important aspect for classification is the question whether any concerning "increase" of anal tissue is always present at the same location or dynamically changes its position by intermittently prolapsing and reducing either spontaneously or by manual manipulation. The former suggests an external pathology, whereas the latter hints at an internal source.

34.3 Differential Diagnosis of "Hemorrhoids"

Hemorrhoids in a strict sense are well-defined anatomical entities. Since the term hemorrhoids is used by patients in a completely nonspecific way, a wide range of differential diagnosis will need to be considered (Table 34.1). The healthcare provider should merge the patient's narrative with likely and possible differential diagnoses in order to formulate a working diagnosis, pending confirmation by the subsequent physical exam.

Table 34.1 Differential diagnosis for reported "hemorrhoids symptoms"

Symptom	DDx
Bleeding	Internal hemorrhoids Rectal prolapse Tumor (anal, rectal, colon) Proctitis/colitis Rectal varices Dieulafoy ulcer of the rectum Anal fissure Ruptured thrombosed external hemorrhoid
Itching	Anal fissure Anal pruritus Anal irritation Skin pathology: Psoriasis, lichen, extramammary Paget disease, AIN/Bowen disease, etc.
Dynamic protrusion	Internal hemorrhoids grade II/III Chronically protruding internal hemorrhoids grade IV (low sphincter tone) Rectal prolapse
Fixed protrusion	Incarcerated internal hemorrhoids grade IV (high sphincter tone) External hemorrhoids Skin tags Tumor Condylomata Secondary fistula opening
Pain	Anal fissure Thrombosed external hemorrhoid Acute incarcerated internal hemorrhoids (grade IV) Perirectal abscess Distal rectal cancer
Drainage	Perirectal abscess Perirectal fistula Rectal adenoma/tumor

34.4 Symptom Analysis

(a) Internal Hemorrhoids

Engorgement of the internal hemorrhoidal plexus leads to the two most common symptoms, that is, bleeding and prolapse. Both are typically painless. Bleeding is typically bright red in color and shows on the toilet paper only or by dripping at the end of bowel movements. Pain, discomfort, or itching is often thought to be caused by hemorrhoids but objectively is more frequently the result of other conditions that are in the differential diagnosis (Tables 34.2 and 34.3). Internal hemorrhoids are only painful when they are prolapsed and cannot be reduced. These incarcerated or grade IV internal hemorrhoids become strangulated by the tightness of the sphincter tone. The pain in this situation is the result of a combination of venous congestion, possible secondary thrombosis, and the sphincter spasticity itself.

(b) External Hemorrhoids

External hemorrhoids (with at least some vascular elements) and skin tags (without vascular component) are typically innocent bystanders (Table 34.4). If large, they may on occasion interfere with maintaining hygiene in the area. If there is pain, it is typically associated with either an acute perianal thrombosis (aka thrombosed hemorrhoid) or a chronic anal fissure hiding underneath and causing some inflammation of the tag.

Table 34.2 Descriptive clinical parameters for hemorrhoids

Grade of prolapse of internal hemorrhoids	
	I No prolapse
	II prolapse, spontaneous reduction
	III prolapse, manual reduction
	IV incarcerated prolapse, reduction impossible
Axial location	
	Internal covered by mucosa
	External covered by skin
	Mixed
Radial location	
	1 pile
	2 piles
	3 piles
	Circumferential
Complications	
	Active bleeding
	Thrombosis, acute (<72 h post onset)
	Thrombosis, subacute to chronic (>72 h post onset)
	Ulceration
	Necrosis/gangrene
Treatment modifiers	
	Pregnancy
	Immunosuppression
	Inflammatory bowel disease
	Liver disease Post radiation

Table 34.3 Internal hemorrhoids: presentation and management

Grade	Description (covered with mucosa)	Symptoms	Treatment options
I	Bulging into anal canal	Painless bleeding	Diet Local and general drugs Rubber band ligation Infrared coagulation Sclerotherapy
II	Protrude out of anal canal with bowel movements; reduce spontaneously	Painless bleeding, swelling	Rubber band ligation Infrared coagulation Sclerotherapy (PPH/stapled hemorrhoidectomy)
III	Protrude and require manual reduction	Above plus possible strangulation	Rubber band ligation PPH/stapled hemorrhoidectomy excisional hemorrhoidectomy
IV	Constant protrusion; irreducible	Above plus high risk of strangulation with pain, necrosis, sepsis	Excisional hemorrhoidectomy (PPH/stapled hemorrhoidectomy)

Table 34.4 External and mixed internal/external hemorrhoids

	Description	Symptoms	Treatment options
External hemorrhoids	Skin-covered protrusions	Discomfort, itching Severe pain if thrombosed	Symptomatic conservative treatment Excisional hemorrhoidectomy
Mixed hemorrhoids	Internal and external components	According to the predominant component	Excisional hemorrhoidectomy PPH/stapled hemorrhoidectomy

34.5 Clinical Examination

The diagnosis of hemorrhoids is a clinical one. Determining whether the presence of hemorrhoids represents the source of the patient's actual problem or rather innocent bystanders entails translating the information from the history into a working diagnosis and performing a clinical examination.

Appropriate hemorrhoid management depends on (1) a correct clinical diagnosis and association with the patient's complaints, (2) the patient's type and severity of symptoms, and (3) the grade, extent, and location of the hemorrhoid at the time of presentation. After the history-taking, the physical exam aims at corroborating the working hypothesis.

Descriptive clinical parameters for hemorrhoids (Table 34.2) should include the extent of prolapse (grades I–IV), the axial location with regard to the dentate line (internal, external, mixed), the radial location and extent in 1–3 of the hemorrhoidal piles, and the presence or absence of complications such as thrombosis, necrosis, ulceration, and active bleeding. Additional modifiers that should be taken into consideration before initiating a treatment are pregnancy, HIV infection, inflammatory bowel disease, and liver disease.

34.6 Due Diligence

Imaging or blood work is not needed except in very rare situations of dramatic blood loss or signs of perineal sepsis. In the overall workup and management of rectal bleeding and other anorectal symptoms, however, it is of vital importance to avoid a tip-of-the-iceberg approach and prematurely assign symptoms to hemorrhoids while missing a critical more proximal pathology (such as a colorectal cancer). It is therefore mandatory to rule out relevant differential diagnoses, specifically colorectal malignancy, anal cancer, or melanoma, and to distinguish a hemorrhoidal prolapse (radial pattern) from a rectal prolapse (circumferential pattern).

A visual evaluation beyond the blind digital rectal exam is strongly advised in every patient. The tools include endoscopic procedures (flexible sigmoidoscopy, full colonoscopy) or radiological studies (CT colonography, contrast enema). The type and extent of such a diagnostic colonic evaluation do not relate to the screening age of asymptomatic individuals, which is currently set at 45. It should be individually risk-stratified depending on the patient's age, familial risk factors, and the symptom evolution, as well as with published guidelines. In some cardiac patients, endocarditis prophylaxis may be necessary.

34.7 Management Overview

The first assessment should decide whether there is an acute or a chronic symptomatology and whether there is a need for an urgent intervention, general counseling, or elective specialist management. The majority of treatment recommendations for hemorrhoids are not urgent and potentially do not need anything more than reassurance. The specifics depend on a patient's individual constellation of symptoms, objective findings, and expectations, rather than on a well-defined matrix. Pillars consist of (1) conservative (nonoperative) treatments (dietary/lifestyle modification, topical treatment), (2) office interventions, and (3) surgical procedures.

Urgent action is needed for

1. Incarcerated internal hemorrhoids, particularly if tissue necrosis is present
2. Acute thrombosed external hemorrhoids, particularly within the first 72 h post onset
3. Nonrelenting bleeding
4. Perirectal suppurations (acute/chronic abscess)
5. Necrotizing soft tissue infections

Furthermore, primary or emergency care physicians may encounter a patient with an immediate recent history of a hemorrhoid or other anorectal surgery who present with

(a) Acute bleeding
(b) Infection and possible perineal sepsis
(c) Constipation
(d) Pain

Other symptomatologies are of elective nature and warrant a referral to a colorectal specialist.

Treatment of internal hemorrhoids is generally geared toward their clinical grade of prolapse (Table 34.3), with individual modifications as needed. External hemorrhoids and skin tags in the absence of thrombosis—medically speaking—do not need to be treated unless the patient desires for cosmetic or hygiene reasons (Table 34.4). Conservative management and office interventions such as banding, infrared coagulation, and sclerotherapy tend to be most successful when applied to relatively small internal hemorrhoids (grades I/II, some grade III). Surgical hemorrhoidectomy, on the other hand, is appropriate for larger, prolapsing, or incarcerated hemorrhoids, as well as for those patients who do not sufficiently respond to nonsurgical treatments. Advances in surgical techniques and pharmacological treatment options have helped correct the negative connotations associated with a surgical hemorrhoidectomy.

1. Avoidance of Overtreatment

Recognizing that (a) only a fraction of "hemorrhoid" symptoms is truly caused by hemorrhoids and (b) many common remedies lack systematic study, it is easily understandable why treatments fail to provide relief. Patients have a low threshold to self-dispense over-the-counter medications for "hemorrhoids," particularly vasoconstrictants, anesthetics, petroleum-based ointments, vitamin or antibiotic ointments, and many more. Unfortunately, nonspecialist healthcare providers not infrequently perpetuate these layman approaches based on an incorrect assessment and a rapid prescription of poorly selected treatments. All of these choices are among the most frequent sources of secondary anorectal pathology. Topical steroids and local anesthetics are among the most frequently dispensed approaches but lack any documented benefit. In reality, they not only fail to address the problem but may in fact worsen it by contributing to chronic thinning of the skin (steroids) or triggering severe contact dermatitis (topical anesthetics).

2. Conservative (Nonoperative) Treatments

Conservative/medical management is the care foundation for all patients with anorectal pathologies or complaints, even if an interventional approach may be needed, or in the postoperative period. In contrast to the prior paragraph, however, appropriately selected conservative treatment options have an excellent track record and may not only address and improve the specific symptoms but often allow avoidance of more invasive interventions, particularly in patients with minor symptoms and relatively small internal hemorrhoids.

These recommendations include optimized stool management by a generally increased daily fluid consumption and enhancing the diet with fluid-saturated high-fiber supplementation. Natural stool optimizers (prunes, dates, figs), pharmacological stool softeners (docusate), or a mild laxatives (e.g., milk of magnesia) may temporarily be used with the goal of achieving a soft-formed stool (4 on a Bristol stool scale).

Overzealous hygiene may be counterproductive. But additional symptomatic relief may result from warm sitzbaths (scheduled and/or after bowel movements) and application of topical barrier creams (zinc oxide based, potentially with menthol enhancement).

Pain management is important when pain is a major complaint. Prior to pulling out the prescription pad, however, a careful root cause analysis should determine whether the pain would better be addressed by a procedure (thrombosed hemorrhoid, incarcerated hemorrhoids, abscess). Furthermore, the components of pain generation will need to be taken into consideration, for example, thrombosis, open wound, infection, constipation, levator ani spasm, functional anorectal pain. Pharmacological pain relief relies on different drug classes including NSAIDS, opiates, neurolytics (e.g., gabapentin), or muscle relaxants (e.g., hyoscyamine, calcium channel blockers, nitroglycerin), whereas topical anesthetics should largely be avoided outside of immediate interventions.

3. Interventional Management for Hemorrhoids

While primary care or emergency room physicians are not typically expected to perform major surgical interventions, it is important to understand options to provide guidance about respective referrals to the on-call surgeon or colorectal specialists. As a general philosophy, very acute presentations need urgent or emergency management versus chronic symptoms are best handled by appropriate assessment and targeted referral to a colorectal surgeon.

(A) Acute Interventions

The two true indications for acute surgical intervention for hemorrhoids entail a thrombosed external hemorrhoid within 72 h post onset and incarcerated grade 4 internal hemorrhoids. Both conditions are associated with significant pain. It is extremely important to distinguish the two as the former may benefit from a lancing and evacuation of the blood clot with local anesthesia, whereas the same approach would carry a high risk of massive bleeding if incorrectly chosen for the incarcerated internal hemorrhoids.

In the absence of any tissue necrosis, incarcerated internal hemorrhoids (with or without an external component) may benefit from an attempt to reduce them. Successful reduction allows for conversion of an acute emergency into a (semi-)elective condition. It may be beneficial to reduce the hemorrhoidal edema by application of topical granular sugar for 15–20 min prior to attempting a reduction maneuver. Occasionally, a pudendal nerve block with injection of a local anesthetic into the ischioanal fossa facilitates a reduction effort by reducing the pain and the sphincter tone but the injection in itself may in the beginning cause pain. The manual reduction requires gentle but persistent concentric pressure of all 5 fingers on the exteriorized hemorrhoidal tissue and ultimately will need to be followed by a push upward/inward. If successful, the patient may frequently feel an immediate relief of pain. Unfortunately, the chronic congestion of the tissue is associated with a high propensity of recurrent prolapse until the edema has resolved. An external pressure dressing in the form of a roll of gauze taped into the anal verge between the two buttocks may help reduce that re-prolapsing.

If there is tissue necrosis or failure to manually reduce the prolapsing tissue, the surgeon on-call should be immediately consulted for a surgical intervention. The surgical approach of choice is an excisional hemorrhoidectomy *(see below)* with removal of the thrombosed and necrotic tissues. A stapled hemorrhoidectomy—the increasingly preferred approach for elective surgical management of internal hemorrhoids—is not typically advisable in urgent or emergency circumstances as the swollen and thrombosed components are not well and precisely enough addressed.

(B) Elective Interventions

Office Procedures

Once internal hemorrhoids increase in size, they start protruding from the anal canal, become irritated, and more friable. This results in more substantial, mostly bright red bleeding episodes, aggravated by congestion during prolapse. Treatment aims at reversing these symptoms by reducing the amount of redundant tissue able to prolapse. Rubber band ligation, injection sclerotherapy, and infrared coagulation have been the mainstays of office treatment for many years and continue to provide excellent results for grades I and II, potentially grade III hemorrhoids. External hemorrhoids are not appropriate targets for banding or other non-excisional therapies.

Sclerotherapy reduces the bulk of the engorged hemorrhoidal plexus but does not eliminate the tissue. The treatment is easy and quick, but typically repeated injections are required for continued relief. Infrared coagulation is an office technique in which the infrared heating device is placed at the base of each hemorrhoidal bundle and delivers energy, causing the dilated veins to coagulate and thrombose. Rubber band ligation is simple, extremely cheap, and generally very well tolerated, does not require major infrastructure or equipment, and has shown an effectiveness of 90–70% in grade I–III internal hemorrhoids in controlling bleeding and symptomatic prolapse.

Other Nonexcisional Internal Hemorrhoid Procedures

Engorged internal hemorrhoids have both a vascular and a laxity component. A transanal hemorrhoid dearterialization, often combined with a hemorrhoidopexy, represents an intermediate intervention beyond office procedures but short of a tissue excision in the form of a hemorrhoidectomy. The effectiveness and benefit of this procedure remain a matter of debate.

Hemorrhoidectomy

Excisional Hemorrhoidectomy

Excisional hemorrhoidectomy is best suited to address both internal and external hemorrhoid components. For thrombosed external hemorrhoids and cosmetic skin tag excision, a limited external hemorrhoid excision may suffice. However, a standard excisional hemorrhoidectomy includes both internal and external hemorrhoid components and is indicated for incarcerated internal hemorrhoids or if the patient desires to trim the external component as well.

The two most commonly performed techniques of excisional hemorrhoidectomy are the Ferguson closed hemorrhoidectomy and the Milligan–Morgan open hemorrhoidectomy. Both procedures are safe and predictable standard approaches, with the overall best long-term results. Excessive tissue removal may result in a stricture or sphincter injury with incontinence. As the excision extends into the sensitive anoderm, postoperative pain is significant and will need to be addressed. Minor bleeding is anticipated, and major bleeding episodes with a need for a balloon tamponade and/or a second look intervention are overall fortunately rare.

Stapled Hemorrhoidectomy

Under elective circumstances, a stapled hemorrhoidectomy is well-suited to address the internal hemorrhoid component only—with the advantage to avoid a wound in the sensitive anoderm and hence causing less postoperative pain. The concept is similar to a hemorrhoid banding but allows for a much more extensive hemorrhoid tissue removal than a single or a few hemorrhoid bandings.

Compared with an excisional hemorrhoidectomy, the stapled hemorrhoidectomy has been described as safe and was consistently associated with less postoperative pain, less operating time, and greater patient satisfaction, with similar but moderately increased complication and recurrence rates.

Postoperative Pain After Excisional Hemorrhoidectomy

Studies exploring perioperative adjuncts to lessen postoperative pain after excisional hemorrhoidectomy have taken several different directions: (1) pharmacological pain control, (2) use of local anesthetics, (3) use of antibiotics, and (4) reduction of the sphincter tone. Ketorolac and Cox-2 inhibitors are increasingly being used for baseline pain control. Various local anesthetics (e.g., the long-lasting ropivacaine) have been found to lessen the pain and the consumption of pain medication for up to 12 h after surgery.

Assuming that part of the postoperative pain could be related to a low-grade infection, the administration of oral metronidazole has been suggested. However, the significant benefit that has been described in a first study could not be substantiated in a more recent report.

Since sphincter spasm is thought to contribute to the postoperative pain after hemorrhoidectomy, strategies to lower the sphincter muscle tone have been explored. Topical 0.2% nitroglycerine ointment, which has been recommended for anal fissures, has been of modest and statistically insignificant benefit in reducing pain, but has been associated with side effects (headaches) in almost half of the patients. The effect of a surgical reduction of the sphincter tone by means of an internal sphincterotomy has been studied in a randomized trial, which showed no difference in the perception of pain after hemorrhoidectomy or in soiling and the control of gas. To our knowledge, no study has yet scrutinized the effect of perioperative Botox injection. However, given the lack of effectiveness of a surgical sphincterotomy, a benefit from a chemical sphincterotomy seems unlikely.

34.8 Modifiers of Hemorrhoid Treatment

There are a few circumstances in which the otherwise straightforward hemorrhoid treatment may need some special considerations and modifications. Examples include pregnancy, immunosuppression (HIV, solid organ or bone marrow transplant, chemotherapy, etc.), post radiation, inflammatory bowel disease, or the presence of chronic liver disease and cirrhosis.

34.8.1 Immunosuppression

Immunodeficient patients are more susceptible to infections and delayed wound healing after contaminated procedures. Conservative management should therefore be chosen where possible. Broader and potentially extended antibiotic prophylaxis may need to be considered should a surgical intervention be inevitable.

34.8.2 Hemorrhoidal Disease in Pregnancy

Both internal and external hemorrhoids are common complaints during pregnancy, particularly in the third trimester. Minor chronic symptoms ultimately resolve after delivery, and therefore hemorrhoid treatment should be very conservative during pregnancy to minimize harm to the fetus. However, acute hemorrhoid presentations (thrombosed external hemorrhoid, incarcerated internal hemorrhoids) may equally benefit from proactive surgical management as in nonpregnant patients. The swift intervention may shorten the time to pain resolution and decrease the potential side effects caused by prolonged symptomatic medications.

34.8.3 Inflammatory Bowel Disease and Hemorrhoids

Inflammatory bowel disease (IBD) may either present hemorrhoid-like symptoms (bleeding) or the underlying diarrhea may exacerbate hemorrhoidal manifestations. Crohn's disease characteristically manifests with a heterogeneous variety of anorectal symptoms, including atypical ulcerations, edematous skin tags, abscess, or fistula formation. In addition to the challenging differential diagnosis, patients with IBD are frequently under treatment with steroids, and traditional or biologic immunosuppressants that alter their healing capacity. Caution should be exerted in patients with even a remote history of Crohn's disease to distinguish a flare of perianal manifestations as opposed to a true classical hemorrhoid presentation. Even well-intended interventions may trigger local complications (7% in ulcerative colitis, 12–42% in Crohn's disease) that may ultimately necessitate a proctectomy. Medical management should be optimized in order to suppress any local disease activity, leaving, if at all, only those residual symptoms that may truly be associated with a hemorrhoidal disease.

34.8.4 Chronic Liver Disease: Hemorrhoids Versus Rectal Varices

Hemorrhoids are not associated with portal hypertension. But chronic liver disease and cirrhosis result in portal hypertension, which may manifest with rectal varices, impaired coagulation, poor nutritional status, and gastrointestinal bleeding episodes. Careful evaluation and generally a conservative approach are preferred, but bleeding may require local interventions (sclerotherapy, etc.). True internal hemorrhoids in patients with liver cirrhosis may occasionally require surgical management, whereby a stapled hemorrhoidectomy is preferred.

34.8.5 Radiation

Radiation therapy for pelvic malignancies has a high incidence of radiation proctitis that occurs as self-limited acute proctitis during the radiation and months to years later as chronic radiation proctitis that depends on the dose of radiation and typically worsens over time. Chronic impairment of microvascular perfusion results in tissue weakening and neo-vascularizations. Those may result in rectal bleeding episodes similar to hemorrhoidal bleeding. Even in the presence of concomitant hemorrhoidal disease, caution should be exerted about interventional treatment as the tissue healing may be dramatically impaired. Primary efforts consist of hyperbaric oxygen, mucosal treatment with topical formalin, argon beam plasma coagulation (APC), or endoscopic radiofrequency ablation represent the most promising approaches.

34.9 Conclusion

In the past few years, there have been significant advances in the understanding and management of hemorrhoidal disease. A wide array of old and new treatment modalities is available and allow a stage and symptom-adjusted approach. Avoidance and control of postoperative pain have been the major impetus in the search for more satisfactory treatments. Rubber band ligation and stapled hemorrhoidectomy are clearly evolving as the standards of operative treatment because of convincing evidence of decreased pain and improved patient satisfaction. Even in the presence of other medical conditions, hemorrhoids can be accurately and safely treated.

Tables 34.5 and 34.6 illustrate the conditions that require an urgent referral (Table 34.5) or may be initially managed by the primary care provider or the emergency room physician, with the plan for an elective referral to a specialist (Table 34.6).

Table 34.5 Urgent action and referrals

	Description	Management by PCP/ER	Tests before referral	Referral/consultation
Incarcerated internal hemorrhoids	No tissue necrosis Tissue necrosis present	Attempt to reduce with sugar –	None None	Surgery (acute care or colorectal) Surgery (acute care or colorectal)
Thrombosed external hemorrhoids	< 72 h post onset > 72 h post onset	– Pain management, warm sitzbaths	None None	Surgery (acute care or colorectal) Colorectal surgery
Nonrelenting spontaneous bleeding		Assure hemodynamic stability	Blood work, transfusion, imaging (e.g. bleeding scan or angiography to rule out more proximal GI bleeding)	ER, GI, surgery
Postoperative bleeding (significant)		Assure hemodynamic stability	Blood work transfusion	Surgeon or covering team Acute care surgery if none other available
Perirectal abscess	Acute Chronic intermittent (w/wo fistula)	Antibiotics do not replace incision/drainage	None None	Surgery (acute care or colorectal) Colorectal surgery
Postoperative perineal sepsis	Fevers, pain, urinary retention	Foley catheter Initiate antibiotics without delaying surgery consult	Possible CT with IV contrast	Surgeon or covering team Acute care surgery if none other available
Necrotizing soft tissue infections	Tissue crepitus Disproportional pain Sepsis	Initiate antibiotics without delaying surgery consult	Possible CT with IV contrast	Surgery

Table 34.6 Initial management by PCP/ER physician and elective referrals

	Description	Management by PCP/ER	Tests before referral	Referral/consultation
Intermittently prolapsing/bleeding hemorrhoids	No tissue necrosis	Bowel management	None	Colorectal surgery
Subacute thrombosed external hemorrhoids	> 72 h post onset	Pain management, warm sitzbaths	None	Colorectal surgery
Anal fissure with sentinel skin tag	Painful "hemorrhoid" and bleeding during/after BM	Bowel management, warm sitzbaths	None	Colorectal surgery
Postoperative constipation	After anorectal procedure	Laxatives until effect	None	Surgeon or covering team Acute care surgery if none other available
Postoperative bleeding (minor)	After anorectal procedure	Laxatives and stool management	None	Surgeon or covering team

Suggested Reading

1. Coughlin OP, Wright ME, Thorson AG, Ternent CA. Hemorrhoid banding: a cost-effectiveness analysis. Dis Colon Rectum. 2019;62:1085–94.
2. Hawkins AT, Davis BR, Bhama AR, et al. The American Society of Colon and Rectal Surgeons Clinical Practice Guidelines for the Management of Hemorrhoids. Dis Colon Rectum. 2024;67:614–23.
3. Ratto C, Parello A, Veronese E, et al. Doppler-guided transanal haemorrhoidal dearterialization for haemorrhoids: results from a multicentre trial. Colorectal Dis. 2015;17:O10–9.
4. McGraw-Hill Manual: Colorectal Surgery. McGraw-Hill Medical. 2009. Accessed 12 June 2025, at https://accesssurgery.mhmedical.com/book.aspx?bookID=425.
5. Nunoo-Mensah JW, Kaiser AM. Stapled hemorrhoidectomy. Am J Surg. 2005;190:127–30.

Anorectal Abscess

35

Paige E. Likes and Robert A. Catania

35.1 Presentation

Patients with anorectal abscesses typically present with acute, severe perianal pain. Presentation may include reports of difficulty sitting, fever, purulent drainage, dyschezia, as well as rectal bleeding. External physical exam may reveal localized erythema, swelling, and tenderness, frequently with associated fluctuance. In certain instances, no external findings may be present, but tenderness, induration, or fluctuance may be appreciated on digital rectal examination. Exam findings typically allow a narrowing of the anorectal pain differential diagnoses, which include anal fissures and external hemorrhoids.

Within anorectal abscesses, the diagnosis may be further classified into four categories dependent on the anatomic space in which they develop. Classifications include perianal, ischiorectal, intersphincteric, and supralevator, with perianal abscesses being the most common presentation (see Table 35.1).

The terms perianal and perirectal are often used interchangeably, but it is important to distinguish between them as it influ-

P. E. Likes
John Peter Smith Hospital, Fort Worth, TX, USA

R. A. Catania (✉)
Southern New Hampshire Medical Center, Nashua, NH, USA

G. P. Kohn et al. (eds.), *The SAGES Manual of Surgical Referral for Primary and Emergency Care*,
https://doi.org/10.1007/978-3-031-92678-5_35

Table 35.1 Classification

Classification of anorectal abscesses	
Perianal	Surrounding the anal verge; lacks tissue penetration deep to the external anal sphincter Most common and most easily visualized on physical exam
Ischiorectal	Surrounding the rectum, through the external sphincter Second most common presentation
Intersphincteric	Between the external and internal anal sphincters
	Presentation: Fluctuant mass protruding into the lumen on digital rectal examination
Supralevator	Located above the levator muscle, cephalad to the anal canal Least common
	Presentation: Perianal pain with no external findings, induration/fluctuance on digital exam above anal canal, fever, +/− urinary retention

ences the approach to management. A perirectal abscess is situated beyond the external anal sphincter and includes ischiorectal, intersphincteric, and supralevator abscesses, while a perianal abscess does not extend through the external sphincter. Patients with a perirectal abscess will require surgical referral for drainage under anesthesia, whereas perianal abscess may not require referral if the evaluating provider has the capability to perform surgical drainage at the bedside.

35.2 Diagnostics

35.2.1 Laboratory Blood Tests

Not routinely recommended for perianal abscess. If concern for a deeper process (perirectal abscess) or systemic infection, a complete blood count (CBC) is indicated. If the patient has diabetes or if there is concern for sepsis or Fournier's gangrene include basic metabolic profile (BMP) and lactic acid (LA).

35.2.2 Culture

Not routinely indicated for perianal abscess.

If significant inflammation and minimal fluctuance, there is a possible *Methicillin*-resistant *Staphylococcus aureus* (MRSA) presence. If MRSA infection is suspected, microbial cultures are indicated. If recurrent infection occurs, microbial cultures are recommended.

35.2.3 Imaging

Dependent on location, many anorectal abscesses are easily diagnosed by physical exam and patient history. A perianal abscess is usually easily identified on physical exam by the presence of erythema and/or fluctuance, whereas the perirectal abscesses can have few external findings on physical exam. For a perianal abscess identified on physical exam, imaging is typically not necessary. If the physical exam is inconclusive or if there is concern for a deeper infection or fistula, additional diagnostic evaluation is warranted. Options include computed tomography of the abdomen and pelvis with IV and rectal contrast (CT), magnetic resonance imaging (MRI), and ultrasound (US) (either transperineal or endoanal).

The choice of initial imaging modality is largely dependent on patient history and presentation. Transperineal ultrasound (TPUS) may be considered for initial diagnostics due to the low cost and accessibility; however, due to the inconsistent quality of TPUS, the widespread choice for first-line imaging is contrast-enhanced CT, with 77% sensitivity in detecting anorectal abscesses.

If the patient has a history of Crohn's disease or other immunosuppressive disease, or if there is significant concern for fistula formation, MRI offers a significant advantage over CT with increased sensitivity and specificity in the diagnosis of anorectal fistula.

35.3 Treatment

35.3.1 Incision and Drainage

The historical method for anorectal abscess treatment is incision and drainage, which remains the primary recommendation; incision and drainage may be performed in the operating room (OR) or at the bedside depending on the specifics of the abscess.

If the abscess is small (<2 cm) and superficial, the procedure can often be completed in the Emergency Department or Primary Care Office and does not require surgical consultation. With increasing abscess size and severity of infection, drainage in the OR is preferred and a surgical referral is indicated. The OR provides the advantage of general anesthesia, allowing more comprehensive rectal examination, improved drainage, and the option of fistulotomy or seton placement if indicated.

35.3.2 Surgical Referral

Surgical drainage is the hallmark of treatment for perianal or perirectal abscess. Surgical referral is indicated any time a drainage procedure cannot be performed by the evaluating provider. The listed criteria can be utilized as indications for surgical referral:

1. Recurrent abscess
2. Known history of inflammatory bowel disease
3. Known history of fistula
4. Known history of diabetes mellitus
5. Failure to resolve following outpatient or ED drainage procedure
6. Findings such as tenderness, induration, or fluctuance on internal rectal examination or imaging suggesting ischiorectal, supralevator, or intersphincteric abscess
7. Patients presenting with sepsis or suspicion of Fournier's gangrene

Table 35.2 Testing and management prior to surgical referral

Acute presentation
NPO
CBC
BMP and LA[a]
Imaging
First line: CT abdomen/pelvis with IV contrast and rectal contrast
Subacute or chronic presentation
MRI[+]

NPO nothing by mouth; [a]For patients with diabetes mellitus or in whom sepsis or Fournier's gangrene is suspected

If a surgical referral is indicated, the recommended testing and management prior to referral can be found in Table 35.2.

35.3.3 Antibiotics

Following incision and drainage, empiric antibiotics are suggested for reduced the risk of fistula formation. Regimen options

- Amoxicillin-clavulanate
- Ciprofloxacin and metronidazole

Antibiotics *without* incision and drainage are not considered an adequate treatment option. The management algorithm is summarized in Fig. 35.1.

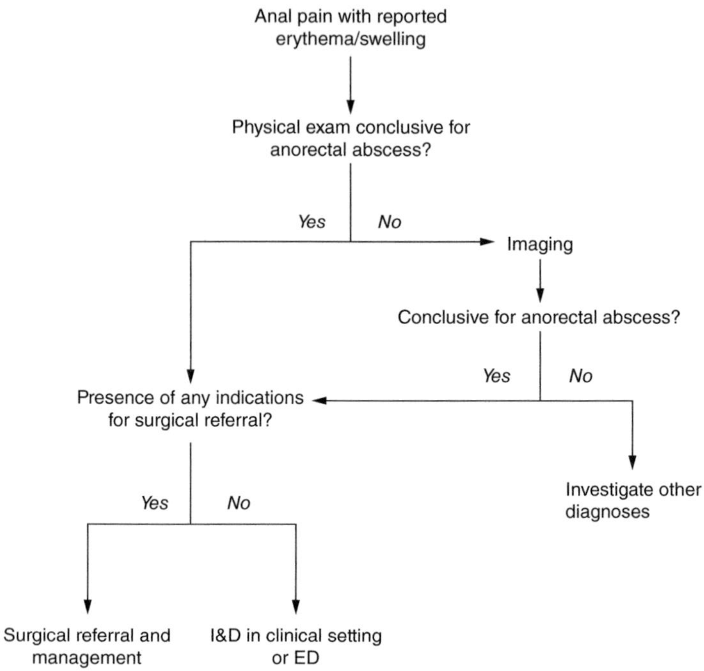

Fig. 35.1 Summary of management of anorectal abscess Key: I&D: Incision and Drainage

Further Reading

1. Abcarian H. Anorectal infection: abscess-fistula. Clin Colon Rectal Surg. 2011;24(1):14–21.
2. Gaertner WB, Burgess PL, Davids JS, Lightner AL, Shogan BD, Sun MY, Steele SR, Paquette IM, Feingold DL. The American Society of colon and rectal surgeons clinical practice guidelines for the management of anorectal abscess, fistula-in-ano, and rectovaginal fistula. Dis Colon Rectum. 2022;65(8):964–85.
3. Goldenshluger M, Margalit C, Kodesh A, Katz E, Hazzan D, Segev L. Bedside drainage of perianal abscesses: is it safe and effective? Isr Med Assoc J. 2023;25(7):473–8.
4. Rizzo JA, Naig AL, Johnson EK. Anorectal abscess and fistula-in-ano: evidence-based management. Surg Clin North Am. 2010;90(1):45–68.
5. Sigmon DF, Emmanuel B, Tuma F. Perianal abscess. StatPearls [internet]. Treasure Island: StatPearls Publishing; 2023.

Part III

Investigation Finding

Esophageal Diverticula

36

Andrew T. Strong

36.1 Introduction

Esophageal diverticula are outpouchings of the esophageal mucosa and submucosa through the muscular layers of the esophagus. Diverticula may form throughout the esophagus, and classification schema separate diverticula by esophageal segment as anatomic location often relates to the causative etiology. Pulsion-type diverticula, wherein intraluminal pressure causes propulsion of the esophageal the mucosa and submucosa outward, are the more common type. Traction-type diverticula also occur when external pulling forces act on the esophagus, often related to prior surgical scar tissue or inflammatory conditions. These are true diverticula that involve all layers of the esophageal wall, different from pulsion type, which are pseudo-diverticula. We used the term diverticula in this chapter to include both types. Diverticula of the proximal and distal esophagus are often pulsion type, while mid-esophageal diverticula often arise from traction.

A. T. Strong (✉)
Digestive Disease Institute, Cleveland Clinic, Cleveland, OH, USA

Cleveland Clinic Lerner College of Medicine of Case Western Reserve University, Cleveland, OH, USA
e-mail: stronga3@ccf.org

G. P. Kohn et al. (eds.), *The SAGES Manual of Surgical Referral for Primary and Emergency Care*,
https://doi.org/10.1007/978-3-031-92678-5_36

Zenker's diverticulum is the most encountered esophageal diverticulum, representing 70% of all esophageal diverticula. This occurs through a naturally weak point in the esophagus known as Killian's triangle within the posterolateral aspect of the cervical esophageal segment. Zenker's diverticulum forms because of a spastic cricopharyngeus muscle that produces over-pressurization of the hypopharynx. Other types of diverticula of the proximal esophagus include Larimer's diverticulum and Killian–Jamieson diverticula, which arise from other anatomic weak points in the hypopharynx.

Diverticula arising in the distal esophagus are called epiphrenic diverticula. Epiphrenic diverticula form in association with hypercontractile disorders of the esophagus, achalasia, or distal esophageal stricture.

Treatment of esophageal diverticula is determined both by the involved esophageal segment and the causative etiology. There are no medical treatments for diverticula, and all treatments are surgical. The objective of treatment is reduction or resolution of symptoms and/or the prevention of aspiration and malnutrition. Operative management traditionally mandated open surgery; however, endoscopic approaches to some diverticula are becoming more common with similar effectiveness and more rapid recovery.

36.2 Presenting Symptoms

The presenting complaint for most esophageal diverticula is dysphagia or difficulty swallowing. Dysphagia becomes an increasingly frequent complaint with increasing age, and as a symptom is relatively nonspecific and relates to several conditions affecting the esophagus and nervous system. Dysphagia should be contrasted from other similar terms, including odynophagia and globus sensation. Odynophagia is pain with swallowing, which may occur with or without dysphagia. Globus sensation is the sensation of a lump or tightness in the chest or esophagus in the *absence* of swallowing. When characterizing dysphagia, distinguishing disorders in the oropharyngeal phase versus the esophageal phase guides diagnostic workup. The oropharyngeal phase of swallowing relates to the formation of a food bolus, manipulation through the upper esophageal sphincter and initiation of a swallow, as well as glottic and epiglottic closure. Oropharyngeal dysphagia thus relates to increased food bolus retention, inadequate transmission, or manipulation into the hypopharynx and/or failure to initiate a swallow. Esophageal phase dysphagia involves the body of the esophagus and is under involuntary neuromuscular control. Esophageal phase dysphagia is more often related to strictures, stenoses, or alteration in the motility of the esophagus. There are several benign, common causes of both oropharyngeal and esophageal dysphagia, of which diverticula are some. However, given that dysphagia may also be a presenting complaint for malignancies, initial evaluation should focus on elucidating risk factors for cancers, including history of smoked or chewed tobacco, alcohol dependence, long-standing history of heartburn, and family history. In addition, characterizing the circumstances under which dysphagia symptoms developed may aid in ruling in or ruling out malignancy as a causative etiology. Factors that may be elucidated in history as it related to swallowing function could include the following descriptors.

- Time course (rapid onset over weeks may imply a rapidly growing tumor or inflammatory process).
- Trouble initiating a swallow (implies oropharyngeal phase).
- Choking or coughing with attempted swallowing (implies oropharyngeal phase).
- Location (oropharyngeal dysphagia typically affects the neck; with esophageal dysphagia lesion is at or below area indicated).
- Regurgitation of undigested food.
- Symptoms with solids vs liquids or both.
- Chest pain (more common with esophageal dysphagia and with motor disorders of the esophagus).

The flow chart (Fig. 36.1) depicts some of the other common causes of dysphagia based on some key characteristics. Some of these etiologies are discussed elsewhere in this text as well.

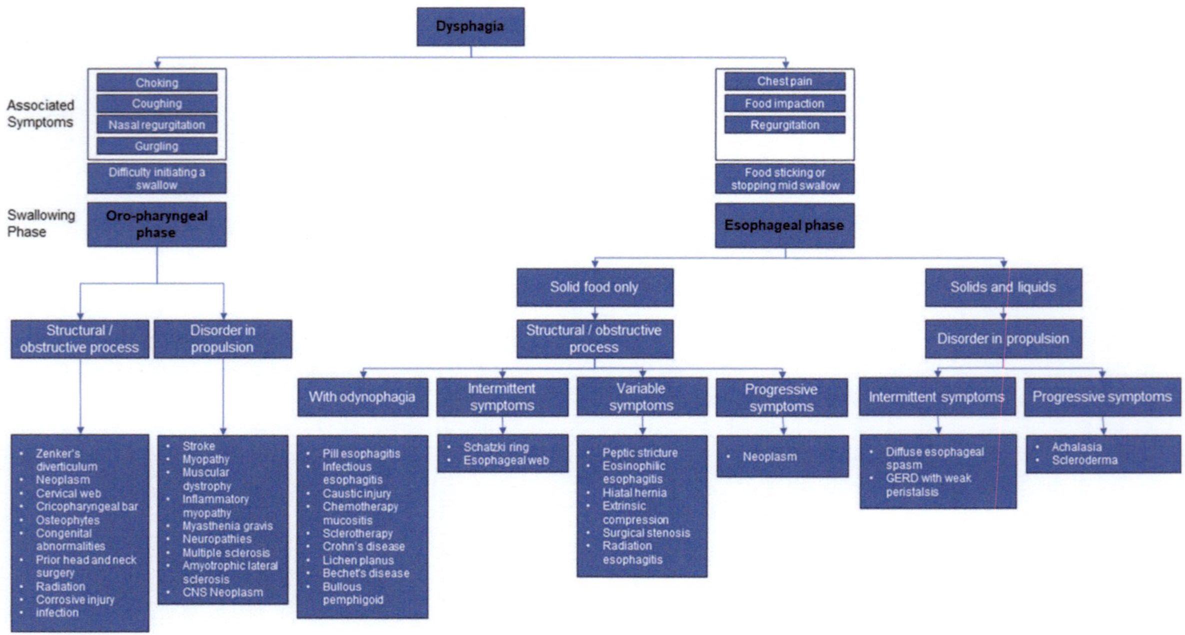

Fig. 36.1 Conceptual framework of dysphagia characteristics and etiologies

Patients with esophageal diverticula may complain of symptoms consistent with both oropharyngeal phase or esophageal phase dysphagia. Other associated symptoms include regurgitation of undigested food or medication tablets, aspiration, recurrent coughing, or halitosis. The symptoms may be related to two separate factors. For pulsion-type diverticulum, localized muscular spasm constricts passage of a food bolus, which may cause symptoms itself. As diverticula enlarge, they fill preferentially and retain ingesting food or medications. Enlargement of the diverticulum may distort and cause a local mass effect further impairing food bolus passage. Regurgitation is related to the emptying of the diverticulum, which may occur hours after food ingestion, yet appear as undigested food. Epiphrenic diverticula are often associated with either achalasia or hypercontractile esophageal motility disorders and symptoms of the underlying disorder typically predominate; however, regurgitation may originate from the diverticulum itself.

For many disorders causing oropharyngeal or esophageal dysphagia, a physical exam will be unrevealing. However, for Zenker's diverticulum, a physical exam may clinch the diagnosis for a patient with oropharyngeal dysphagia symptoms. Boyce's sign is the physical exam finding of a gurgling mass in the lateral neck (typically left sided) and is pathognomonic for a proximal esophageal diverticulum. For patients with prior neck surgery, including anterior approaches to the cervical vertebral bodies, or patients with prior intrathoracic surgery, scar tissue can cause traction-type diverticula, so the presence of surgical scars in those locations provide an additional clue.

36.3 Evaluation and Workup

For the patient with dysphagia, testing initially includes multiple complementary testing modalities (see Tables 36.1 and 36.2). Initial evaluation should be concerned with defining the urgency of evaluation. Any patient presenting with dysphagia in association with dyspnea, stridor, high fever, new neurological deficits, or caustic ingestion should be diverted to an emer-

Table 36.1 Urgency of evaluation by presenting symptoms

Urgency and location of evaluation	Presenting patient factors
Prompt emergency room presentation and evaluation	Dysphagia associated with dyspnea or stridor Dysphagia with esophageal food impaction Dysphagia related to caustic ingestion Dysphagia associated with other new neurological deficits dysphagia related to foreign body ingestion
Urgent surgical evaluation	Dysphagia with limited ability to tolerate liquid intake Dysphagia with significant weight loss (>10% total body weight) Rapidly progressive dysphagia over weeks or less Dysphagia with a noted anterior neck mass on physical exam (e.g., goiter)
Expedited imaging and or endoscopic evaluation for diagnosis and differentiation	Dysphagia with significant risk factors for gastrointestinal cancer, including history of biopsy-proven Barrett's esophagus Progressive dysphagia, but with retained ability to tolerate liquid Dysphagia with recurrent aspiration
Nonurgent surgical evaluation (outpatient follow-up)	Dysphagia with intermittent regurgitation Dysphagia with intermittent symptoms Incidentally noted small esophageal diverticula with attributable symptoms Dysphagia in a patient with prior neck or thorax radiation Recurrent dysphagia with prior attributable cause (prior peptic strictures or Schatzki's rings, Any incidentally noted epiphrenic diverticulum
Management by primary care provider	Incidentally noted small proximal or mid esophageal diverticula without attributable symptoms

Table 36.2 Pre-referral workup and evaluation

Presenting symptom or sign	Pre-referral evaluation and testing	
Oropharyngeal dysphagia	Ambulatory history and physical exam	Evaluation for prior, current, or evolving neurological disorder Evaluation of history of aspiration pneumonia Evaluation for risk factors or oropharyngeal cancer including exposure to HPV if known, tobacco use (smoked or smokeless) Evaluation of anterior and lateral neck for masses
	Testing	Modified barium swallow If no pathology noted, consider biphasic esophagram If masses present, ultrasound or CT scan
	Management	Pathology noted on MBS → speech therapy referral, possible referral to dietitian Pathology noted on esophagram → referral to appropriate specialist, (gastroenterology, surgeon) If no pathology noted, consider referral for endoscopic oropharyngeal evaluation
Esophageal phase dysphagia	Ambulatory history and physical exam	Evaluation for cancer risk factors including unexplained weight loss, history of heartburn, smoking, family history of upper gastrointestinal cancers. Evaluation for progression from solids to liquids General assessment of nutritional status
	Testing	Biphasic esophagram Possible referral for upper gastrointestinal endoscopy
	Management	Testing guides referral, no additional outpatient management

(continued)

Table 36.2 (continued)

Presenting symptom or sign	Pre-referral evaluation and testing	
Incidentally noted esophageal diverticulum on cross-sectional imaging	Ambulatory history and physical exam	Assessment of dysphagia symptoms Surgical history related to esophagus and nearby structures
	Testing	Biphasic barium esophagram
	Management	Diverticula under 2 cm and asymptomatic can be serially monitored annually with biphasic esophagram; Diverticula with attributable symptoms or > 2 cm warrant surgical evaluation All epiphrenic diverticula warrant evaluation for causative esophageal dysmotility disorder
Incidentally noted esophageal diverticulum on routine upper endoscopy	Ambulatory history and physical exam	Assessment of dysphagia symptoms Surgical history related to esophagus and nearby structures
	Testing	Biphasic esophagram For epiphrenic diverticulum consider high-resolution manometry
	Management	Diverticula under 2 cm and asymptomatic can be serially monitored annually with biphasic esophagram Diverticula with symptoms or > 2 cm warrant surgical evaluation All epiphrenic diverticula warrant evaluation for causative esophageal dysmotility disorder

gency room for prompt evaluation. For the majority of other potential causes of dysphagia, further evaluation can occur in the outpatient setting (see Table 36.1). Contrast-enhanced radiographic evaluation is often first, but may be paired with videoscopic luminal inspection with upper gastrointestinal endoscopy, and/or esophageal manometry. The American College of Radiology ACR Appropriateness Criteria® for Dysphagia lists several variants for evaluation for dysphagia. In the ambulatory care setting, imaging recommendations for "unexplained oropharyngeal dysphagia initial imaging" are the most applicable section of the ACR Appropriate Criteria. Under that guideline, a biphasic fluoroscopic esophagram is the best first test. Other potentially appropriate studies include fluoroscopic barium swallow and fluoroscopic single-contrast esophagogram. CT scan is rarely indicated. Local diagnostic facilities or radiology departments may use slightly different terminology for these studies.

	Fluoroscopic barium swallow	Single-contrast esophagram	Biphasic esophagram
Assessment	Oral cavity, pharynx, and cervical esophagus	Includes full column distension, mucosal relief views and observation of esophageal motility Can include both videofluoroscopic and static views	Includes full column distension, mucosal relief views and observation of esophageal motility, double-contrast views Can include both videofluoroscopic and static views
Contrast agent(s)	Barium and barium impregnated food of varying consistency	Barium or water-soluble contrast	Barium and water-soluble contrast; barium-impregnated tablet
Special considerations	Performed in conjunction with speech therapist Can also evaluate compensatory maneuvers in improve swallowing function	Better suited to patients with limited ability to cooperate with study, including elderly patients	Provides greater mucosal detail Patients must be able to cooperate with multiple position changes to complete study

With contrast-enhanced X-ray, an esophageal diverticulum will appear as an outpouching that alters the normal esophageal contour and confirms the diagnosis. Some projections may be able to also visualize the tissue septum between the diverticulum and the native esophagus as well (Fig. 36.2).

For patients who have symptoms of a dysmotility disorder, a timed esophagram would also confirm the diagnosis of a diverticulum. Patients with less specific symptoms often undergo an upper gastrointestinal series, which includes contrast-enhanced video fluoroscopy of the esophagus and stomach would also confirm the presence of an esophageal diverticulum. Importantly,

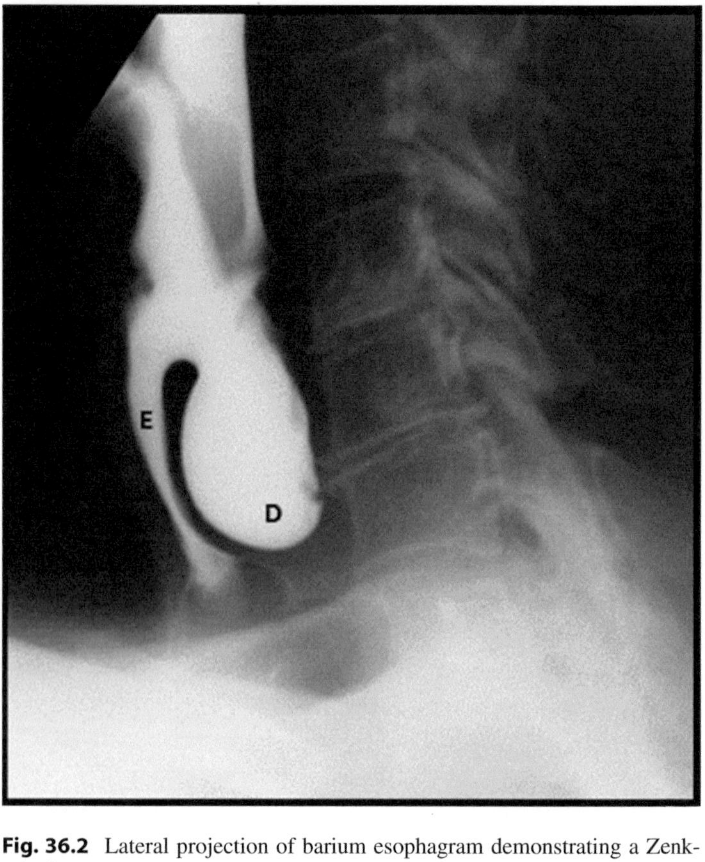

Fig. 36.2 Lateral projection of barium esophagram demonstrating a Zenker's diverticulum. D marks diverticulum, E marks esophageal lumen

these studies may also reveal alternate etiologies for dysphagia, including esophageal webs or strictures, diffuse esophageal spasm, achalasia, hiatal hernia, gastroesophageal reflux disease, and masses of the esophagus or gastroesophageal junction.

Cross-sectional imaging, such as CT scan, is not necessary for diverticula of the cervical segment. However, with increasing use of CT scan and MRI, the incidental identification of esophageal diverticula is increasing. Routine upper endoscopy obtained for alternative indications may also incidentally reveal esophageal diverticula. Incidentally noted diverticula are often smaller and either only mildly symptomatic or asymptomatic. If they have not been characterized by one of the contrast-enhanced imaging studies above, then repeat imaging with that modality is recommended.

Radiographic identification of an esophageal diverticulum should be followed by endoscopic assessment. While rare, the chronically inflamed state of mucosa within esophageal diverticula may give rise to squamous cell cancer. If radiographic imaging is suggestive of an esophageal dysmotility disorder, then timed esophagram and referral for high-resolution esophageal manometry should be made.

Once the diagnosis of a diverticulum of the esophagus is made, referral for surgical evaluation is appropriate. Asymptomatic diverticula do not need surgical treatment, but referral to a specialist can facilitate prospective monitoring, so that intervention may be pursued once symptoms develop, when diverticula are smaller in size. Esophageal diverticula may be managed by multiple surgical and interventional subspecialities depending on local practice environments and expertise:

- Diverticula of the hypopharynx may be managed by otolaryngologists, general surgeons, or interventional gastroenterologists.
- Diverticula of mid esophagus are most frequently managed by thoracic surgeons.
- Diverticula of the distal esophagus are most often epiphrenic diverticula, related to an underlying esophageal dysmotility disorder such as achalasia. These may be managed by interventional gastroenterologists, thoracic surgeons, or general surgeons.

36.4 Treatment of Esophageal Diverticula

Surgical or endoscopic treatment of esophageal diverticula is reserved for symptomatic or large diverticula. The principles of management of pulsion-type esophageal diverticula are to treat the underlying muscular or neuromuscular disorder, and to prevent filling of the diverticulum. Treatment of muscular or neuromuscular disorders is accomplished most often by myotomy. Taking Zenker's diverticulum as a prototypical example, this implies division of the cricopharyngeus muscle. To prevent filling of the diverticulum, various techniques have been proposed. Historically these included resection of the diverticulum (diverticulectomy), inversion of the diverticulum so that it is in an antidependent position (diverticulopexy). Increasingly, division of the septum between the diverticulum to incorporate the diverticulum into the esophageal lumen is being adopted (diverticulotomy). Techniques and devices allowing diverticulotomy to be completed from a rigid or flexible endoscopic platform are driving increasing adoption of this approach. Division of the common wall also accomplishes a simultaneous myotomy. For traction-type diverticulum, the same principles apply; however, removal or division of the tissue causing the traction force may be indicated as well.

36.5 Conclusion

Esophageal diverticula are becoming increasingly common as more are incidentally noted on cross-sectional imaging or endoscopic studies obtained for other reasons. Esophageal diverticula are also benign causes of dysphagia, a frequent presenting symptom in the ambulatory care setting. Evaluation includes radiographic and endoscopic evaluation prior to surgical referral. Local practice patterns and expertise will dictate management by one of several interventional or surgical subspecialists. Surgical management is focused on palliating symptoms and prevention of serious complications such as malnutrition and aspiration.

Selected Readings

1. Strong AT, Ponsky JL. Esophageal diverticula. Benign Esophageal Dis Mod Surg Approaches Tech: Springer; 2021. p. 173–210.
2. Radiology ACR Appropriateness criteria: Dysphagia 2021.
3. Shebrain S. Evaluation of esophageal diverticula. SAGES Man. Foregut Surg. Springer International; 2019. p. 513–23.
4. Hirano I, Kahrilas PJ. Dysphagia. Harrisons Princ. Intern. Med. 21st ed. McGraw Hill Education; 2022.

37 Barrett's Esophagus

Paul J. Nguyen-Lee, Julie E. Kim,
and Ivy N. Haskins

37.1 Introduction

Barrett's esophagus (BE) is associated with gastroesophageal reflux disease (GERD) and is defined as the replacement of the normal squamous mucosa of the distal esophagus with at least 1 cm of columnar mucosa. While suspicion for BE may be heightened with the visual identification of salmon-colored mucosa of the distal esophagus during esophagogastroduodenoscopy (EGD), the diagnosis of BE requires tissue sampling and pathologic confirmation. The diagnosis of BE, particularly in at-risk patients, is important as BE is the only known precursor to esophageal adenocarcinoma (EAC).

37.2 Risk Factors for Barrett's Esophagus

There are several modifiable and nonmodifiable risk factors for BE. Nonmodifiable risk factors for BE include older age (> 50 years of age), white race, male sex, a family history of BE or EAC in at least one first-degree relative, and diagnosis of GERD

P. J. Nguyen-Lee · J. E. Kim · I. N. Haskins (✉)
Department of Surgery, University of Nebraska Medical Center,
Omaha, NE, USA

G. P. Kohn et al. (eds.), *The SAGES Manual of Surgical Referral for Primary and Emergency Care*,
https://doi.org/10.1007/978-3-031-92678-5_37

before the age of 30. Modifiable risk factors for BE include tobacco use, central obesity, uncontrolled GERD symptoms, long-standing (> 5 years) GERD symptoms, presence of a hiatal hernia, and long-segment BE. Long-segment BE is defined as BE >3 cm, whereas short-segment BE is defined as BE <3 cm.

37.3 Classification of Barrett's Esophagus

There are both endoscopic and pathologic classifications of BE. The endoscopic classification of BE is known as the Prague C & M classification system. In order to use the Prague C & M classification system, the esophagogastric junction (EGJ) must first be identified. The EGJ is defined as the proximal extent at which all gastric mucosal folds are lost with minimal to moderate insufflation during esophagogastroduodenoscopy (EGD). It is important to note that identification of the EGJ in a patient with BE may be more challenging if there is a concomitant hiatal hernia because the EGJ no longer corresponds with the squamocolumnar junction (SCJ) or the Z-line. The C & M values correspond to the circumferential length of BE (C) and the length of the longest tongue or segment of BE (M). In this classification system, the M length must always be equivalent to, or greater than, the C length. The Prague C & M classification system is used because it is easily reproducible between endoscopists and can be used to track the progression and regression of visible BE over time.

The pathologic diagnosis of BE refers to the degree of dysplasia present in tissue samples obtained, including no dysplasia, low-grade dysplasia (LGD), high-grade dysplasia (HGD), and indefinite for dysplasia (IND). The degree of dysplasia present is important to determine as it impacts the risk of progression to EAC. Because of interobserver variability in the interpretation of the degree of dysplasia, the American College of Gastroenterology recommends that the presence and degree of dysplasia be confirmed by two pathologists, at least one of whom specializes in gastrointestinal diseases. In patients with BE without dysplasia, the risk of progression to EAC is approximately 0.2–0.5% annually while the risk of progression to EAC in patients with BE with HGD is approximately 7%

per year. These differences in the risk of progression to EAC help guide the recommendations for eradication therapy (EET) and the frequency of surveillance EGD for patients with BE. Endoscopic eradication therapy uses endoscopic resection and ablation methods to replace dysplastic epithelium with neo-squamous epithelium in an effort to reduce the risk of EAC.

37.4 Summary of Screening, Surveillance, and Treatment of Barrett's Esophagus

The screening, surveillance, and treatment of BE are quite complex and differ between countries and gastrointestinal and surgical societies. While the intricate details of these recommendations are outside the scope of this chapter, a basic understanding of these recommendations may impact the decision to refer a patient to a surgeon. The recommendations for screening, surveillance, and treatment of BE by the American College of Gastroenterology are briefly summarized below. Outside of the United States, please refer to your national gastroenterology or surgical society for your country's specific recommendations.

37.5 Screening of Barrett's Esophagus

The general population should not be screened for BE. Men with long-standing (> 5 years) or frequent (at least weekly) GERD symptoms with two or more additional risk factors for BE should undergo screening EGD. Women with multiple risk factors for BE may also be considered for screening EGD. If visual inspection of the esophageal mucosa is concerning for BE, four-quadrant biopsies every 2 cm of the area of concern (or at least 8 total biopsies if the area of concern is <2 cm) should be obtained. If Los Angeles Classification Grade B, C, or D esophagitis is present at the time of screening EGD, repeat EGD should be performed in 8–12 weeks following treatment of GERD with a proton pump inhibitor (PPI). Finally, if the SCJ/Z-line appears normal during EGD, biopsies for screening of BE should not be obtained.

37.6 Surveillance and Treatment of Barrett's Esophagus

The purpose of surveillance EGD following a diagnosis of BE is to reduce the risk of progression of BE to EAC.

Patients with BE with no dysplasia should undergo surveillance EGD every 3 years in the setting of long-segment disease and every 5 years in the setting of short-segment disease.

In patients with BE that is indefinite for dysplasia, a repeat EGD should be performed 3–6 months after the index EGD and following optimization of GERD therapy with a PPI. If indefinite for dysplasia persists, patients should undergo surveillance EGD annually.

While it is recommended that patients with BE with low-grade dysplasia undergo EET, some patients do not wish to undergo this procedure. In these scenarios, an alternative to EET is surveillance EGD annually.

For patients with BE with HGD, is it recommended that they undergo EET. There is no surveillance EGD period recommended for patients with BE with HGD who have not undergone EET. The goal of EET is complete eradication of intestinal metaplasia (CEIM).

For patients with BE with LGD who achieve CEIM, surveillance EGD is recommended every six months for the first year following EET and then annually thereafter.

For patients with BE with HGD who achieve CEIM, surveillance EGD is recommended every three months for the first year following EET, every six months for the second year following EET, and annually thereafter. The American College of Gastroenterology recommends that surveillance EGD for BE focus on the areas of previous BE in addition to the high cardia (top of the gastric folds) through the neo-squamous epithelium near the EGJ.

37.7 Role of Surgery in the Management of Barrett's Esophagus

Currently, antireflux surgery in the form of surgical or endoscopic fundoplication is not recommended as an antineoplastic measure in the treatment algorithm for BE. While some data suggest that antireflux surgery aids in preventing the progression of BE to EAC, there is no strong evidence to support this notion. Rather, the role of antireflux surgery in patients with BE would be to address some of the modifiable risk factors for BE, including the presence of a hiatal hernia and improved control of frequent GERD symptoms despite maximal PPI therapy and lifestyle modification. Depending upon the practice patterns in your area, these operations are performed by general surgeons, minimally invasive foregut surgeons, and thoracic surgeons. In patients with either a hiatal hernia or breakthrough GERD symptoms despite maximal PPI therapy and lifestyle modification with associated central obesity, referral to a bariatric surgeon may also be considered. Should a patient with known BE be found to have EAC on surveillance EGD, consideration of esophagectomy and referral to a minimally invasive, oncologic, or thoracic surgeon (or a combination of these surgeon types) should be performed, dependent on the practice patterns in your area.

37.8 Conclusions

Barrett's esophagus is the only known precursor to esophageal adenocarcinoma. While surgery for BE is not indicated as an antineoplastic measure, surgeons and surgery continue to play a role in the management of BE through endoscopic screening, surveillance, and treatment and through risk factor modification, including antireflux surgery, hiatal hernia repair surgery, and bariatric surgery.

What constitutes an emergency related to BE requiring emergency room presentation?	Patients with BE may also have severe esophagitis. Any hematemesis warrants evaluation in the emergency room. Following EET, any concern for esophageal perforation or development of an esophageal stricture with inability to tolerate oral intake also warrants an evaluation in the emergency room
What requires urgent surgical review for BE?	BE is not a surgical emergency. However, if a patient presents to the emergency room with hematemesis, esophageal perforation, or inability to tolerate oral intake from an esophageal stricture following EET, urgent evaluation by an interventional gastroenterologist or surgeon is warranted
What requires nonurgent surgical review for BE?	Persistent GERD symptoms in the presence of BE despite lifestyle modifications and maximal PPI therapy, presence of a hiatal hernia in the setting of BE, and/or presence of central obesity in the setting of BE
What features would mean that the condition can be managed by the PCP and what should be referred elsewhere?	Education regarding lifestyle modifications and titration of a patient's antacid regimen may be performed by their PCP. Initial management of a patient's weight through lifestyle modifications and/or medical therapy may also be performed by their PCP. It is important that any physician caring for a patient with BE reviews their previous EGDs as there are times that a patient is not aware of their history of BE. In these cases, the PCP should refer the patient to the person in their area (i.e., PCP, gastroenterology, or surgery) who performs diagnostic EGD. Endoscopic eradication therapy for BE and surveillance endoscopy following EET should be managed either by an interventional gastroenterologist or a surgeon. Surgical management of esophageal cancer should be managed by a minimally invasive gastrointestinal, thoracic, or oncologic surgeon (or a combination of the above surgeons)

(continued)

What management should be instituted prior to referral to a surgeon?	Lifestyle modification of GERD and titration of one's antacid regimen should be performed prior to referral to a surgeon. While weight loss efforts for patients with central obesity may have been initiated, it is possible that patients may not have lost any weight prior to referral to a surgeon.
What tests should be performed prior to referral to a surgeon?	Esophageal manometry testing is an additional test often performed prior to antireflux or hiatal hernia repair surgery to help guide the type of fundoplication performed. Some surgeons also obtain a barium esophagram, which may better characterize an esophageal or gastric abnormalities and is used as a roadmap for the esophagus and the stomach during these types of operations. It is not unreasonable, however, to refer a patient to a surgeon without obtaining either of these tests. Further, for patients being considered for bariatric surgery or oncologic surgery, the testing required for these patient populations is usually institution and insurance specific and we would encourage you to have a discussion with the surgeon who you plan to refer them to prior to obtaining any additional tests

Suggested Readings

1. Shaheen NJ, Falk GW, Iyer PG, Gerson LB. American College of Gastroenterology. ACG Clinical Guideline: Diagnosis and Management of Barrett's Esophagus [published correction appears in Am J Gastroenterol. 2016;111(7):1077]. Am J Gastroenterol. 2016;111(1):30–51. https://doi.org/10.1038/ajg.2015.322.
2. Shaheen NJ, Falk GW, Iyer PG, et al. Diagnosis and management of Barrett's esophagus: an updated ACG guideline. Am J Gastroenterol. 2022;117(4):559–87. https://doi.org/10.14309/ajg.0000000000001680.
3. Sharma P, Dent J, Armstrong D, et al. The development and validation of an endoscopic grading system for Barrett's esophagus: the Prague C & M criteria. Gastroenterology. 2006;131(5):1392–9. https://doi.org/10.1053/j.gastro.2006.08.032.
4. Slater BJ, Collings A, Dirks R, et al. Multi-society consensus conference and guideline on the treatment of gastroesophageal reflux disease (GERD). Surg Endosc. 2023;37(2):781–806. https://doi.org/10.1007/s00464-022-09817-3.

Esophageal Varices 38

Nicholas Dalkie and Mehrdad Nikfarjam

Abbreviations

ACLD	Advanced chronic liver disease
CP	Child–Pugh
CSPH	Clinically significant portal hypertension
EVL	Endoscopic variceal ligation
HVPG	Hepatic venous pressure gradient
LSM	Liver stiffness measurement
MELD	Model for end-stage liver disease
NSBB	Nonselective beta-blocker

38.1 Introduction

Esophageal varices are a notable complication of portal hypertension. If left untreated, the thin-walled esophageal varices become prone to rupture as the portal pressure continues to increase. This poses a substantial risk of life-threatening bleeding, with a 6-week

N. Dalkie · M. Nikfarjam (✉)
Department of Surgery, University of Melbourne, Austin Health, Heidelberg, VIC, Australia
e-mail: m.nikfarjam@unimelb.edu.au

G. P. Kohn et al. (eds.), *The SAGES Manual of Surgical Referral for Primary and Emergency Care*,
https://doi.org/10.1007/978-3-031-92678-5_38

mortality rate ranging from 15% to 20%. Primary prophylaxis against variceal hemorrhage is effective treatment; consequently, it is vital to identify patients who are at risk of this condition and referral for specialist management. Although there are other non-hepatic factors that might contribute to portal hypertension, such as portal vein thrombosis, the vast majority is the result of cirrhosis or advanced chronic liver disease (ACLD).

The presence or absence of esophageal varices in a patient with ACLD is dependent on the magnitude of the portal vein pressure. The hepatic venous pressure gradient is the benchmark for measuring this pressure and is achieved by inserting an intravascular pressure-sensing catheter into the distal hepatic veins and comparing the reading to the pressure in the right atrium, to gain a reading termed the hepatic venous pressure gradient (HVPG). The HVPG has a normal pressure range of 1–5 mmHg and a value greater than 5 mmHg is diagnostic of portal hypertension and defined as clinically significant portal hypertension (CSPH) once it reaches a value of ≥10 mmHg. Complications and decompensation occur once CSPH develops, with a higher pressure correlating with a high probability a patient will have varices.

The goal of the primary physician is to identify patients with ACLD at risk of portal hypertension and initiate urgent referral for those with CSPH. Direct measurement of HVPG to confirm and grade portal hypertension is, however, not readily available and is performed in a minority of cases. The primary physician must undertake a standard medical history, clinical examination, and perform investigations that indicate the likelihood of a patient with ACLD having portal hypertension, particularly CSPH. Referral to a specialist for endoscopic variceal screening or treatment should then follow.

38.2 History

1. Assess for underlying chronic liver disease

   Knowledge of the etiology and management of ACLD is critical as it plays a crucial role in the progression of

CSPH. Treatment based on etiology attempts to resolve the root cause of ACLD. Illustratively, nutritional adjustments to manage metabolic-associated steatotic liver disease; alcohol abstinence in the case of alcoholic liver disease; or antiviral treatment for hepatitis B or C. Potentially reducing portal hypertension, these interventions may impede or halt the progression of the disease. The development of or progression of varices can be expected if treatment has been withheld or is ineffective.

2. Assess for prior bleeding events or endoscopic examination

   Patients presenting with symptoms of gastrointestinal bleeding, either reporting melena or hematochezia, can both indicate the presence of CSPH or other sources of bleeding and should be referred with urgency. A review of prior hospitalizations for decompensation events should also prompt consideration of potential varices. As varices increase in size at a rate of 7% per year, with a 1-year rate of hemorrhage of 5% for small varices and 15% for large varices, it is important to know if a patient has undergone prior endoscopic examination. Any prior endoscopy reports should be reviewed for comment of variceal presence, size, or mention of high-risk features as these will help determine the timing of next endoscopy.

3. Assess social factors

   Social circumstances are important when considering referring a patient for variceal screening for various reasons. Patients with strong social support are more likely to adhere to the treatment of underlying ACLD and appointments. Patients with a history of continued alcohol or substance abuse are more likely to have progression of ACLD and require more frequent screening. Social determinants such as education, income, and transportation can also affect the patient's ability to understand the management of their condition and access healthcare services, including endoscopy.

38.3 Clinical Examination

A thorough clinical examination should be performed, with particular attention to findings of decompensated cirrhosis that indicates CSPH.

1. Ascites

   Ascites is the most common first presentation of CSPH and is associated with concurrent esophageal varices in 70–80% of patients. If there is clinical evidence of ascites, with associated abdominal pain or tenderness elicited on examination, then consideration should be given to spontaneous bacterial peritonitis, an infection of the ascites that may precipitate variceal hemorrhage.
2. Hepatic encephalopathy

   A wide variety of neurological findings may be present from changes in tone or reflexes, to abnormalities in examination of higher function. The neuropsychiatric changes of the hepatic encephalopathy spectrum can often be only slight and may involve attaining collateral history from relatives or caregivers for any slight changes in personality or behavior. However, it is important to recognize new-onset encephalopathy as variceal bleeding may be the precipitating event.
3. Caput medusae

   Caput medusae are a rare finding on clinical examination and result from the recanalization of the umbilical vein and increased blood flow through paraumbilical collaterals. Infrequently this finding will be seen in the absence of clinically evident ascites, but their presence is strongly associated with coexisting varices in around 90% of patients.

38.4 Investigations

1. Laboratory investigations

   Basic blood tests should be requested to assist the decision in referral, as well as support likely of CSPH and potential varices. From this respect, a platelet count of $<150 \times 10^9/L$ is a strong predictor of CSPH. A significant reduction in hemoglobin may also suggest unrecognized blood loss.

While liver enzymes are useful in the diagnosis of liver disease, they have no diagnostic value when it comes to CSPH or esophageal varices.

2. Abdominal ultrasound

   Abdominal ultrasound is an easily accessible noninvasive investigation that can provide valuable information in the assessment of CSPH and its sequelae. Patients with known cirrhosis will be undergoing regular ultrasound as part of hepatocellular carcinoma surveillance. Findings of portal vein size and flow, umbilical vein recanalization, upper abdominal collaterals, and splenic size are all useful in providing supportive information.

3. Transient elastography

   Some ultrasound providers may also be able to assess for liver stiffness measurement (LSM) by way of transient elastography. This is, however, more commonly performed through specialist gastroenterology services. The LSM of greater than 20 kPa correlates well with the degree of fibrosis and CSPH.

38.5 Severity Scoring Systems

Severity scoring of ACLD, used in addition to the investigations noted, can help guide the urgency of referral endoscopic variceal assessment.

1. Child–Pugh (CP)

   This is the most well-known severity scoring system and combines blood test markers of synthetic liver function (bilirubin, albumin, INR) with clinical findings of decompensated disease (ascites, encephalopathy), and will give a class of A, B, or C. Patients with CP A cirrhosis are generally in a compensated state of ACLD and rarely have varices, whereas CP B and C frequently do and may require either medical or endoscopic intervention.

2. Model for end-stage liver disease (MELD)

   The MELD score is a newer scoring system that removes the subjective assessments of ascites and encephalopathy severities, as well as albumin that can fluctuate for a number of reasons aside from intrinsic liver function, and uses a complex equation involving bilirubin, INR, creatinine, sodium, and need for dialysis to provide a score between 6 and 40. Its use is generally more among specialist gastroenterologists and hepatologists, but also has utility in patient risk stratification.

Both scoring systems provide valuable information on referral as they stratify patients into different risk and probability groups. Patients with CP C cirrhosis have a very high 6-week mortality risk following variceal hemorrhage, and all benefit from primary prophylactic treatment of the varices if present. They do have a very low 1-year survival and may opt for no invasive procedures. An in-depth discussion about patient wishes and expectations should be had prior to referral.

38.6 Management

While most of the management of esophageal varices is undertaken and guided by specialist gastroenterologists/hepatologists or surgical endoscopists, primary care also plays a crucial role in the long-term management. The role of primary care in this setting is to ensure patients are undergoing endoscopy at the recommended time intervals and maintain and prescribe medical therapy.

1. Primary prophylaxis

   Primary prophylaxis refers to the management of varices before the first episode of variceal hemorrhage. Following identification of a patient at risk of CSPH and varices, a referral will be made for endoscopy, and based on those findings may be recommended for primary prophylaxis if CSPH is confirmed. Previously the decision of endoscopic or medical therapy would be at the discretion of the specialist; however, recent data support use of nonselective beta-blockers (NSBB), in particular carvedilol. Endoscopic variceal ligation (EVL) is reserved for patients who cannot tolerate or have a contraindication to NSBB.

Patients with confirmed CSPH who can tolerate NSBB do not require routine endoscopic surveillance. If patients require EVL for primary prophylaxis, then they will undergo an eradication phase of endoscopy every 4–8 weeks and at 6 months, and then yearly. If there are none or only small varices that cannot be banded, then repeat endoscopy will be every 2 years.

2. Secondary prophylaxis

   If a patient has suffered a previous variceal hemorrhage, then treatment will be secondary prevention to prevent further events, which occur at a rate of up to 60% within a year if there is no further treatment. Dual modality therapy with both NSBB and EVL is still recommended in this setting, with evidence showing dual therapy has superior survival compared to either alone. Frequency of endoscopy in secondary prophylaxis is the same as for primary prophylaxis, that is, eradication phase, then 6-month check, then yearly endoscopic surveillance. If at surveillance there are any varices that require EVL, then a patient falls back into an eradication phase as previously until these varices are again eradicated.

Patients in whom either primary or secondary prophylaxis management with EVL is unsuccessful, that is, require frequent, and multiple procedures without eradication, or recurrent varices despite the above measures, then the treating specialist will need to consider other interventions. Given that this may reflect progression of the liver disease or development of a complication that can worsen portal pressures, such as a portal vein thrombosis or hepatocellular carcinoma, investigations and management will be instigated by the treating specialist and are outside the scope of this document.

Carvedilol has now become the NSBB of choice for use in portal hypertension. The benefits it has over prior generations, such as propranolol and nadolol, include data demonstrating reduced number of decompensation events, increased survival, improved ascites, and lower risk of spontaneous bacterial peritonitis. From a monitoring perspective in primary care, it does not need to be titrated to heart rate, and is generally started at a dose of 6.25 mg daily and increased to 12.5 mg daily after 3 days if the patient is tolerating. Higher doses may be used if indicated for nonhepatic indications.

38.7 Referral to Specialist

Any concern regarding a patient at the primary care level should prompt a consideration of referral to specialist for further management. While patients may be referred to anyone qualified to perform upper gastrointestinal endoscopy for assessment solely of esophageal varices in patients with CSPH, long-term care of a patient with ACLD should be under the care of a gastroenterologist or hepatologist, and therefore referral should be directed toward these specialists.

The urgency of this referral is dependent on the clinical scenario and patient condition, and in the case of a newly decompensated patient, or one with signs of acute gastrointestinal bleeding, may even warrant referral directly to emergency for immediate assessment and treatment. Table 38.1 outlines a general guidance that may be used to inform the decision on urgency. Note that these are for guidance only, and some features in one category may be deemed to be more or less urgent, particularly in the case of what may prompt a referral directly to the Emergency Room. Table 38.2 contains information that should be conveyed on referral or investigations that should be arranged and included in the case of outpatient referrals.

Table 38.1 Suggested information from history, clinical examination, and investigations that may be used to guide decision on urgency of referral of a patient with cirrhosis for specialist assessment

Criteria	Requires emergency presentation to hospital	Urgent outpatient referral	Nonurgent outpatient referral
History	Hematemesis or melena acutely Syncope Severe abdominal pain Confusion or altered mental status	Hematemesis or melena in recent history but resolved New development of abdominal distension without pain	New diagnosis of cirrhosis Untreated viral hepatitis Persistent alcohol intake in a known cirrhotic
Clinical examination findings	Hypotension Tachycardia Ascites with abdominal tenderness or fever Overtly altered mental status (overt hepatic encephalopathy) Melena on rectal exam	New ascites Acutely worsening jaundice Mild changes in mental status or personality (covert hepatic encephalopathy)	Worsening ascites Peripheral stigmata of chronic liver disease
Laboratory investigations	Acute drop in hemoglobin Acute kidney injury Marked deterioration in liver synthetic function (bilirubin and INR)	Acute deterioration of bilirubin or INR	New abnormalities in liver function tests Slowly deteriorating liver function tests or coagulopathy in a known cirrhotic
Radiological investigations	Occlusive portal venous system thrombosis	New findings of Ascites Liver lesion Nonocclusive portal venous system thrombosis	Features of cirrhosis or portal hypertension without complications

Table 38.2 Information that should ideally be included in referral for outpatient review of patient with cirrhosis and/or concern of clinically significant portal hypertension in whom esophageal varices is suspected

Category	Information to include
History	Etiology of cirrhosis (if known) Prior complications of cirrhosis Prior treatments for cirrhosis or underlying etiology Metabolic disease risk factors Alcohol history Social supports and functional status
Examination	Vital signs Presence (or absence) of ascites Assessment of hepatic encephalopathy Peripheral signs of chronic liver disease
Investigations	Full blood count Liver function tests Coagulation profile Basic metabolic panel Abdominal ultrasound Liver stiffness measurement (if available)
Liver severity score	MELD score Child–Pugh score

38.8 Summary

Esophageal varices are a serious complication of CSPH, with high mortality if undiagnosed and untreated in patients with ACLD. While most treatment will be completed by specialists, it is important for nonspecialists to recognize which patients are at risk, what factors contribute to that risk, and refer appropriately.

Once a patient has undergone index endoscopy, they may require medical therapy oversight at the nonspecialist level and guidance for ongoing surveillance if appropriate. Figure 38.1 provides an overview to guide nonspecialists.

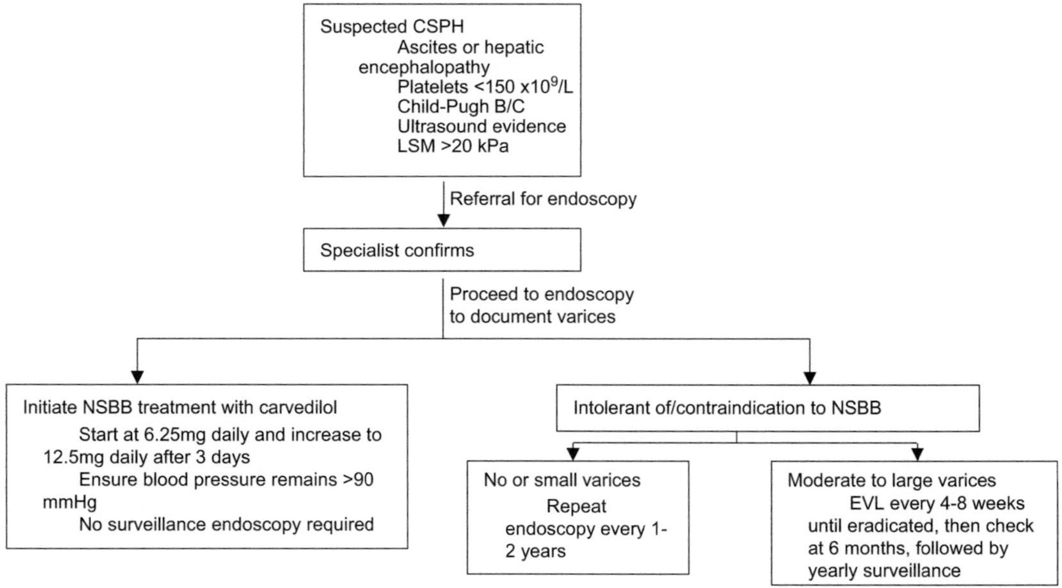

Fig. 38.1 Approach to clinically significant portal hypertension (CSPH) assessment in the non-specialist setting, and expected management, adapted from Baveno VII guidelines and AASLD practice guidance (De Franchis 2022 [2], Kaplan 2023 [4]). *NSBB* Non selective beta-blockers, *LSM* Liver stiffness measurement

Disclosure Statement The authors have no conflict of interests in relation to this paper.

Suggested Readings

1. Diaz-Soto M, Garcia-Tsao G. Management of varices and variceal hemorrhage in liver cirrhosis: a recent update. Ther Adv Gastroenterol. 2022;15:1–12.
2. De Franchis R, Bosch J, Garcia-Tsao G, et al. Baveno VII—Renewing consensus in portal hypertension. J Hepatol. 2022;76:959–74.
3. Garcia-Tsao G, Bosch J. Management of varices and variceal hemorrhage in cirrhosis. N Engl J Med. 2010;362:823–32.
4. Kaplan D, Bosch J, Ripoll C, et al. AASLD practice guidance on risk stratification and management of portal hypertension and varices in cirrhosis. Hepatol. 2023; https://doi.org/10.1097/hep.0000000000000647.
5. Villanueva C, Albillos A, Genescà J, et al. ß blockers to prevent decompensation of cirrhosis in patients with clinically significant portal hypertension (PREDESCI): a randomised, double-blind, placebo-controlled, multicentre trial. Lancet. 2019;393:1597–608.

Gastroparesis

39

Elizabeth D. Winter
and William S. Richardson

39.1 Relevant History

Gastroparesis is a complex and often debilitating condition that is challenging for even the experienced provider to treat. In many cases, management can be successful using simply lifestyle interventions and medications. However, this is not always the case. In the refractory gastroparesis patient, consideration for surgical intervention is important. When I was a medical student, the only surgical treatment for gastroparesis offered was subtotal or total gastrectomy. This intervention has been found to be a morbid and invasive procedure often without much symptomatic or functional improvement. Thankfully, today there are multiple alternative interventions offered both endoscopically and surgically for these refractory patients. In fact, this field continues to evolve, with more minimally invasive options available. These options include gastric stimulators and pyloric procedures, which have increased the interest in surgery as a treatment for gastroparesis.

For definition purposes, we will label a patient with gastroparesis if they have appropriate symptoms, a positive gastric emptying study, are not taking medications that could contribute to

E. D. Winter · W. S. Richardson (✉)
Oschner Medical Center, New Orleans, LA, USA
e-mail: wrichardson@ochsner.org

G. P. Kohn et al. (eds.), *The SAGES Manual of Surgical Referral for Primary and Emergency Care*,
https://doi.org/10.1007/978-3-031-92678-5_39

delayed gastric emptying and have no anatomic reason for delayed gastric emptying. A stepwise approach is widely adopted for the treatment of these patients starting with lifestyle changes and nutritional support followed by medical treatment, and finally, surgery.

This guideline is evidence-based and accurate as of the time of writing, but this is an evolving field, and recommendations may change.

39.2 Clinical Examination

When clinically examining a patient who presents with concern for gastroparesis, it is important to first start with a thorough medical and surgical history. Second, you will obtain a complete evaluation of their symptomatology and disease severity.

Gastroparesis is most commonly idiopathic (unrelated to an underlying illness) or diabetic. It can be post-surgical or linked to other diseases such as neurological disorders like Parkinson's disease, collagen, and vascular disorders. Postsurgical gastroparesis is most often a consequence of vagal nerve injury during upper GI procedures but also can be caused by distal gastrectomy and other gastric procedures. A complete history of related diagnoses and surgery is important to diagnose a cause for gastroparesis. Keep in mind as well that many common medications can worsen gastroparesis symptoms or even cause gastroparesis itself, including opioids, certain antidepressants, blood pressure medications, and weight loss medications.

Most patients with gastroparesis will have the symptoms of nausea and vomiting, along with some epigastric pain and occasional severe bloating. Symptoms may be accompanied by reflux as gastroparesis is a known contributor to GERD, and in some cases abdominal muscle spasming. Unfortunately, these are common symptoms for many GI problems such as IBS, SIBO, fibromyalgia, food allergies, as well as anatomic sources such as ulcer disease, hernias, and even cancer (Table 39.1). For example, there is a considerable overlap with functional dyspepsia (FD). Recently

Table 39.1 Differential diagnoses for nausea and vomiting

CNS	GI	Infectious	Meds/toxins	Metabolic	Psychiatric
Increased intracranial pressure	IBD, IBS	Acute otitis media	Antiarrhythmics	Adrenal disorders	Eating disorders
Migraine	Obstruction	Spontaneous bacterial peritonitis	Antibiotics	DKA	Conversion disorder
Seizure d/o	Malignancy	Adenovirus	Anticonvulsants	Paraneoplastic syndromes	Depression
Vestibular d/o	Hernia	Norwalk	Chemotherapeutics	Parathyroid disorders	Anxiety
	Volvulus	Rotavirus	Digoxin	Pregnancy	
	Motility disorders		NSAIDS	Thyroid disorders	
	Mesenteric ischemia		Opiates	Uremia	
			Toxins		

published ENSM consensus statement differentiates the two disease processes with their cardinal symptoms—early satiation, postprandial fullness, and epigastric pain/burning in FD, with nausea and vomiting as cardinal symptoms of gastroparesis. Further imaging studies can help differentiate these disease processes, as will be discussed below.

Finally, and arguably the most important aspect of your approach, patient-reported symptom scales are essential in evaluating the patient with gastroparesis. The Gastroparesis Cardinal Symptom Index (GCSI), as seen in Table 39.2, developed by the American Neurogastroenterology and Motility Society is a patient-based symptom severity assessment that has been validated by a number of studies (1). It or similar scoring should be used consistently in this patient population to follow symptom development and treatment outcomes. While it is difficult to standardize imaging and functional studies, this is a way for providers to communicate and share information on the success or failure of treatment.

Table 39.2 Gastroparesis Cardinal Symptom Index (GCSI)

Gastroparesis cardinal symptom index Please mark the severity and frequency of your symptoms based on this scale	
Severity	Frequency
0 = absent	0 = absent
1 = mild (*not influencing normal activities*)	1 = rare (*1 times/week*)
2 = moderate (*diverting from, but not urging modification of usual activities*)	2 = occasional (*2–4 times/week*)
3 = severe (*influencing usual activities severely enough to urge modification*)	3 = frequent (*5–7 times/week*)
4 = extremely severe (*requesting bed rest*)	4 = extremely frequent (*>7 times/week*)

(continued)

Table 39.2 (continued)

Gastroparesis cardinal symptom index Please mark the severity and frequency of your symptoms based on this scale		
Symptom	Severity	Frequency
1. Vomiting: *Forceful expulsion of stomach content from the mouth. It should be distinguished from retching, which is defined as "heaving as if to vomit."*		
2. Nausea: *Feeling sick to your stomach as if you were going to vomit.*		
3. Early satiety: *A feeling that the stomach is over-filled after starting to eat, so that you are unable to finish a normal-sized meal.*		
4. Bloating: *Feeling like you need to loosen your clothes. Stomach or belly is visibly larger.*		
5. Postprandial fullness: *Feeling excessively full after meals.*		
6. Epigastric pain: *The epigastrium can be identified as the area about the size of one hand in the central part of the upper abdomen. The pain should be distinguished from discomfort, which is defined as subjective, negative, and unpleasant feeling, but one that "does not hurt."*		
7. Epigastric burning: *Burning is a special time of pain that can be described as an "inside flame."*		

39.3 Diagnostic Studies

As an adjunct to your thorough history, there are multiple aspects to the evaluation of gastroparesis patients including both imaging and functional studies. Gastroparesis patients can be malnourished, so weight history as well as basic labs are important to obtain. There is no current blood lab to rule-in gastroparesis but malnourished patients may need J-tube feeding or TPN until symptoms can be controlled. The typical workup includes CT, upper endoscopy, and gastric emptying study.

An abdominal CT should be obtained to rule out anatomic causes of obstruction. This can identify hiatal hernias, evidence of prior upper abdominal surgery, pyloric obstruction or thickening, or an enlarged stomach. However, in gastroparesis patients there are commonly no significant findings on imaging. Keep in mind, there may be a bezoar in the stomach, which may be rarely interpreted by radiology as poor flow of contrast through the stomach.

Esophagogastroduodenoscopy may also identify obstruction, ulcer disease, hiatal hernia, and esophagitis. It can also help rule out other causes of symptoms, including celiac disease.

Gastric emptying scintigraphy is the main study utilized to diagnose gastroparesis. An abnormal gastric emptying test is required in both US and European guidelines for establishing a diagnosis. However, there is a lack of standardization across institutions for this test that presents issues for providers when interpreting studies from other institutions. There are several conditions under which it may be falsely positive. Confounding factors giving false positives include medications, obstructions (hiatal hernia, achalasia), and ulcer disease. Before the study, patients are counselled to hold medications that may lead to delayed gastric emptying (DGE).

Gastric scintigraphy most commonly utilizes radio-labeled solid food—usually low-fat egg whites. A true positive is over 10% retention at 4 h. The relationship between the degree of DGE and symptom severity has been controversial.

39.4 Medical Treatment

Most patients with gastroparesis can be managed medically. First, if possible, eliminating medications that can cause symptoms is especially important. Some of these patients are on chronic narcotics or other medications that significantly worsen their symptoms.

Diet modification can be helpful, but difficult for patients to implement. A high-protein, low-fat, low-carbohydrate, and low-fiber diet has been found to improve symptoms, along with decreasing size and increasing the frequency of meals to about six small meals per day. However, many patients are not able to do this, and many are overweight or gain weight due to overconsumption of comfort foods, which they still absorb well. Other dietary changes such as low lactose or gluten may be helpful in select patients.

It is important to also consider the lower GI tract in these patients as constipation worsens the symptoms of gastroparesis and can also signal you to a broader intestinal dysmotility in these patients.

Gastroparesis has been found to be associated with psychosocial comorbidities such as anxiety and depression. Patients may be helped with anxiolytics and referral to psychiatry.

Promotility agents are most frequently used in both symptomatic and functional treatment for gastroparesis. Metoclopramide, a D2 antagonist is highly effective, and is the only US FDA-approved medication. Domperidone, another D2 antagonist, has also been found to be efficacious and has similar side effects but is not FDA approved in the United States. Erythromycin, a motilin analog, is sometimes effective, but is frequently not covered by insurance. Many other medications have been trialed for gastroparesis, and a full review is beyond the scope of this chapter. Patients with severe gastroparesis frequently require multiple antinausea medications to control their symptoms.

In severe cases, patients may require hospital visits for periodic IV hydration.

When the regimen has been optimized several times without improvement, and all medication and lifestyle changes have been made, we will call this refractory gastroparesis.

39.5 Surgical Treatment

When patients have no significant response to standard medical regimen or are precluded from taking these medications due to side effects, we can begin discussing the involvement of gastroenterology and surgery for more invasive treatment options.

First, it is important to address malnutrition in the case of severe weight loss or intractable vomiting. If these patients are unable to tolerate anything PO over extended periods, they may benefit from the implementation of enteral access like a jejunostomy tube. Furthermore, if your patient is experiencing severe nausea and vomiting, a gastrostomy tube or PEG may be placed for venting. While enteral access and gastric venting do not treat or improve gastric emptying, they can significantly improve quality of life.

Gastroparesis patients have also recently been shown to benefit from minimally invasive pyloric procedures. Endoscopic pyloric procedures include endoscopic myotomy, sometimes called gastric peroral endoscopic myotomy (G-POEM). Improvement in symptoms in the short term with these procedures is about 80% but far-fewer get near-complete relief and many have no improvement in symptoms.

Transabdominal procedures include pyloromyotomy and pyloroplasty. These are well-established procedures performed most commonly either laparoscopically or robotically. Both function to expand or relax the pylorus, thereby increasing gastric emptying. It has been suggested that these surgical procedures are less morbid and less invasive to first attempt when treating a clinically challenging patient as opposed to gastrectomy. These have been found to be effective and safe procedures that have been reported to improve or even normalize gastric emptying.

Pyloric Botox injections have also been utilized for relaxation of the pylorus but are not recommended for the treatment of gastroparesis and have been found to show no improvement in GE in at least two independent randomized controlled studies.

Another minimally invasive surgical intervention uses gastric stimulation. This includes laparoscopically placing a pacemaker with leads to the stomach, helping regulate motility. It can be placed using minimally invasive techniques. Postoperatively a stimulator will require follow-up with surgery to adjust settings for symptomatic improvement. Additionally, unlike a pyloric procedure, it will eventually require additional procedures in the future for battery replacement. Some of these devices are not MRI compatible, so it is important to discuss with the patient's surgeon regarding the model used. Controlled trials in the past for gastric stimulators at large institutions have reported no significant improvement in symptoms; however, there is strong anecdotal evidence and many open-label studies that have reported significant improvement in total symptom severity. Additionally, a new large, multicenter randomized crossover study showed that electrical stimulation significantly reduced the frequency of refractory vomiting.

There also exist several more invasive options performed with the intent of improvement in gastric emptying. These range from injections to endoscopic procedures to major abdominal surgeries aimed at rerouting the GI tract. Surgical options include but are not limited to gastric sleeve, Roux-en-Y gastric bypass (RYGB), partial or subtotal gastrectomy.

In conclusion, the step-wise approach to the gastroparesis patient includes first lifestyle and medical interventions that may need to be combined with more invasive interventions in the case of refractory gastroparesis. A combined approach is typically required, utilizing subspecialties such as gastroenterology, especially those specializing in motility disorders, as well as general surgery for both symptomatic interventions and interventions that may improve gastric emptying itself.

Tests and management prior to referral to surgery
Optimization of comorbid conditions (diabetes, constipation, depression/anxiety)
Elimination of medications that may worsen or contribute
Prokinetic agents
Nutritional labs
Imaging:
CT abdomen pelvis with IV contrast
EGD
Upper GI contrast study
Gastric emptying study

(continued)

What constitutes an emergency requiring ER presentation?	· Dehydration · Intolerance to PO intake
What requires urgent surgical review?	· History of multiple recent hospitalizations for dehydration · Significant intolerance to PO intake
What requires nonurgent surgical review?	· Symptomatic gastroparesis resistant to medical management
What features of gastroparesis may be managed by the PCP and what should be referred elsewhere?	PCP Coaching in lifestyle modifications Management of comorbidities (e.g., DMII, constipation, psychosocial) Promotility agents Referral: Endoscopic evaluation: Gastroenterology -Resistant to medical management: Gastroenterology and surgery

Suggested Readings

1. American College of Gastroenterology Clinical Guidelines for Gastroparesis.

   Camilleri M, Kuo B, Nguyen L, Vaughn VM, Petrey J, Greer K, Yadlapati R, Abell TL. ACG Clinical Guideline: Gastroparesis. Am J Gastroenterol. 2022 Aug 1;117(8):1197–1220. https://doi.org/10.14309/ajg.0000000000001874. Epub 2022 Jun 3. PMID: 35926490; PMCID: PMC9373497.
2. European Society of Neurogastroenterology and Motility (ESNM) Consensus Statement.

   Schol J, Wauters L, Dickman R, Drug V, Mulak A, Serra J, Enck P, Tack J; ESNM Gastroparesis Consensus Group. United European Gastroenterology (UEG) and European Society for Neurogastroenterology and Motility (ESNM) consensus on gastroparesis. United European Gastroenterol J. 2021 Apr;9(3):287–306. https://doi.org/10.1002/ueg2.12060.

Erratum in: United European Gastroenterol J. 2021 Sep;9(7):883–884. PMID: 33939892; PMCID: PMC8259275.

3. Efficacy and Safety of Drugs for Gastroparesis: Systematic Review and Network Meta-analysis.

   Ingrosso MR, Camilleri M, Tack J, Ianiro G, Black CJ, Ford AC. EGastroenterology. 2023 Apr;164(4):642–654. https://doi.org/10.1053/j.gastro.2022.12.014. Epub 2022 Dec 26. PMID: 36581089.

Gastritis with Ulcer

40

Léa Tessier and Yung Lee

Abbreviations

PPI	Proton pump inhibitor
GI	Gastroenterologist
NSAID	Nonsteroidal anti-inflammatory drug
MALT	Mucosa-associated lymphoid tissue
PUD	Peptic ulcer disease
ED	Emergency department
CBC	Complete blood count

40.1 History

"Gastritis" describes inflammation to the gastric mucosa. It can be classified by time course (acute versus chronic).

Acute gastritis is a temporary inflammation secondary to stress on the gastric mucosa that can arise from a wide range of factors.

L. Tessier · Y. Lee (✉)
Department of Surgery, Division of General Surgery, McMaster University, Hamilton, ON, Canada
e-mail: yung.lee@medportal.ca

G. P. Kohn et al. (eds.), *The SAGES Manual of Surgical Referral for Primary and Emergency Care*,
https://doi.org/10.1007/978-3-031-92678-5_40

These include medications [nonsteroidal anti-inflammatory drugs (NSAIDs), aspirin, corticosteroids], corrosive agents, radiation, ischemia or shock, trauma or severe burns, sepsis, or certain infections such as enteroviruses. Acute gastritis may manifest with acute-onset epigastric pain, bloating, dyspepsia, nausea, and vomiting, or signs of upper gastrointestinal bleeding.

Chronic gastritis is most commonly caused by *Helicobacter pylori* infection. Acute *H. pylori* infection may initially be asymptomatic. Without treatment, *H. pylori* infection typically leads to chronic gastritis and peptic ulcer disease (PUD), which may be asymptomatic in up to 70% of patients, or may manifest with abdominal pain and dyspepsia (e.g., postprandial fullness, early satiation, burning sensation). Patients may present with complications of chronic gastritis and PUD, including symptoms of upper gastrointestinal (GI) bleeding (e.g., melena) and anemia. Constitutional symptoms should be assessed as patients may have progression to gastric cancer and mucosa-associated lymphoid tissue (MALT).

Another cause of chronic gastritis is autoimmune gastritis; these patients are often asymptomatic, though may have similar gastrointestinal symptoms. These individuals may present with megaloblastic, pernicious, or iron-deficiency anemias. Symptomatic anemia, including neurological symptoms from vitamin B12 deficiency, should be screened for.

A review of medical history should include a history of *H. pylori* infection (including treatment and evidence of eradication). Patients with systemic or inflammatory conditions, such as sarcoidosis, Crohn's disease, or eosinophilic gastroenteritis, may develop gastritis or ulcers from gastric or duodenal involvement of these processes. Other autoimmune disorders may be present in patients with autoimmune gastritis, including Hashimoto thyroiditis, Addison disease, chronic spontaneous urticaria, myasthenia gravis, type 1 diabetes, vitiligo, and erosive oral lichen planus.

Family history should include that of systemic, inflammatory, autoimmune diseases, as well as malignancies (e.g., gastric, esophageal). Bacteriology and epidemiological studies have found intrafamilial clustering of *H. pylori* infection, suggesting increased risk of infection in an individual living amongst family or spouse with a history of *H. pylori*.

Social history should include a history of cigarette smoking and excessive alcohol use.

40.2 Clinical Exam

Physical exam findings for gastritis and peptic ulcer may reveal epigastric abdominal tenderness. Complications of chronic gastritis and PUD may reveal themselves on exam. Upper GI bleed may present as melena stool on digital rectal exam or signs of anemia (e.g., pallor, weakness). A patient presenting with malignancy may have frailty or cachexia. Vitamin B12 deficiency can manifest as decreased reflexes, gait abnormalities, peripheral neuropathy, and loss of vibratory sense and proprioception, and cognitive deficits. Perforation of a peptic ulcer should be suspected in patients with abnormal vital signs, severe tenderness, and peritonitis. These patients should be sent to the emergency department (ED) for urgent surgical consultation. Table 40.1 presents a general guide for referral based on patient presentation.

Table 40.1 General guide for referral based on patient presentation

Presentation	Referral
Symptoms of gastritis (abdominal pain and dyspepsia) without alarm signs	Management by primary care provider: Acid suppression, diagnosis, and eradication of *H. pylori*, elimination of NSAIDs, smoking cessation
<60 years of age with alarm symptoms Persistent symptoms after management by primary care provider	Nonurgent referral to general surgery or gastroenterologist
>60 years of age with alarm symptoms	Urgent surgical referral

(continued)

Table 40.1 (continued)

Presentation	Referral
Signs or symptoms of perforation Severe pain refractory to PPI or analgesia, or patients with transfusion-dependent anemia, should also be transferred to the ED	Emergency department presentation

Alarm symptoms: >60 years of age with weight loss, signs or symptoms of bleeding, dysphagia, vomiting, fever, or a family history of esophageal or gastric cancer
Signs and symptoms of perforation: peritonitis, severe pain, hemodynamic instability, and free air on imaging

Table 40.2 Investigations and treatments prior to specialist referral

Investigations	Treatments
Complete blood count Noninvasive *H. pylori* testing (urea breath test or stool antigen test)	Elimination of NSAIDs Smoking cessation Acid suppression (PPI) Eradication of *H. pylori* if diagnosed

40.3 Investigations

Investigations should follow a stepwise process to identify the underlying etiology minimizing unnecessary invasive testing. Table 40.2 presents a list of investigations to consider prior to referring the patient to a specialist.

40.3.1 Laboratory Assessments

Patients with uncomplicated peptic ulcers often have normal laboratory values. In the case of a bleeding ulcer, patients may have an iron-deficiency anemia. Leukocytosis on a standard complete blood count (CBC) may be present in the setting of a perforated ulcer. Patients under the age of 60 without alarm features of weight loss, signs or symptoms of bleeding, dysphagia, vomiting, fever, or a family history of esophageal or gastric cancer should undergo noninvasive *H. pylori* testing (urea breath test or stool antigen test).

40.3.2 Imaging

Plain films and abdominal computed tomography (CT) scans are not sensitive and are generally of limited use in uncomplicated peptic ulcer disease. The patient should be transferred to a nearby tertiary center if perforation is suspected. Urgent imaging should then be obtained, such as an upright abdominal X-ray or a CT scan of the abdomen with IV contrast.

40.3.3 Upper Endoscopy

Endoscopic evaluation by a specialist (e.g., gastroenterologist, general surgeon) is the most accurate test for peptic ulcer disease. Endoscopic biopsies are done to determine the etiology of gastritis (e.g., *H. pylori* infection, systemic or inflammatory conditions) and investigate malignancy in suspicious–appearing lesions.

Patients >60 years of age with alarm symptoms warrant an upper gastrointestinal endoscopic evaluation with biopsy. Patients with a history of complications (such as a history of perforation) or recurrence of symptoms despite appropriate treatment (acid suppression with PPI, *H. pylori* eradication, elimination of risk factors including NSAIDs and smoking) also warrant endoscopic evaluation.

40.4 Referrals

Most patients with benign peptic ulcers are treated appropriately (acid suppression with a PPI, diagnosis and eradication of *H. pylori*, elimination of NSAIDs, smoking cessation) and do not require surgical consultation. Confirmation of healing of a gastric

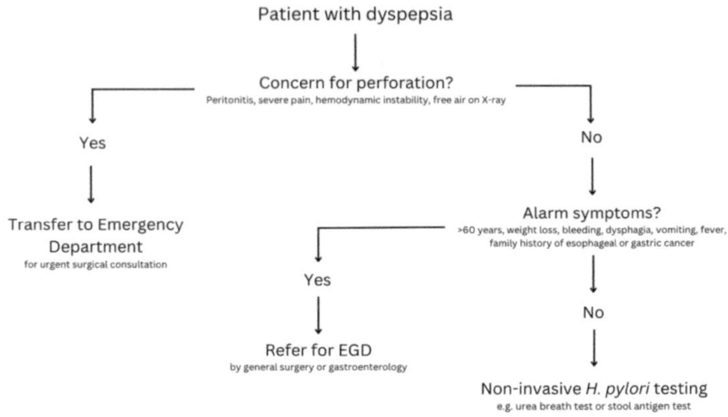

Fig. 40.1 Algorithm for referral to general surgery

ulcer is suggested by repeat endoscopy after treatment. Figure 40.1 demonstrates an algorithm for referral to general surgery.

While endoscopy and biopsy are the gold standard for ruling out malignancy, they are expensive and come with a small risk of serious morbidity and mortality. Current guidelines by the American College of Gastroenterology (ACG) and the Canadian Association of Gastroenterology (CAG) recommend endoscopic evaluation only in individuals at high risk for malignancy. As such, referral to an endoscopist (e.g., general surgeon, gastroenterologist) is warranted in patients with advanced age (>60 years) with alarm symptoms (weight loss, signs or symptoms of bleeding, dysphagia, vomiting, fever, or a family history of esophageal or gastric cancer).

The value of endoscopy in young patients (<60 years) with alarm features to rule out neoplasia is controversial; current evidence suggests that alarm symptoms in young patients have limited utility in detecting an organic pathology, and the risk of a GI malignancy is <1% in this population. East Asian individuals have increased prevalence of atrophic gastritis and higher incidence of gastric cancer. The threshold for referral to an endoscopic specialist may therefore be adjusted, although there are no established Eastern guidelines for investigating gastritis. Nonetheless, endoscopic evaluation may be appropriate and cost effective, even in patients who immigrate from high to low gastric cancer incidence countries.

Patients who present with signs or symptoms concerning for perforation, including peritonitis, severe pain, hemodynamic instability, and free air on imaging, should be sent to the ED for broad-spectrum intravenous antibiotics and intravenous proton pump inhibitor (PPI) in addition to urgent consultation by a general surgeon. Patients with severe pain refractory to PPI or analgesia, or patients with transfusion-dependent anemia, should also be transferred to the ED.

Suggested Readings

1. Sugano K, Tack J, Kuipers EJ, et al. Kyoto global consensus report on Helicobacter pylori gastritis. Gut. 2015;64(9):1353–67. https://doi.org/10.1136/gutjnl-2015-309252.
2. Moayyedi PM, Lacy BE, Andrews CN, Enns RA, Howden CW, Vakil N. ACG and CAG clinical guideline: management of dyspepsia. Am J Gastroenterol. 2017;112(7):988–1013. https://doi.org/10.1038/ajg.2017.154.
3. Chey WD, Leontiadis GI, Howden CW, Moss SF. ACG Clinical Guideline: treatment of helicobacter pylori infection. Am J Gastroenterol. 2017;112(2):212–39. https://doi.org/10.1038/ajg.2016.563.

Gastric Masses

41

Saamia Shaikh, Oscar Paredes Torres,
and Sophia K. McKinley

Abbreviations

GERD	Gastroesophageal reflux disease
GI	Gastrointestinal
CBC	Complete blood count
IV	Intravenous
GIST	Gastrointestinal stromal tumor
NET	Neuroendocrine tumor
EUS	Endoscopic ultrasound
EGD	Esophagogastroduodenoscopy
GOO	Gastric outlet obstruction

S. Shaikh
St. Joseph's University Medical Center, Paterson, NJ, USA

O. P. Torres
Department of Abdominal Surgery, National Institute of Neoplastic Diseases, Lima, Peru

S. K. McKinley (✉)
Department of Surgery, Harvard Medical School, Massachusetts General Hospital, Boston, MA, USA
e-mail: skmckinley@mgh.harvard.edu

G. P. Kohn et al. (eds.), *The SAGES Manual of Surgical Referral for Primary and Emergency Care*,
https://doi.org/10.1007/978-3-031-92678-5_41

41.1 Initial Evaluation of Asymptomatic Gastric Masses

Gastric masses can be asymptomatic and may be found incidentally during upper endoscopy performed for another reason (e.g., gastritis, GERD). Gastric masses may also be found incidentally on imaging such as CT scan or MRI. Masses noted during endoscopy should be biopsied by the endoscopist to attain a tissue diagnosis, and the management of the mass depends on the specific histology. If a small mass (<2 cm) is noted on axial imaging, we recommend initial referral to an endoscopist to perform an EGD and biopsy of the mass. Again, the histology of the mass will dictate surgical referral. For larger tumors that are identified on imaging (>2 cm), it is appropriate to place referral for endoscopy while simultaneously requesting surgical evaluation as tumors of this size are more likely to require surgical treatment.

Endoscopic examination with biopsy is the diagnostic modality of choice for gastric lesions as it allows for tissue diagnosis in addition to localization and direct visualization of the tumor. Multiple biopsies must be taken to obtain an adequate sample for molecular and histologic examination. Depending on the appearance of the lesion, the endoscopist may employ endoscopic ultrasound (EUS) to differentiate between intramural lesions and extrinsic compression, detect whether a mass is homogeneous or heterogeneous, evaluate its borders or margins, evaluate for the enlargement of regional lymph nodes, and assess the depth of invasion. EUS with fine-needle aspiration (EUS-FNA) or fine-needle biopsy (EUS-FNB) permits sampling of deeper portions of a gastric mass relative to the standard mucosal biopsy.

41.2 Initial Evaluation of Symptomatic Gastric Masses

Nearly all patients with symptomatic gastric masses will require surgical referral (Table 41.1). The most common presenting symptoms of gastric masses include gastrointestinal bleed and

Table 41.1 Emergency department and surgical referral for gastric masses

Scenario		
Symptoms of gastric mass that warrant emergency department evaluation	Obstruction that prevents adequate oral intake or causes persistent nausea/vomiting GI bleeding including lower and upper GI bleeding that results in hemodynamic changes or syncope Gastric perforation, which manifests as peritonitis and shock Severe abdominal pain Any signs/symptoms of shock and abdominal sepsis Any sign/symptom associated with hemodynamic instability Any sign/symptom considered acutely life-threatening by the referring physician All of the above scenarios should prompt surgical consultation	
Gastric masses warranting urgent surgical evaluation	Nearly all gastric masses warrant urgent surgical evaluation given the risk of malignancy (within 2–3 weeks), including All symptomatic tumors All tumors >2 cm	Notable exception: Gastric lymphoma is managed by medical oncology unless symptoms necessitate emergency room referral, in which case surgical consultation is recommended
Gastric masses warranting nonurgent surgical evaluation	Very few gastric masses qualify for nonurgent surgical referral (>3 weeks before evaluation). These include Endoscopically unresectable polyps Gastric polyposis syndromes Type 1 neuroendocrine tumors that cannot be endoscopically managed	

(continued)

Table 41.1 (continued)

Scenario		
Gastric masses that can be managed by primary care physician	All gastric masses should be referred for specialist care	
Gastric masses that can be managed by nonsurgical specialists	Gastroenterology: Small type I neuroendocrine tumors (every 6–12- month endoscopic surveillance) Gastric polyps (endoscopic resection and surveillance depending on polyp histology)	Medical oncology Gastric lymphoma, management depends on subtype of lymphoma

associated anemia, abdominal pain, nausea, early satiety, obstruction, and weight loss. These symptoms should prompt a complete history and physical examination, including abdominal examination, digital rectal examination, and lymph node examination. Family history of GI cancers and risk factors for stomach cancer, including history of *H. pylori* infection, smoking, alcohol use, and East Asian ancestry, are important in the evaluation of all gastric tumors. Upper GI endoscopy and axial imaging are the most commonly used initial evaluations for patients with symptoms of a gastric mass (Table 41.2). GI bleeding and anemia require upper GI endoscopy as an initial test, and symptoms of pain, nausea, and obstruction will typically prompt axial imaging, usually a CT abdomen/pelvis with IV and oral contrast. Both endoscopy and axial imaging can identify a gastric mass. Just as for asymptomatic gastric masses, visualization of a symptomatic gastric mass on a CT scan or MRI should trigger a referral to endoscopy for endoscopic evaluation and biopsy. If a tumor is symptomatic, simultaneous referral to a surgeon with experience in stomach surgery would be advisable as well.

Table 41.2 Initial workup of gastric masses prior to specialty referral

Clinical scenario	Initial workup and referral
Gastric mass noted on endoscopy	The most important test is biopsy of the mass, which should occur at the time of endoscopy Additional tests to order at the time of surgical referral include a complete blood count (white blood cell count, red blood cell counts, platelets) and basic metabolic panel (sodium, potassium, carbon dioxide, chloride, blood urea nitrogen, creatinine, and glucose) Necessity of axial imaging depends on tumor histology and will be ordered by the gastroenterologist or gastric surgeon
Gastric mass noted on imaging	All gastric masses noted on imaging should prompt referral to gastroenterology for biopsy. Surgical referral can be placed simultaneously if the mass is symptomatic or greater than 2 cm Small, asymptomatic tumors may be referred to gastroenterology alone with additional surgical referral depending on final histology of the mass Additional tests to order at the time of GI or surgical referral includes a complete blood count (white blood cell count, red blood cell counts, platelets) and basic metabolic panel (sodium, potassium, carbon dioxide, chloride, blood urea nitrogen, creatinine, and glucose) Further testing is dictated by the gastric mass histology and will be ordered by the gastroenterologist or gastric surgeon
Symptomatic gastric mass	Initial workup of suspected gastric mass depends on symptoms but may include referral to gastroenterology for upper GI endoscopy, basic labs, or axial imaging, including CT abdomen/pelvis with IV and oral contrast All confirmed gastric masses associated with symptoms should be referred to a gastric surgeon Further testing is dictated by the gastric mass histology and will be ordered by the gastroenterologist or gastric surgeon.

41.3 Indications for Emergent Surgical Evaluation

Although rare, patients with gastric masses can present with life-threatening gastrointestinal bleeding, which requires urgent intervention (Table 41.1). These patients should undergo standard treatment for GI bleeding, which begins with an endoscopic evaluation that should identify the gastric mass as a source of bleeding, and endoscopic maneuvers to control the hemorrhage, including injection, clips, and coagulation, should all be attempted. Interventional radiology consultation for consideration of angioembolization may be necessary if bleeding persists despite endoscopic treatment. Surgical resection is the treatment of last resort for a hemodynamically unstable patient with a bleeding gastric mass, and as such, it is appropriate to obtain surgical consultation as soon as the bleeding mass is identified so that the surgical team can be involved in the ongoing management of the patient. Even if endoscopic maneuvers or angioembolization are successful, surgical follow-up will be required, and so it is prudent to involve the surgical team early.

Patients may also emergently present with a perforated gastric mass. In this scenario, patients usually present with peritonitis, hemodynamic instability, and free air on imaging. These patients should undergo emergent surgical evaluation and will likely require immediate exploration. Depending on the intraoperative findings, the surgeon may choose to perform a Graham patch repair or resection. If the surgeon performs a repair, they must obtain a biopsy of the perforated mass to identify the underlying pathology to inform future care.

Finally, any gastric mass that causes gastric outlet obstruction (GOO) warrants immediate surgical consultation for evaluation and management. The initial management of a patient with a suspected gastric outlet obstruction is placement of a nasogastric tube for gastric decompression, and workup should begin with axial imaging with CT abdomen/pelvis with IV contrast. Oral contrast is likely not to be tolerated in this setting. Once the gastric outlet obstruction is confirmed, endoscopy is again required for endoscopic evaluation and biopsy. While surgical intervention for GOO will likely not occur on an emergent basis, it is important to involve a surgeon early to assist in the management of the obstruction. Management of gastric outlet obstruction depends on the underlying pathophysiology and can range from endoscopic bypass, surgical bypass, placement of a feeding jejunostomy tube, or even parenteral nutrition and chemotherapy. A surgeon with expertise in stomach pathology provides an essential perspective in selecting the optimal treatment strategy for GOO, and so should be consulted once GOO is diagnosed.

41.4 Specific Gastric Mass Histology and Need for Surgical Referral

41.4.1 Gastric Adenocarcinoma

All patients with gastric adenocarcinoma should be referred to be seen by a surgical oncologist or general surgeon with expertise in gastric tumors within 1–2 weeks of diagnosis. While some patients with very early gastric cancer can be treated with endoscopic resection, the majority of patients in the United States and North America with gastric cancer present with later-stage disease that is not amenable to endoscopic treatment. Referring physicians should obtain a CT chest, abdomen, and pelvis with IV and oral contrast as part of the staging of gastric cancer. Further staging studies, including endoscopic ultrasound, PET, and diagnostic laparoscopy with peritoneal washings, will be completed per the expertise of the gastric cancer surgeon and multidisciplinary team.

41.4.2 GI Stromal Tumor (GIST)

Gastrointestinal stromal tumors (GISTs) are a type of sarcoma arising from the muscularis propria and originate from the interstitial cells of Cajal. GISTs may be found incidentally or present with bleeding, early satiety, bloating, and pain. National guidelines recommend surgical resection of tumors larger than 2 cm. All patients with gastric GIST, including those that are <2 cm, should be referred to a surgical oncologist or general surgeon with expertise in gastric tumors to discuss management. Referring physicians can consider obtaining a CT chest, abdomen, pelvis with IV, and oral contrast to obtain baseline scans prior to surgical referral or can defer obtaining staging imaging to the consulting surgeon. The urgency of referral depends on the size and symptoms of the tumor. Smaller (<5 cm), asymptomatic tumors can be referred to be seen within a month, whereas larger, symptomatic tumors should be seen within 1–2 weeks. Patients who are admitted to the hospital due to symptoms of GIST should be seen by a gastric surgeon during their initial inpatient hospitalization.

41.4.3 Gastric Lymphoma

The cornerstone of treatment for primary gastric lymphomas is primarily medical, and surgical intervention is reserved for cases of obstruction, perforation, and hemorrhage. The treatment for gastric MALT-lymphoma, for example, is eradication of *H. pylori* using triple therapy with a proton pump inhibitor and antibiotics. Furthermore, gastric diffuse B-cell lymphoma is usually treated with cytotoxic chemotherapy. Gastric lymphoma does not require surgical referral but should be referred to medical oncology for evaluation and management within 1 week of diagnosis.

41.4.4 Gastric Neuroendocrine Tumor (NET)

Gastric neuroendocrine tumors (carcinoids) originate from enterochromaffin cells. They are divided into three groups based on proliferation rate and malignant potential. Type I gastric NETs are related to hypergastrinemia in the setting of atrophic gastritis and are typically multiple and < 1 cm. These lesions are indolent and treated by endoscopic polpyectomy/resection by a gastroenterologist who performs endoscopic surveillance every 6–12 months. Type II gastric NETs occur in the setting of hypergastrinemia due to Zollinger–Ellison syndrome and are treated similarly to type I carcinoids and are also typically indolent in behavior. Type III gastric NETs are sporadic tumors that are treated similarly to gastric adenocarcinoma due to their malignant potential. Patients with type III gastric NET should always be referred to a surgeon with expertise in stomach tumors, preferably within several weeks. Patients with type 1 and II gastric NET only require surgical referral for endoscopically unresectable lesions or symptoms.

41.4.5 Gastric Polyps

Gastric polyps rarely cause symptoms and are almost always found incidentally on endoscopy. Hyperplastic polyps, fundic gland polyps, and adenomas are generally endsocopically treated, and surgical referral is only indicated for patients with endoscopically unresectable polyps, polyps with malignant potential or high-grade dysplasia, or symptoms. Patients with polyposis syndromes who are found to have dysplastic gastric polyps also warrant surgical referral for discussion of radical surgery versus continued endoscopic surveillance and management. Some patients with gastric polyposis syndromes require gastrectomy for cancer prophylaxis. Otherwise, they will typically require endoscopic surveillance every 6–12 months depending on the number of polyps and history of any dysplastic polyps.

41.4.6 Miscellaneous Gastric Tumors

In addition to the masses listed above, there are rare gastric masses such as leiomyoma, leiomyosarcoma, plexiform neurofibroma, or glomus tumor. These rare histologies should always be referred to a surgeon with expertise in stomach tumors for further evaluation and management. For benign histology such as a gastric lipoma, surveillance is not necessary and surgical referral is only mandated for symptomatic tumors.

41.5 Conclusion

Surgical referral for gastric masses is dictated by tumor type and symptomology. Emergent surgical evaluation is necessary for patients with perforation, obstruction, or significant bleeding due to a gastric mass. In the outpatient setting, it is still prudent to refer any patient with a symptomatic gastric mass for surgical evaluation within 1–2 weeks. While some notable tumor types do not require surgical consultation, such as gastric lymphoma, most gastric masses will require surgical evaluation. Therefore, it is appropriate to refer any patient with any tumor histology to a gastric surgeon for history and physical and confirmation that no additional testing or intervention is necessary.

Recommended Readings

1. NCCN Clinical Practice Guidelines in Oncology: Gastric Cancer. https://www.nccn.org/guidelines/category_1
2. Blay J-Y, Kang Y-K, Nishida T, et al. Gastrointestinal stromal tumours. Nat Rev Dis Primers. 2021;7:22.
3. Ajani JA, Lee J, Sano T, et al. Gastric adenocarcinoma. Nature Reviews Disease Primers. 2017;3:1–19.

Gallbladder Polyps

42

Qais AbuHasan and Dimitrios Stefanidis

42.1 Introduction

Gallbladder disorders are prevalent among the population, with many patients initially presenting to their primary care physician for related symptoms. A right upper quadrant ultrasound (US) is the best initial diagnostic study for the evaluation of gallbladder symptoms as the presence of gallstones, which the US is highly sensitive in picking up, typically confirms the diagnosis and prompts surgical referral for a cholecystectomy. Nevertheless, in up to 4.5% of USs, gallbladder polyps are incidentally detected, which raises the question of whether surgical referral is warranted, especially in the absence of gallstones.

Gallbladder polyps are growths originating from the mucosal wall of the gallbladder. They are predominantly benign but can have malignant potential when certain features or risk factors are present. It is, therefore, essential that the primary care physician identifies these high-risk patients and refers them for cholecystectomy in a timely fashion to prevent the advancement of polyps to a malignant state.

Q. AbuHasan · D. Stefanidis (✉)
Department of Surgery, Indiana University School of Medicine, Indianapolis, IN, USA
e-mail: dimstefa@iu.edu

G. P. Kohn et al. (eds.), *The SAGES Manual of Surgical Referral for Primary and Emergency Care*,
https://doi.org/10.1007/978-3-031-92678-5_42

42.2 Evaluation and Management of Gallbladder Polyps

Gallbladder polyps are usually asymptomatic and are mostly found incidentally during imaging of the gallbladder for other reasons. They could, however, present with nonspecific dyspeptic pain or even biliary colic. Transabdominal US represents the modality of choice to identify and characterize gallbladder polyps. Other modalities include abdominal computed tomography (CT) with or without oral contrast, CT cystoscopy, and endoscopic US. However, these studies have lower sensitivity for the detection of gallbladder polyps compared to US, and the associated radiation, invasiveness, and expense make them less-than-ideal diagnostic options. Of note, the use of US can be limited in its inability to differentiate between dysplastic and non-neoplastic lesions, but this does not change the management plan.

The assessment of gallbladder polyps takes multiple factors into account that dictate the next step of management. It is important to evaluate the size of the polyp, any growth and/or rate of growth, the type of polyp, and cancer risk factors. When identified, polyps should be followed up to rule out any risk of malignancy. If risks or concerning features are present, this would require referral to a surgeon for a cholecystectomy. After the initial imaging, if concerning polyp characteristics are not present, a repeat US should be performed at 6 months, and then annually for 3 years. It is safe to discontinue monitoring the polyp if it disappears or has no growth during the follow-up period. Increased size, growth rate, or features as defined below require surgical referral.

Surgical referral is not warranted for patients with gallbladder polyps if:

(a) The patient is asymptomatic *AND*.
(b) The polyp does not exceed 5 mm in size *AND*.
(c) The absence of risk factors for gallbladder cancer.

42.3 When Should You Refer to a Surgeon?

The indications for surgical referral are based on patient demographics, risk factors, and polyp features associated with gallbladder cancer. These factors can be apparent on presentation, history of related disorders, or imaging findings. Any of the following can be an indication for referring to a surgeon. The flow chart summarizes the referral indications (Fig. 42.1).

Patient Demographics Age and race/ethnicity play an important role in assessing the risk of gallbladder carcinoma. Individuals aged 60 and above face an elevated risk of developing gallbladder cancer. Additionally, certain ethnic backgrounds exhibit higher

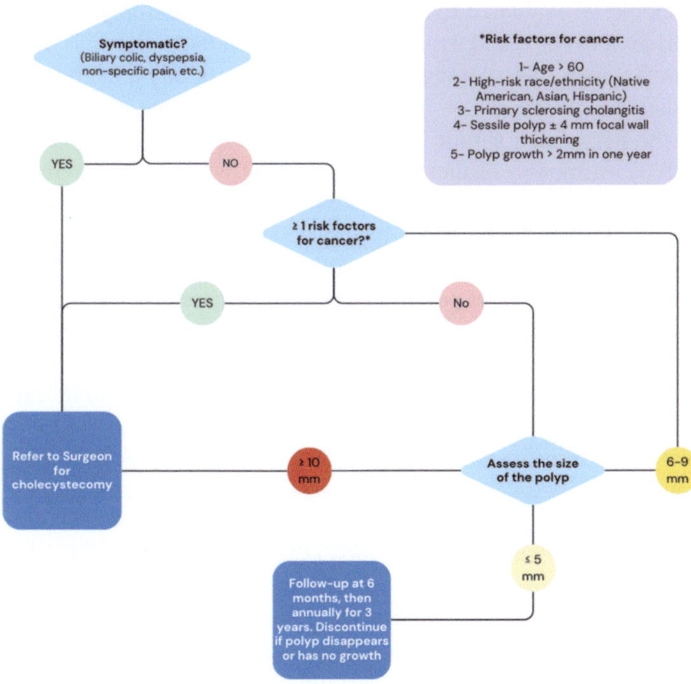

Fig. 42.1 Decision tree flow chart for the referral of patients with gallbladder polyps to a surgeon

susceptibility, with Native American, Japanese, Hispanic, and Asian populations showing a particularly increased risk compared to other ethnicities. When additional indications are present, individuals from these high-risk racial and ethnic groups should be referred to a surgeon for further evaluation.

Symptoms Most gallbladder polyps do not cause significant symptoms; however, some patients might present with biliary colic, nonspecific pain, or dyspepsia due to the polyp. Careful assessment for gallstones and/or other causes of pain should be conducted. If, by exclusion, symptoms are attributed to the gallbladder polyp and are causing a significant impact on the patient's well-being, cholecystectomy could be indicated.

Size and Growth It is important to note the size of the polyp on initial imaging. If the polyp size reaches the threshold of 10 mm, it should be evaluated by a surgeon for cholecystectomy. Smaller polyps between 6 and 9 mm can be referred if the patient has other risk factors for developing gallbladder cancer or any other referral indications discussed in this section. During follow-up, changes in the polyp size should also be monitored, while disappearing polyps warrant no further surveillance, a growth of >2 mm over a 1-year period requires a consultation for gallbladder removal.

Type Polyps have various macroscopic shapes and growth patterns that have been associated with different risks of malignant potential. Gallbladder polyps can be pedunculated, where the outgrowth is attached to the mucosal wall by a stalk, often referred to as ball-on-wall, or they can present as a sessile polypoid lesion that has a wide base attached as opposed to the thin and long stalk of the pedunculated type. Sessile lesions have higher odds of malignant transformation, particularly with associated focal gallbladder wall thickening of more than 4 mm and require a surgical referral.

Primary Sclerosing Cholangitis (PSC) Patients with PSC have an inherently increased risk of developing cancer of the biliary tract, whether it is the common bile duct or the gallbladder. Even benign-appearing gallbladder polyps of any size should raise concern in a patient with PSC and should be referred to a surgeon for cholecystectomy.

Managing gallbladder disorders polyps is a fundamental part of general surgery training and can be further developed through specialized training. For the management of gallbladder polyps, care providers can refer patients to general, hepatobiliary, or gastrointestinal surgeons. They are equipped with the training and experience to provide care for at-risk patients and perform a cholecystectomy if required (Tables 42.1 and 42.2).

Table 42.1 Management and surgical review requirements for gallbladder polyps

Emergent surgical review	Gallbladder polyps do not typically lead to surgical emergencies necessitating an emergency room (ER) visit. However, immediate ER presentation is imperative if concurrent biliary emergencies such as acute cholecystitis or acute cholangitis are present
Urgent surgical review	Patients exhibiting imaging features suggestive of gallbladder cancer, such as mural thickening or calcification, or infiltration into the liver, warrant urgent surgical assessment. Moreover, symptoms not tolerated by the patient warrant prompt surgical review
Nonurgent review	Evaluation can be conducted nonurgently in symptomatic patients, or asymptomatic patients in the presence of cancer risk factors (age >60, native American, Asian, or Hispanic ethnicity, primary sclerosing cholangitis, sessile polyp type with or without 4 mm focal wall thickening, polyp growth of >2 mm in one year) and for polyps larger than 5 mm
Primary care provider (PCP) management	Patients who have no symptoms, with a polyp 5 mm or smaller (with no concerning imaging findings), and lack risk factors for gallbladder cancer, should undergo an ultrasound assessment at six months, followed by annual evaluations for three years. If there are no changes observed, monitoring can be discontinued

Table 42.2 Tests and management of gallbladder polyps prior to surgical referral

Blood tests	Laboratory blood tests are not specific for gallbladder polyps or cancer. Tests that *can* be ordered prior to referral include: alkaline phosphatase (ALP), gamma-glutamyl transferase (GGT), alanine aminotransferase (ALT), aspartate aminotransferase (AST), and bilirubin
Imaging	Transabdominal ultrasound is needed prior to surgical referral. The imaging should describe the number of polyps (if more than one), the size and type of the polyp, and other gallbladder features such as wall thickening, calcifications, and biliary stones.

42.4 Conclusion

Gallbladder polyps present most often as an incidental finding and are benign in the vast majority of cases. However, some features and risk factors for gallbladder carcinoma warrant referral for surgery. This includes any polyp larger than 10 mm, sessile polyps with focal wall thickening, rapidly growing polyps, or patients with primary sclerosing cholangitis, patients aged >60, and those of Native American, Asian, and Hispanic ethnicities. Patients with smaller asymptomatic polyps can be followed up with semiannual to annual transabdominal US for up to 3 years and discontinued if the polyp disappears or no change is noted.

Suggested Readings

1. Foley KG, Lahaye MJ, Thoeni RF, Soltes M, Dewhurst C, Barbu ST, Vashist YK, Rafaelsen SR, Arvanitakis M, Perinel J, Wiles R. Management and follow-up of gallbladder polyps: updated joint guidelines between the ESGAR, EAES. EFISDS and ESGE. European Radiology. 2022;1:1–1.
2. Kamaya A, Fung C, Szpakowski JL, Fetzer DT, Walsh AJ, Alimi Y, Bingham DB, Corwin MT, Dahiya N, Gabriel H, Park WG. Management of incidentally detected gallbladder polyps: society of radiologists in ultrasound consensus conference recommendations. Radiology. 2022;305(2):277–89.
3. Valibouze C, El Amrani M, Truant S, Leroy C, Millet G, Pruvot FR, Zerbib P. The management of gallbladder polyps. J Visc Surg. 2020;157(5):410–7.

Gallstones

43

Dean C. Spilias

43.1 Overview

Gallstones are a common clinical problem in primary care, emergency departments, and inpatient hospital settings. Gallstone prevalence increases with age, from below 1% under the age of 20, to 11.5% in the over-70-year-old population. While there are genetic differences in gallstone prevalence, gallstones are common enough in all populations that ethnic differences do not play a role in diagnosis or management. Approximately 15% of individuals with gallstones are thought to develop symptoms, the remainder staying asymptomatic for prolonged periods.

Gallstones (cholelithiasis) can form within any part of the biliary tree—typically the gall bladder (cholecystolithiasis), but also in the bile duct (choledocholithiasis) or intrahepatic biliary tree (hepatolithiasis), particularly in areas of stasis such as choledochal cysts or above biliary strictures.

D. C. Spilias (✉)
Monash Medical Centre, Clayton, VIC, Australia

Melbourne Upper GI Surgical Group, Melbourne, VIC, Australia
e-mail: dspilias@uppergi.net

G. P. Kohn et al. (eds.), *The SAGES Manual of Surgical Referral for Primary and Emergency Care*,
https://doi.org/10.1007/978-3-031-92678-5_43

Gallstones can be primarily made of cholesterol; bile salts; or a mixture of the two. 15–20% of gallstones calcify, becoming radio-opaque; the remainder are not seen on plain X-ray studies.

Cholesterol stones, with >50% cholesterol composition, and mixed stones with 20–50% cholesterol are the most common. They represent 80% of gallstones in Western populations and result from supersaturation of bile with cholesterol (as opposed to elevated blood lipid levels). They are associated with "Western" diet (high calorie, high refined sugar, low fiber, low unsaturated fat), sedentary lifestyle, obesity, rapid weight loss, total parenteral nutrition (TPN), pregnancy, exogenous estrogens, female sex, and increasing age.

Pigment stones (<20% cholesterol content) can be "black" stones that form in the gall bladder. These can be spontaneous, but also may be associated with pre-existing conditions, including hemolysis, hemoglobinopathies, cirrhosis, or intestinal malabsorption. "Brown" primary bile duct stones, by contrast, typically form in the bile duct or intrahepatic biliary tree and often are associated with bacterial or parasitic infections, or biliary strictures—surgical (injury or anastomosis), autoimmune (primary biliary cholangitis/cirrhosis (PBC), sclerosing cholangitis, autoimmune cholangiopathy), or ischemic being the most common stricture etiologies.

43.2 Clinical Presentations

Gallstones can cause symptoms in the gall bladder, bile duct, or elsewhere in the body.

In the gall bladder:

- Biliary colic
- Acute cholecystitis

In the bile duct:

- Biliary colic (with uncomplicated choledocholithiasis)
- Obstructive jaundice
- Cholangitis
- Pancreatitis

Elsewhere:

- Gallstone ileus
- Intra-abdominal abscess from perforated gall bladder or stones spilled at the time of surgery

43.3 Initial Investigations

If clinical signs suggest local inflammation (tenderness, Murphy's sign), initiation of antibiotic therapy should not be delayed while waiting for investigation results.

If clinical signs suggest systemic inflammation or sepsis, particularly if jaundice is also present, antibiotics should be started without delay and the patient should be referred for same-day surgical review or transferred to the emergency department.

Initial investigations aim to confirm the clinical suspicion of gallstone disease; diagnose complications of gallstone disease such as choledocholithiasis, obstruction, cholangitis, or pancreatitis; and assess the severity of diseases, particularly in the setting of sepsis.

Initial blood tests:

- Leucocyte count: assess for sepsis
- C-reactive protein: assess for inflammation
- Liver enzymes and bilirubin: assess for hepatic injury or obstructive jaundice
- Prothrombin time (PT-INR): assess for hepatic dysfunction
- Lipase: assess for pancreatitis

Initial imaging:

- Upper abdominal ultrasound: confirm the diagnosis; assess for cholecystitis, choledocholithiasis, or liver abscess

Pancreatitis and obstructive jaundice generally require transfer to the emergency department.

In cases of acute biliary infections, an assessment of severity is required, along with a definitive diagnosis (acute cholecystitis, cholangitis, pancreatitis).

If the initial investigations and clinical picture do not suggest biliary infection (acute cholecystitis or cholangitis), obstruction, or pancreatitis, treatment can be symptomatic and an elective surgical referral can be made.

43.4 Diagnosing Acute Pancreatitis, Acute Cholecystitis, and Cholangitis

The severity and rate of progression of acute biliary sepsis can, unfortunately, be under-recognized. In particular, cholangitis does not always present with Charcot's triad of pain, fever, and jaundice. The Tokyo Guidelines 2018 are a series of evidence-based consensus statements that have been widely adopted as the standard of care for acute biliary infections. Initial treatment is based on severity, with investigations differentiating between cholangitis and cholecystitis.

Acute cholecystitis is characterized by

- Local signs of inflammation (tenderness, Murphy's sign)
- Systemic inflammation of variable severity (fever, elevated CRP, leucocytosis)
- Imaging findings (usually ultrasound) characteristic of acute cholecystitis

Specific factors that should be considered in unwell patients (or if suspected on ultrasound) include perforation of the gall bladder, gangrenous cholecystitis, bleeding into a gangrenous gall bladder (hemorrhagic cholecystitis), and liver abscesses (which can mimic or accompany cholecystitis). Contrast-enhanced CT scan is useful in making these diagnoses.

Cholangitis is characterized by

- Systemic inflammation, with local signs of inflammation being inconsistent
- Cholestasis—elevated bilirubin is not required for the diagnosis, abnormal liver enzymes are enough

- Imaging findings (typically ultrasound or ERCP) of biliary dilation
- Evidence of a cause of biliary dilation

Acute pancreatitis is characterized by

- Pain
- Local or systemic signs of inflammation, of variable severity
- Biochemical or radiological evidence of pancreatic inflammation (typically, pancreatic lipase elevated to five times normal level)

43.5 Severity Grading for Acute Cholecystitis and Cholangitis

Biliary infections are graded from grade I (mild) to III (severe).

Grade III represents organ dysfunction. The priority in grade III disease is urgent initiation of intravenous antibiotics and urgent decompression of the affected organ—the gall bladder in the case of cholecystitis, the bile duct in the case of cholangitis. Urgent transfer to inpatient surgical care, along with facilities for organ support, is required.

Grade II represents compensated sepsis. The patient will show signs of a clinically significant systemic infection, but without significant organ dysfunction. Intravenous antibiotics and decompression as soon as is practical are appropriate.

Grade I disease meets the diagnostic criteria, but not the criteria of grade II or III disease. These patients are systemically well. Grade I cholecystitis can be managed in the ambulant setting, with review to ensure improvement, and semi-elective surgical referral (cholecystectomy within 7 days is still desirable; otherwise surgery is generally delayed 6–8 weeks to allow inflammation to resolve).

Cholangitis of any grade should be managed in hospital.

Acute pancreatitis of any severity should be managed in hospital.

43.6 Antibiotic Choice in Biliary Sepsis

The majority of bacteria isolated from patients with biliary infections are enteric gram-negative bacilli and gram-positive cocci. Anaerobic bacteria are less common, but should be suspected with gangrenous cholecystitis or if there has been previous biliary surgery or instrumentation (such as ERCP).

Empirical antibiotic selection should reflect local factors as well as the likely organisms—for example, antibiotic availability or local patterns of antibiotic resistance. If a single organism is cultured, then targeted antibiotic selections can be made.

Suitable empirical oral antibiotic choices include

- Amoxicillin/clavulanic acid
- Ciprofloxacin (+/− metronidazole)
- Cefalexin (+/− metronidazole) is commonly used; however, efficacy against *Enterobacter* spp. is poor. If cefalexin is chosen, early clinical review is required to assess response

Suitable empirical intravenous antibiotic choices include

- Piperacillin/tazobactam
- Ceftriazone +/− metronidazole (again assessing response early and frequently, as efficacy against gram-positive cocci is poor)
- Meropenem
- Cefipime + metronidazole or clindamycin

43.7 Radiological Investigation of Gallstone Disease

Investigations are used to

- Confirm the presence of cholelithiasis
- Differentiate between different causes of acute biliary/pancreatic inflammatory conditions
- Assess for severity and complications
- and ultimately to guide management decisions

Different investigations have different strengths and weaknesses. In particular, contrast-enhanced CT scanning is a useful modality when assessing patients with undifferentiated abdominal pain. However, when gallstone disease is suspected, ultrasound is often the better initial investigation.

43.8 Ultrasound

Upper abdominal ultrasound is the initial investigation of choice for suspected cholelithiasis. It is sensitive (>95%) and specific for the detection of stones in the gall bladder, and has acceptable sensitivity for bile duct stones.

Findings consistent with acute cholecystitis include gall bladder wall thickening (≥3 mm), pericholecystic fluid, and positive sonographic Murphy's sign (tenderness from probe pressure over the gall bladder). Ultrasound can also demonstrate "sludge" (microlithiasis) or hematoma, and polyps or masses arising from the gall bladder wall.

43.8.1 Traps and Exceptions

- Bile duct diameter. 7 mm is generally considered the upper limit of normal bile duct diameter; however, this range applies to an intact biliary tree in adult patients across all ages. The bile duct commonly dilates following cholecystectomy, often to 9 or 10 mm; or with increasing age, with 1 mm per decade of life is a reasonable estimate of normal bile duct diameter. Take this into consideration if radiological findings are discordant with the clinical picture.
- Non-distended gall bladder. A distended gall bladder is required for accurate sonography, and is the state in which normal measurements are validated. Recent food intake, gall bladder carcinoma, xanthogranulomatous cholecystitis (acute cholecystitis with granuloma formation and fibrosis), and perforation of the gall bladder can all result in a nondistended gall bladder and reduce the accuracy of sonography.

- Pericholecystic fluid. Cirrhosis, ascites, congestive cardiac failure, and tricuspid regurgitation can all result in pericholecystic fluid or borderline thickening of the gall bladder wall.

43.9 Magnetic Resonance Cholangiopancreatography (MRCP)

MRCP is a noncontrast MRI study of the gall bladder, pancreas, and biliary tract. T2-weighted imaging sequences are employed, using the fluid as an intrinsic contrast medium; this results in rapid, low-risk acquisition of images, at the expense of decreased imaging information about the soft tissues and blood vessels. Images are therefore obtained of the fluid-filled structures, allowing assessment of diameter, filling defects (such as stones or polyps) and abnormal fluid collections (such as cysts).

43.9.1 Traps and Exceptions

- Implanted devices, metal foreign bodies. The usual contraindications to MRI scanning apply to MRCP. Some pacemakers have MRI-conditional leads, allowing MRI with special precautions taken; however, this should be considered carefully and other imaging modalities should be explored first.

43.10 Endoscopic Retrograde Cholangiopancreatography (ERCP)

ERCP is an endoscopic procedure requiring cannulation via the duodenal ampulla of Vater and thereby carries a clinically significant procedural risk of pancreatitis, perforation, bleeding, cholangitis, and an associated (low) mortality rate. It is generally reserved for therapeutic, not diagnostic, purposes. Therapeutic ERCP is an option for the management of choledocholithiasis; however, it is often possible to remove bile duct stones at the time of cholecystectomy.

43.10.1 Traps and Exceptions

- Cholangitis, obstructive jaundice. In these conditions, the primary intervention required is decompression of the biliary tree, and ERCP is often the preferred modality for achieving decompression.
- Previous upper gastrointestinal tract surgery. Disruption of the continuity of the gastrointestinal tract by gastrectomy, gastric bypass, or other gastric surgery can make ERCP difficult or impossible to achieve.
- Biliary spasm, sphincter of Oddi dysfunction. The risk of pancreatitis is increased in patients with biliary spasm. The need for ERCP and potential alternatives should be considered before proceeding.

43.11 Computerized Axial Tomography (CT Scan)

Abdominal-protocol CT (oral contrast and portal venous phase intravenous contrast) is a common modality used in the investigation of undifferentiated abdominal pain. It has limited utility in the assessment of suspected gallstones as most gallstones are radiolucent. However, it is useful in selected cases for assessing for complications such as perforated gall bladder, gangrenous or hemorrhagic cholecystitis, or for assessing the severity of acute pancreatitis (typically at the 72-hour interval after diagnosis).

43.12 CT Cholangiography (CT-IVC)

CT cholangiography uses meglumine iotroxate, an intravenously administered contrast agent that is excreted in the biliary tree, to provide contrast images similar to MRCP. This contrast agent is not available in all locations. It has largely been replaced by MRCP in the initial assessment of the biliary tree, but remains useful when MRCP is unavailable or contraindicated. It is also useful in assessing for or localizing extravasation of bile from the biliary tree, such as when investigating a bile leak post cholecystectomy, biliary reconstruction, or liver surgery.

43.12.1 Traps and Exceptions

- Allergy to iodinated contrast media, hyperthyroidism, and severe hepatic or renal dysfunction are contraindications to the administration of the contrast agent.
- Biliary obstruction or cholestasis, with a total bilirubin level >30 μmol/L (>1.754 mg/dL), impairs biliary excretion of the contrast agent and may result in inadequate images.

43.13 Cholescintigraphy (Hepatic IDA or DDA Scan; HIDA Scan)

Cholescintigraphy is a nuclear medicine technique using Tc99m IDA (iminodiacetic acid) analogs to investigate the liver and biliary tract. HIDA scan is of limited use in the assessment of gallstone disease, but is sometimes used to confirm the diagnosis of cholecystitis if an ultrasound is equivocal. It is useful in the investigation of congenital biliary abnormalities, functional disease of the gall bladder and bile ducts, and diagnosis and localization of postoperative bile leaks.

43.14 Management

43.14.1 Prevention

There are no consensus recommendations on measures to prevent cholelithiasis. Observational studies favor lower calorie, alcohol and refined sugar intake; increased unsaturated fat and fiber intake; and avoidance of obesity, or gradual weight loss to treat obesity.

Ursodeoxycholic acid may be considered for prophylaxis in the setting of rapid weight loss.

Cholecystectomy is sometimes performed concurrently with some metabolic-bariatric operations to prevent the future development of symptomatic gallstones.

43.14.2 Asymptomatic Gallstones

Asymptomatic gallstones do not require follow-up or intervention, provided they are limited to the gall bladder (not the biliary tree) and are not associated with gall bladder polyps.

43.14.3 Biliary Colic

Self-resolving biliary colic is managed with analgesia, antispasmodics, low-fat diet, and elective surgical referral.

Hyoscine butylbromide is useful in relieving biliary spasm (including opiate-induced spasm) at an adult dose of 20 mg (single dose).

Severe pain may require a single dose of opiate analgesia.

Nonresolving pain indicates progression toward cholecystitis. Blood flow within the gall bladder wall is impaired due to increased intraluminal pressure. This causes mucosal damage, bile-induced inflammation ("chemical cholecystitis") and ultimately transmigration of intestinal organisms across the damaged mucosa. Nonresolving biliary colic should be managed as mild cholecystitis, with initiation of antibiotics and early (within 7 days, preferably within 72 hours) cholecystectomy.

43.14.4 Choledocholithiasis

Uncomplicated choledocholithiasis requires semi-urgent referral for (1) removal of the stone(s) within the bile duct before cholangitis or pancreatitis develop; and (2) cholecystectomy to prevent further episodes in the future.

In many cases, bile duct stones can be removed at the time of cholecystectomy, without the need for separate ERCP.

43.14.5 Acute Biliary Infections: Acute Cholecystitis, Cholangitis

Initial supportive measures and treatment of sepsis may in some cases precede a definitive diagnosis; however, it is important to continue investigations until a definitive diagnosis has been made.

43.14.6 Acute Cholecystitis

Treatment of cholecystitis consists of

- Antibiotics to treat local and systemic sepsis
- Assessment of severity
- Supportive care and symptom relief
- Source control: drainage or resection (cholecystectomy) for *treatment* and to *prevent recurrence*

Source control is generally through laparoscopic cholecystectomy.

In selected patients unfit for surgery, options include

- ERCP and sphincterotomy, preferably with a long stent placed into the gall bladder via the cystic duct
- Lumen-apposing stents to form a semi-permanent communication between the gall bladder and the stomach or duodenum via endoscopic ultrasound (EUS-guided cholecysto-duodenostomy or -gastrostomy)
- Or occasionally, antibiotics alone, although this will not prevent recurrent cholecystitis

43.14.7 Grade I Cholecystitis

Early source control with laparoscopic cholecystectomy provides optimal treatment in fit patients with access to surgical care. Oral antibiotics, antispasmodics, analgesics, and low-fat diet are appropriate initial treatment in the ambulatory setting, and allow bridging to surgery when early surgical referral is unavailable.

Suitable empirical antibiotic choices include

- Amoxicillin/clavulanic acid
- Ciprofloxacin (+/– metronidazole)
- Cefalexin (+/– metronidazole) is commonly used; however, efficacy against *Enterobacter* spp. is poor. If cefalexin is chosen, early clinical review is required to assess response

Surgical referral should be semi-urgent as cholecystectomy is ideally performed within 7 days (and preferably within 72 hours).

If early access to surgical care is unavailable, antibiotics are continued until symptoms have resolved. Low-fat diet is required, and cholecystectomy should be delayed for 6–8 weeks to allow resolution of local inflammation.

43.14.8 Grade II Cholecystitis

These patients have systemic infection, and treatment should be initiated with intravenous antibiotics in an inpatient setting.

Suitable antibiotic choices include

- Piperacillin/tazobactam
- Ceftriazone +/– metronidazole (again assessing response early and frequently, as efficacy against gram-positive cocci is poor)

Surgical referral should be semi-urgent or through the emergency department. There is no role for ongoing management in the outpatient setting.

In appropriate centers, early laparoscopic cholecystectomy (within 72 hours and as early as is practical) is preferred. If advanced laparoscopic cholecystectomy facilities (and skills) are unavailable, an alternative is delayed cholecystectomy (after 6–8 weeks). If the patient is unfit for surgery, interim source control is achieved through a radiologically guided (ultrasound-guided) percutaneous cholecystectomy tube, with external drainage.

43.14.9 Grade III Cholecystitis

These patients are unwell and require stabilization, and often interim drainage of the gall bladder, prior to cholecystectomy.

Gangrenous or perforated cholecystitis is more common. Antibiotic selection should cover anaerobic organisms as well as the more likely upper gastrointestinal tract pathogens, as synergistic infections can occur.

Suitable antibiotic choices include

- Piperacillin/tazobactam
- Meropenem
- Cefipime + metronidazole or clindamycin

Urgent surgical referral and intensive care unit assessment are required.

Fit patients, who respond to initial antibiotic and supportive therapy, in a center with advanced laparoscopic cholecystecomy facilities and experience, can proceed to laparoscopic cholecystectomy after the initial period of stabilization.

If these criteria are not met, interim drainage of the gall bladder with a radiologically-placed cholecystectomy tube is safer. Cholecystectomy is then performed after a delay of 6–8 weeks in patients who make a good recovery and have an adequate performance status and risk profile for surgery.

43.14.10 Acute Cholangitis

Cholangitis is managed in an inpatient setting. Surgical referral is urgent and through the emergency department.

Treatment is initiated with intravenous antibiotics and supportive care.

Suitable antibiotic choices include

- Piperacillin/tazobactam
- Meropenem
- Cefipime +/– metronidazole or clindamycin

Grade I acute cholangitis can initially be treated with antibiotics, with biliary drainage via ERCP or percutaneous transhepatic cholangiography (PTC) only required if there is a failure to improve.

Patients with grade II cholangitis generally require early drainage, while grade III cases require urgent biliary decompression.

Laparoscopic cholecystectomy *prevents recurrence* of acute cholangitis, rather than directly treating it; *treatment* of cholangitis is with antibiotics and biliary decompression.

43.14.11 Acute Biliary Pancreatitis

Acute pancreatitis management is largely supportive; however, if cholangitis is also present, this must be managed with antibiotics and biliary decompression. Once the episode of acute pancreatitis has settled, measures to prevent recurrence need to be addressed. For gallstone pancreatitis, laparoscopic cholecystectomy should be undertaken as soon as is practical, preferably the same hospital admission. Delays up to 8 weeks are sometimes appropriate in patients recovering from severe pancreatitis.

43.15 Post-Cholecystectomy Care

43.15.1 Normal Recovery Following Laparoscopic Cholecystectomy

Cholecystectomy can generally be achieved laparoscopically or robotically, with current rates of open surgery below 2% of procedures performed. Ambulant surgery is common, with many patients discharged the day of surgery. Most patients require opiate analgesia for 1–3 days and simple analgesia for up to a week. Low-fat diet (<40 g/day, or as low as is practical) is recommended for 6 weeks after surgery (or indefinitely if symptoms of fatty food intolerance are present—bloating, diarrhea). Avoidance of heavy lifting is recommended for 4–6 weeks.

If a biliary stent has been placed during surgery or at ERCP, endoscopic retrieval is usually required at 6–12 weeks following the index procedure.

If a cholecystectomy tube has been used to drain the gall bladder, instead of cholecystectomy, this must be left for a minimum of 6 weeks to allow adequate formation of adhesions around the tube. A cholangiogram must then be performed before considering tube removal; the tube must not be removed if the gall bladder is obstructed and unable to drain normally into the bile duct and then into the duodenum.

43.15.2 Postoperative Problems

In addition to general postoperative concerns, problems specific to biliary surgery include bile leak, damage to the biliary tree, retained or recurrent stones, fatty food intolerance, and late strictures.

Leakage of bile, whether from a disruption of or injury to the bile duct, or from the cystic duct stump or liver with the biliary tree intact, should be suspected if pain increases, or fails to improve, beyond the expected 2–3 days. Initial investigations are ultrasonography or upper abdominal CT (either CT cholangiography, or abdominal-protocol IV and oral contrast) looking for undrained fluid collections; and leucocyte count, total bilirubin, and liver enzymes to assess for hyperbilirubinemia and infection. The presence of a collection or hyperbilirubinemia, residual bile duct stones, or infection not attributable to other causes mandates return to surgical care for further management, which is beyond the scope of this chapter.

Late recurrent pain or jaundice should be initially be investigated with ultrasound, total bilirubin, and liver enzymes, looking for dilation of the biliary tree, bile duct stones, or biochemical evidence of liver injury. MRCP is usually the most useful modality if further imaging is required.

Fatty food intolerance is managed by the restriction of dietary fat intake. Investigations are usually not required, but fecal microscopy looking for oil or fat crystals is useful in selected cases. If symptoms continue, a therapeutic trial of cholestyramine or oat bran fiber can be undertaken.

43.16 Summary Table

Initial blood tests:

- Leucocyte count: assess for sepsis
- C-reactive protein: assess for inflammation
- Liver enzymes and bilirubin: assess for hepatic injury or obstructive jaundice
- Prothrombin time (PT-INR): assess for hepatic dysfunction
- Lipase: assess for pancreatitis

Initial imaging:

- Upper abdominal ultrasound: confirm the diagnosis; assess for cholecystitis, choledocholithiasis, or liver abscess

Initial management and when to refer:

Condition	Criteria	Urgency	Management overview
Grade III acute biliary infection (severe cholecystitis or cholangitis)	Systemic sepsis with signs of decompensation or organ dysfunction	Immediate referral (transfer to ER)	Systemic antibiotics Organ support Urgent biliary drainage/ cholecystectomy
Grade II acute biliary infection (moderate cholecystitis or cholangitis)	Systemic signs of inflammation, but well-compensated with no organ dysfunction	Urgent (same-day) surgical referral, or transfer to ER	Antibiotics Analgesia Early biliary drainage if cholangitis present Laparoscopic cholecystectomy within 72 hours
Grade I acute biliary infection (mild cholecystitis or cholangitis)	Local signs of inflammation No systemic signs suggesting sepsis	Semi-urgent (within 72 hours) surgical referral	Antibiotics Analgesia Laparoscopic cholecystectomy within 7 days (preferably within 72 hours)
Biliary colic	Pain with no sepsis or jaundice	Elective / nonurgent surgical referral	Low-fat diet Antispasmodics Analgesia Elective cholecystectomy to prevent recurrence
Choledocholithiasis with obstructive jaundice	Acute pain and jaundice	Urgent (same-day) surgical referral, or transfer to ER	Further imaging if cause not demonstrated on ultrasound Semi-urgent (within 72 hours) ERCP or laparoscopic bile duct exploration to remove stones Cholecystectomy to prevent recurrence

(continued)

Condition	Criteria	Urgency	Management overview
Acute gallstone pancreatitis	Acute pain with biochemical or imaging evidence of pancreatitis	Urgent (same-day) surgical referral, or transfer to ER	Inpatient management of acute episode Early cholecystectomy to prevent recurrence (if gallstones present)
Asymptomatic gallstones		Reassure	No need for surgical review unless gall bladder polyps or choledocholithiasis are demonstrated on ultrasound

Selected Resource

1. Tokyo Guidelines 2018 for acute cholangitis and cholecystitis (TG18): http://www.jshbps.jp/modules/en/index.php?content_id=47

Liver Lesions

44

Juan S. Malo and D. Rohan Jeyarajah

44.1 Benign Liver Lesions

In the absence of chronic liver disease, the vast majority of lesions correspond to benign liver tumors and can include both solid and cystic lesions. Solid lesions can be classified according to their histological origin: epithelial and mesenchymal. The most common epithelial lesions are focal nodular hyperplasia (FNH) and hepatocellular adenoma (HCA). Mesenchymal benign tumor classification is based on their origin from blood vessels (Hemangioma), adipose tissue (angiomyolipoma), and muscle tissue (leiomyoma).

J. S. Malo
Methodist Richardson Medical Center, Richardson, TX, USA

D. Rohan Jeyarajah (✉)
Methodist Richardson Medical Center, Richardson, TX, USA

TCU Burnett School of Medicine, Fort Worth, TX, USA
e-mail: rohanjeyarajah@gmail.com

G. P. Kohn et al. (eds.), *The SAGES Manual of Surgical Referral for Primary and Emergency Care*,
https://doi.org/10.1007/978-3-031-92678-5_44

44.1.1 Focal Nodular Hyperplasia (FNH)

Described by Edmonson in 1958, focal nodular hyperplasia is thought to be the result of increased hepatocyte number caused by hypoperfusion or hyperperfusion from anomalous arteries within the hepatic lobule (Table 44.1).

Incidence is higher in women (female-to-male ratio 9:1), suggesting a direct relationship with estrogen levels. However, recent literature showing oral contraceptives as a cause of developing focal nodular hyperplasia is not proven (4).

44.1.1.1 Radiological Features

Several findings are associated with FNH regardless of the imaging modality: lack of capsule, often with lobulated contours; lesion homogeneity except for the characteristic central scar. MRI

Table 44.1 Management and surgical consultation for benign liver lesions

	Management	Surgical consultation
FNH	Conservative. 6-month triple-phase CT/MRI with contrast to prove stability.	HPB surgery if clearly symptomatic or undefined lesions
Hemangioma	Conservative. Follow-up triple-phase CT/MRI with/ without if symptomatic.	HPB surgery if symptomatic
HCA	OC cessation, weight loss. Follow-up MRI with gadoxetate disodium 6–12 months if asymptomatic or <5 cm in size.	HPB surgery if >5 cm, symptomatic, or no regression after OC cessation
Simple cysts	Conservative. No follow-up imaging required. If symptomatic, US first to assess size/compression.	HBP surgery if symptomatic or complicated cyst
Pyogenic abscess	Based on clinical presentation. Broad-spectrum antibiotics.	HPB surgery at the time of diagnosis
Amebic abscess	If uncomplicated: amebicidal (e.g., metronidazol)	HPB surgery if large in size, sepsis, or rupture
Hydatid cyst	Anthelmintics prior to surgery.	HPB surgery at the time of diagnosis

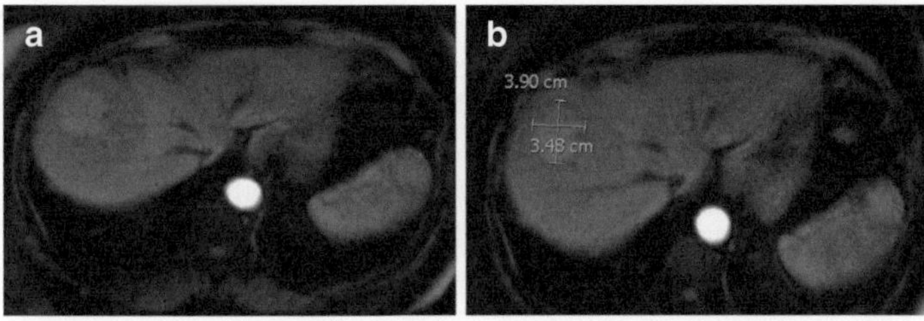

Fig. 44.1 (**a**, **b**) T1-weighted images of segment VIII FNH. (HPB Clinic. Methodist Richardson Medical Center (MRMC). Richardson, Texas)

(Fig. 44.1a, b) has a sensitivity of close to 70% and almost 100% specificity to make a differential diagnosis from other benign liver lesions.

44.1.1.2 Management and Surgical Consultation

Conservative management is indicated. Initial 6-month imaging follow-up is recommended to prove stability. There are no reports to date regarding malignant transformation of this lesion.

Symptomatic Lesions Consultation with a hepatopancreaticobiliary (HPB) surgeon is advised for further management. Liver-directed therapies can be considered, and surgical resection remains the gold standard for those lesions that are clearly symptomatic or with an unclear diagnosis (6).

44.1.2 Hemangioma

Hemangiomas, also known as cavernous hemangiomas, are the most common benign liver tumors accounting for approximately 70% of these lesions. It can be present in all ages, with a mean age at presentation of 50 years. Some hemangiomas carry estrogen receptors with growth related to oral contraceptives (OC) and pregnancy. This most likely explains a higher incidence in women with a female-to-male ratio of 5:1. They can present equally in either lobe of the liver and are usually <5 cm in size.

The majority of hemangiomas are asymptomatic, and following the line of benign lesions, their diagnosis is usually incidental during imaging studies, obtained for other reasons. If symptomatic, these can range from mild abdominal discomfort or pain to mass effect to surrounding organs (those localized on the left side), bile duct compression with resulting jaundice or vascular compression of inferior vena cava, hepatic veins, or portal vein. These symptoms are very rare.

Though extremely rare, complications can mostly occur in larger lesions. Inflammation can occur with resulting thrombosis of a portion of the hemangioma causing fever, abdominal pain, weight loss, and reactive thrombocytosis. A very rare but severe complication is the Kasabach–Merritt syndrome characterized by the presence of a liver hemangioma associated with thrombocytopenia, microangiopathic hemolytic anemia, and coagulopathy.

44.1.2.1 Radiological Features

On ultrasound, it presents as a homogeneous hyperechoic mass with no vascular pattern on color Doppler.

CT criteria for the diagnosis include: These lesions are best seen on triple-phase CT scan, or on MRI contrasted with a gadolinium intravenous contrast. CT should be triple-phase with intravenous (IV) contrast.

MRI, whether with or without contrast, has demonstrated a sensitivity of 98% and a specificity of 99% (Fig. 44.2a, b).

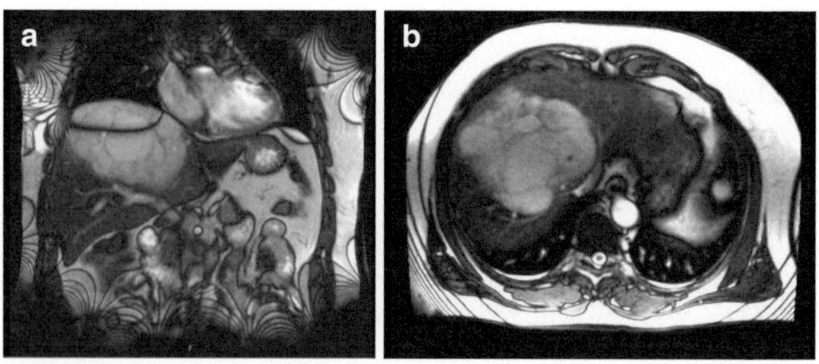

Fig. 44.2 (**a**, **b**) T2-weighted MRI of giant asymptomatic hepatic hemangioma. (HPB Clinic. MRMC. Richardson, Texas)

44.1.2.2 Management and Surgical Consultation

Due to the benign and uncomplicated history of hemangiomas, conservative management is recommended. Postoperative complications outweigh the benefits if resection is opted for asymptomatic lesions. Every effort should be made to avoid surgery.

Symptomatic Lesions Referral to an HPB surgeon is advised. Surgical resection constitutes the ultimate treatment of choice; nonetheless, embolization and ablative therapies have been described. Surgical resection can be achieved by enucleation, leaving all normal liver tissue intact.

44.1.3 Hepatocellular Adenoma (HCA)

Hepatocellular adenoma (HCA) is a very rare, benign solid liver lesion and mostly, as the other benign lesions, is found incidentally during imaging studies obtained for other reasons. What makes HCA different from the rest of benign lesions is its small potential for malignant transformation and complications such as rupture or bleeding. Bleeding is a more life-threatening issue in this lesion, as opposed to hemangioma, as HCAs are arterially supplied. HCAs have a higher incidence in women, and a causal role has been linked to estrogen levels due to increased size during pregnancy (mostly third trimester) and decreased in diameter after oral contraceptive cessation. Other associated risk factors include obesity, metabolic syndrome, and nonalcoholic steatohepatitis (NASH). Most HCAs are asymptomatic, and more than half of the patients present with two or more lesions.

44.1.3.1 Radiological Features

Due to the high accuracy of MRI (Fig. 44.3a, b) for diagnosing HCAs, the usefulness of biopsy results for decision-making is limited to cases that are not clearly defined by imaging. If a differential diagnosis between FNH and HCA is required, MRI with gadoxetate disodium or contrast-enhanced ultrasound (CEUS) are useful tools.

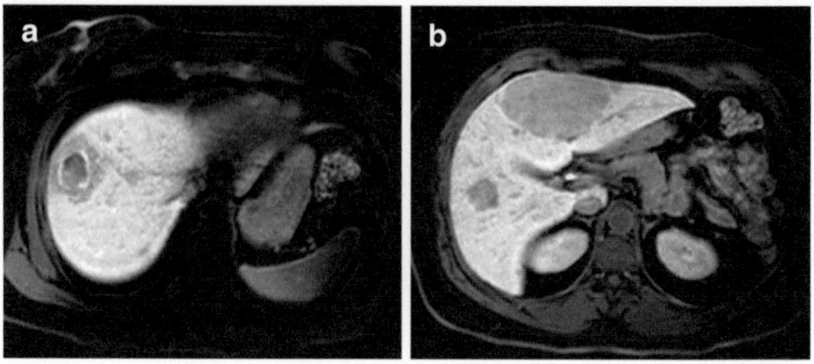

Fig. 44.3 (**a**, **b**) Postcontrast MRI. Patient with OC treatment with multiple HCAs and baseline liver steatosis. (HPB Surgery Service. MRMC. Richardson, Texas)

44.1.3.2 Management and Surgical Consultation

The paradigm of treatment for HCA has shifted from aggressive resection of all lesions to a more conservative approach. Once the diagnosis is made, risk factors should be addressed, including cessation of oral contraceptives and/or weight loss. Lesions that are asymptomatic and small in size (<5 cm) can be managed with serial imaging every 6–12 months. HCA does no longer imply a contraindication for pregnancy; nonetheless, close observation is recommended.

Surgical Consultation HPB consultation for lesions >5 cm, symptomatic, or lesions that do not regress in size after retrieval of OC. To note, all men with HCA will require resection regardless of the size due to the increased risk of malignant transformation.

44.1.4 Simple Cysts

Simple cysts, also known as benign hepatic cyst, constitute serous-filled lesions with no communication with the biliary tree, which allows for differentiation from other benign and malignant cystic lesions. They are usually asymptomatic and diagnosed as an incidental finding on imaging studies. Symptomatic simple cysts are usually larger in size, can cause abdominal pain, nausea, anorexia by compression to adjacent organs, or cholestasis secondary to compression of the biliary tract. Simple cysts can be complicated by infection, hemorrhage, or even rupture into the biliary tree or the peritoneal cavity.

44.1.4.1 Radiological Features

Ultrasound constitutes the most cost-effective radiological tool and has an ability to differentiate between simple cysts. MRI will demonstrate that a cyst is simple fluid. There should be no uptake on contrast injection (Fig. 44.4).

44.1.4.2 Management and Surgical Consultation

Small, asymptomatic simple cysts do not require further follow-up and treatment regardless of size. If patients become symptomatic, imaging (ultrasound first) will assess the size and look for complications and compression (10).

Surgical referral to an HPB surgery specialist will be advised for symptomatic and complicated cysts for further management.

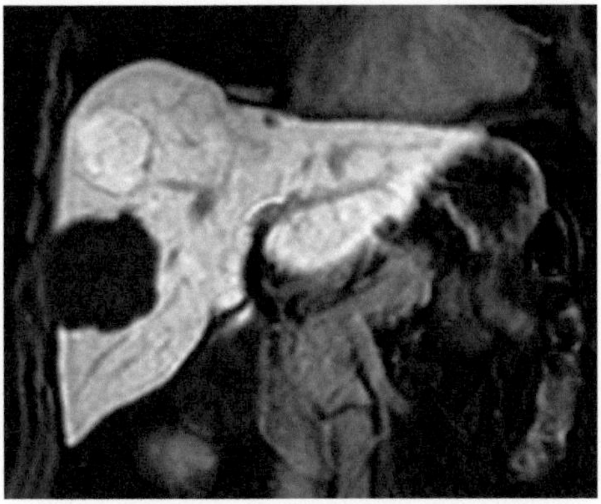

Fig. 44.4 T1-weighted image. Large simple cyst along with other small cysts and with associated FNH on segment VII. (HPB Clinic. MRMC. Richardson, Texas)

44.1.5 Infection-Related Liver Lesions

Due to the pragmatic nature of this manual, it is important to provide a general overview regarding liver lesions that arise from an infectious source.

44.1.5.1 Pyogenic Liver Abscess

Accounts for approximately 80% of liver abscesses in the USA. It is the most common type of visceral abscess. The most common causes are diseases of the biliary tract, infectious gastrointestinal disorders spreading via the portal vein (acute diverticulitis, appendicitis), hematogenous spread via the hepatic artery, direct extension from an intra-abdominal infection, and trauma. They are usually polymicrobial, but some organisms are seen more commonly in them, such as *E. coli, Klebsiella, Streptococcus, Staphylococcus*, and anaerobes. Patients can present with a myriad of symptoms; therefore, a thorough history and physical examination are crucial for the diagnosis. Associated important risk factors include diabetes, cirrhosis, male gender, elderly, immunocompromised states, and people with proton pump inhibitor usage (11). One must ensure that there is no untreated source such as diverticulitis, appendicitis, or biliary disease. Most patients are systemically ill and have fevers. A recent travel history should raise the possibility of an amoebic liver abscess (see below).

Radiological Features

US: Preferred initial diagnostic method. It has an accuracy close to 90% to detect abscesses >2 cm in diameter (12).

CT: Can detect lesions >0.5 cm in diameter.

Management and Surgical Consultation

Diagnosis is usually made in the acute or subacute setting. Initial management will be based on the patient's clinical presentation and should include broad-spectrum empiric antibiotic therapy. Surgical consultation with an HPB surgeon is advised, and percutaneous drainage may be warranted.

44.1.5.2 Amebic Liver Abscess

This entity is present in tropical and subtropical areas and in areas with poor sanitation, related to infestation of *Entamoeba histolytica*. The right lobe is most commonly affected with symptoms similar to pyogenic abscess. Patients often have a travel history and may have had a diarrheal illness. Spiking high fevers are common. Serology is the best method to confirm the diagnosis, but presumptive treatment with metronidazole is advised. Complications include bacterial secondary infection and rupture.

Radiological Features

US and CT will both likely demonstrate the lesion.

Management and Surgical Consultation

First-line treatment of uncomplicated lesions are amebicidal drugs (e.g., metronidazole). Surgical consultation should be advised for larger amebic abscesses, complicated with bacterial infection or rupture, as they may require percutaneous or surgical drainage.

44.1.5.3 Hydatid Cyst

Echinococcosis is a zoonosis caused by *Echinococcus granulosus* with endemic areas in Central America, South America, and some Mediterranean regions. Contamination is via fecal oral route. The etiology is thought to be related to eating raw pork or lamb. Cysts are slowly growing and symptoms present due to compression effects or complications such as rupture with secondary infection or anaphylactic shock.

Radiological Features

US is particularly useful. CT best demonstrates cyst wall calcification and cyst infection.

Management and Surgical Consultation

Anthelmintics (albendazole, mebendazole) must be used and are felt to decrease the risk of anaphylaxis at the time of operation. Surgery is warranted, either laparoscopic or open.

44.2 Malignant Liver Lesions

The large spectrum of malignant liver lesions can be divided according to their localization in primary and secondary liver lesions. Primary tumors based on their histological origin can be classified into hepatocellular, biliary, and mesenchymal tumors. Among secondary lesions, we will direct our focus to metastatic liver lesions.

44.2.1 Hepatocellular Carcinoma (HCC)

Hepatocellular carcinoma (HCC) constitutes the most common primary tumor of the liver and accounts for approximately 90% of these lesions and constitutes the fifth most common cancer worldwide. Significant risk factors include viral hepatitis (hepatitis B and C), alcoholic liver disease, NASH, and nonalcoholic fatty liver disease (NAFLD), the latter being the most common cause of HCC, particularly in Western countries (17). The annual incidence of HCC in patients with cirrhosis is 2–4% (18). HCC not associated with cirrhosis is rare in the West, but can occur. This is more commonly the fibrolamellar variant of HCC (Table 44.2).

Table 44.2 Management and surgical consultation for malignant liver lesions

	Management	Surgical consultation
HCC	US every 6 months for high-risk patients. If $\geq$10 mm multiphase CT/MRI.	HPB or transplant surgery at the time of diagnosis
IHCC	Surgery referral.	HPB or transplant surgery at the time of diagnosis
Metastatic lesions	MRI with gadoxetate disodium.	HPB or transplant surgery at the time of diagnosis

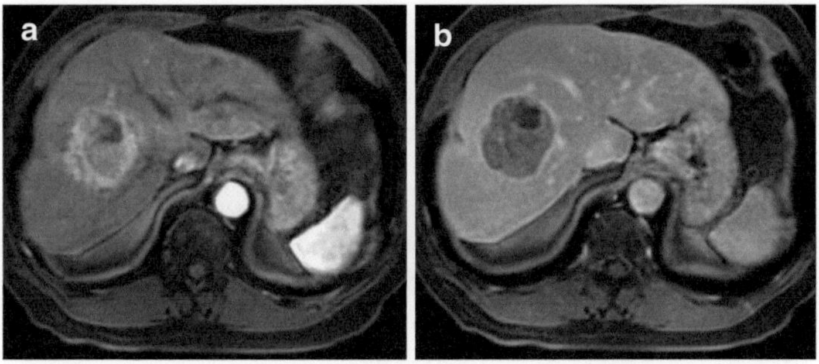

Fig. 44.5 (**a**, **b**) T1-weighted images of heterogeneously arterial hyperenhancing mass with washout and apparent pseudocapsule. (HPB Surgery Service. MRMC. Richardson, Texas)

44.2.1.1 Radiological Features

Ultrasound, computed tomography, and MRI can all be useful tools for diagnosing HCC. Ultrasound is noninvasive and widely used for surveillance. High-risk patients should be US surveilled every 6 months. Once a lesion is found, it must be investigated. Small lesions follow the algorithm mentioned above. Patients with lesions ≥10 mm will require further assessment with multiphasic CT or MRI (Fig. 44.5a, b).

44.2.1.2 Management and Surgical Consultation

Based on epidemiology and patient baseline characteristics, if a suspicion of HCC is made, surgical consultation to an HPB/transplant practice is advisable for further management. Resection or liver transplantation are definitive measures. However, liver-directed therapy and chemotherapy/immunotherapy options are available.

44.2.2 Intrahepatic Cholangiocarcinoma (IHCC)

Intrahepatic cholangiocarcinoma is considered a primary adenocarcinoma of the liver and is the second most common primary tumor of the liver after HCC. It is a biologically aggressive disease and most of the time presents itself with symptoms related to advanced local or metastatic disease. It has a higher incidence in males and presents later in life around the seventh or eighth decades. Many widely known risk factors for IHCC include primary sclerosing cholangitis (PSC) and liver fluke (*Opisthorchis viverrini* and *Clonorchis sinensis)* mostly in Southeast Asia.

For screening and monitoring, CA 19-9 and CEA provide the highest sensitivity and specificity for ICHH.

44.2.2.1 Radiological Features

The most common imaging modalities used to diagnose and stage intrahepatic cholangiocarcinoma include ultrasound (US), computed tomography (CT) , magnetic resonance imaging/magnetic resonance cholangiopancreatography (MRI/MRCP), and positron emission tomography (PET) (Fig. 44.6a, b) (20).

44.2.2.2 Management and Surgical Consultation

At the time of diagnosis or as soon as there is a clinical/radiological suspicion of IHCC, the patient should be referred to an HPB surgeon for further management.

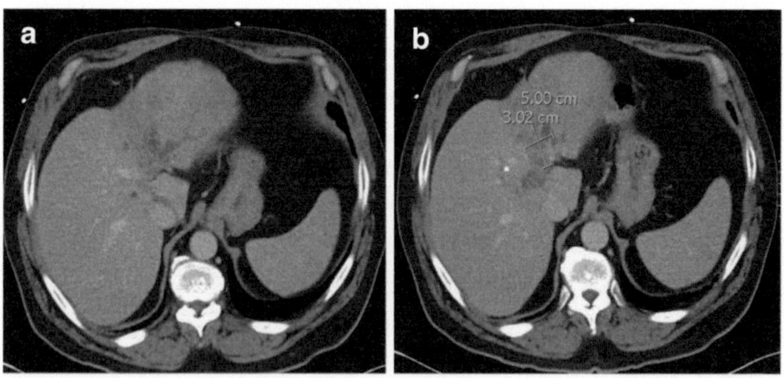

Fig. 44.6 (**a**, **b**) T1-weighted images of centrally obstructing mass with left intrahepatic ductal dilatation. (HPB Surgery Service. MRMC. Richardson, Texas)

44.2.3 Metastatic Lesions

The liver constitutes the site for metastatic disease of cancer originating from different organs, including the colon and rectum, breast, esophagus, stomach, lung, kidney, and skin. Of these, colorectal liver metastases (CRLM) are the most common, with approximately 25% of patients developing them during the course of their illness. The management for this disease has changed significantly over the last decades in regards to diagnosis, surveillance, and treatment (21).

44.2.3.1 Radiological Features

US: Transabdominal US MRI has a limited role in preoperative management. Its sensitivity is low compared with other imaging modalities.

CT: The portal venous phase is the most reliable.

MRI: MRI has superior soft tissue contrast compared to CT.

44.2.3.2 Management and Surgical Consultation

Multidisciplinary management is recommended for these patients. The diagnosis of CRLM will prompt an early referral for HPB surgery evaluation. It is always best if these patients can be seen at the time of diagnosis to develop a plan of treatment for them from the outset.

44.3 Too Small to Characterize Lesions (TSTC)

Oftentimes, during routine imaging studies, we often encounter incidental liver lesions that, due to their small size and unusual features, cannot be confidently categorized, leading to them being termed TSTC. Managing these lesions depends on the patient's individual characteristics. For patients without a known malignancy, research indicates that TSTCs are typically benign, requiring no further follow-up.

However, in patients with a documented primary malignancy, such as breast cancer, the likelihood of metastatic disease varies depending on the type of malignancy: 4% in lymphoma, 14% in colorectal cancer, and 22% in breast cancer. Therefore, meticulous analysis of imaging findings becomes crucial.

Contrast-enhanced MRI has emerged as a reliable tool for characterizing TSTCs. Should further evaluation be necessary, a multiphasic CT scan with intravenous contrast 3 months later is recommended.

Suggested Readings

1. Blumgart's Surgery of the Liver, Biliary Tract and Pancreas, Seventh edition, 2023. Chapters: 87, 88.
2. AASLD guidelines: www.aasld.org/practice-guidelines/management-hepatocellular-carcinoma.
3. Patel S, Cheek S, Osman H, Jeyarajah DR. MRI with gadoxetate disodium for colorectal liver metastasis: is it the new "imaging modality of choice"? J Gastrointest Surg. 2014;18(12):2130–5. https://doi.org/10.1007/s11605-014-2676-0. Epub 2014 Oct 16. PMID: 25319036.

Pancreatic Lesions

45

Abdelazeem Hamed and Ziad T. Awad

45.1 Pancreatic Cystic Neoplasms

Pancreatic cystic neoplasms compromise a heterogeneous group that includes intraductal papillary mucinous neoplasm, serous cystic neoplasm, mucinous cystic neoplasm, pseudocyst, and other rare cystic lesions.

45.2 Intraductal Papillary Mucinous Neoplasms (IPMNs)

Presentation: IPMNs are mucinous cysts of the pancreas with communication to the main pancreatic duct (PD), branch duct, or both. Patients may present with vague abdominal pain/discomfort, weight loss, satiety, or obstructive jaundice. IPMNs may also be found incidentally on imaging performed for other reasons.

Diagnosis: CT and MRI will demonstrate poorly demarcated lobulated mass with dilation of the main or branch ducts.

A. Hamed · Z. T. Awad (✉)
Department of Surgery, University of Florida College of Medicine-Jacksonville, Jacksonville, FL, USA
e-mail: ziad.awad@jax.ufl.edu

G. P. Kohn et al. (eds.), *The SAGES Manual of Surgical Referral for Primary and Emergency Care*,
https://doi.org/10.1007/978-3-031-92678-5_45

Table 45.1 IPMN high-risk features and worrisome features

Worrisome features	Main duct 5–9 mm Cyst size >3 Thickened, enhancing cyst wall Nonenhancing mural nodule Pancreatitis Lymphadenopathy Abrupt caliber change in the main duct with upstream atrophy Elevated CA 19-9
High-risk features	Main duct ≥1 cm Enhancing solid component Jaundice

Endoscopic ultrasound (EUS) with fine needle aspiration (FNA) helps with better evaluation of the cystic neoplasm. Cystic fluid analysis demonstrates high carcinoembryonic antigen (CEA), high amylase, and positive for mucin.

Management: IPMNs have a malignant potential; thus, surveillance imaging and early referral for surgical resection are important. Patients who are symptomatic and with high-risk features of IPMN (see Table 45.1) should be referred to HBP/surgical oncology for pancreatic resection and management by algorithm (Fig. 45.1). Patients with worrisome features (see Table 45.1) should be referred to for endoscopic ultrasound (EUS).

Low- to intermediate-risk cysts: surveillance (Table 45.2) can be limited to 5 years if there is no change in cyst size or characteristics.

Cysts stable for at least 5 years: surveillance can be discontinued in patients older than 75 years with cysts <30 mm or older than 65 years with cysts ≤15 mm.

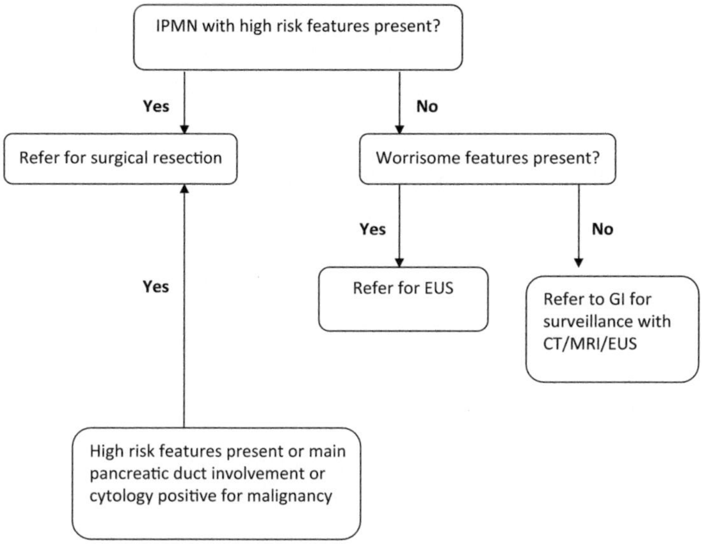

Fig. 45.1 IPMN management algorithm

Table 45.2 IPMN surveilance protocol

<10 mm: asymptomatic IPMNs should be checked annually
10–20 mm: should be checked every 6–12 months
20–30 mm: should be checked every 2 years with EUS or MRI

45.3 Serous Cystic Neoplasm (SCN)

SCN arises from the pancreas with no communication to the main PD. Patients present with vague abdominal pain, discomfort, and early satiety.

Diagnosis: Cystic fluid analysis shows low carcinoembryonic antigen (CEA), low amylase, and negative for mucin. CT and MRI pancreas demonstrate multiple cysts with internal septations (honeycomb pattern). EUS with FNA for further characterization of the cyst and cyst fluid sampling is usually indicated.

Management: Observation is the gold standard for the asymptomatic patient. Indications for surgical resection include symptomatic patients, rapidly growing lesions, and cyst size >4 cm.

45.4 Mucinous Cystic Neoplasm (MCN)

MCNs are mostly benign, but it has a malignant potential. Patients likely present with abdominal pain, early satiety, and weight loss.

Diagnosis: Cystic fluid analysis shows high CEA, low amylase, and positive for mucin. CT and MRI demonstrate thick-wall cyst with solid component (eggshell calcification). EUS with FNA for further characterization of the cyst and cyst fluid sampling is required.

Management: MCN has a malignant potential; thus, referral to HBP/surgical oncology for surgical resection is indicated.

45.5 Pancreatic Pseudocyst

Pancreatic pseudocyst is an encapsulated fluid collection located outside of the pancreas as a complication of acute or chronic pancreatitis. Patients present with feeling unwell, vague abdominal pain, or vomiting. Physical exam will be positive for abdominal tenderness and palpable abdominal mass.

Diagnosis: Contrast-enhanced CT abdomen is the modality of choice for the detection of a pseudocyst.

Management: Spontaneous resolution of pseudocysts is common; thus, the best option for asymptomatic patients is expectant management. Invasive therapies are indicated in symptomatic patients (abdominal pain, satiety, fever). Patients with symptomatic pseudocysts should be referred to advanced endoscopist/IR for endoscopic and percutaneous drainage. Referral for surgical evaluation and possible resection is warranted in selected cases with recurrent pseudocysts after endoscopic drainage, pseudocysts that are difficult to access endoscopically or suspicion of malignancy.

45.6 Exocrine Pancreatic Neoplasm

Exocrine pancreatic tumors are the most common tumors of the pancreas with high malignant potential that include pancreatic adenocarcinoma, acinar cell carcinoma, solid pseudopapillary tumor, and pancreatic lymphoma.

Presentation: Patients present with weight loss, itching, back pain, epigastric pain, and jaundice.

Diagnosis: Elevated CA 19-9. CT pancreas protocol is the modality of choice for pancreatic tumor evaluation as it helps determine tumor location, duct dilation, and relationship of the tumor to critical vessels. Endoscopic ultrasound will help tumor staging, and FNA biopsy is needed for tissue diagnosis. Endoscopic retrograde cholangiopancreatography with brushing (ERCP) might help in the diagnosis and provide biliary decompression in patients with a pancreatic head tumor causing biliary obstruction (Fig. 45.2).

Management: Patients with pancreatic cancers should be referred to surgical oncology and medical oncology and to be discussed in a multidisciplinary team, with management outlined in Fig. 45.2.

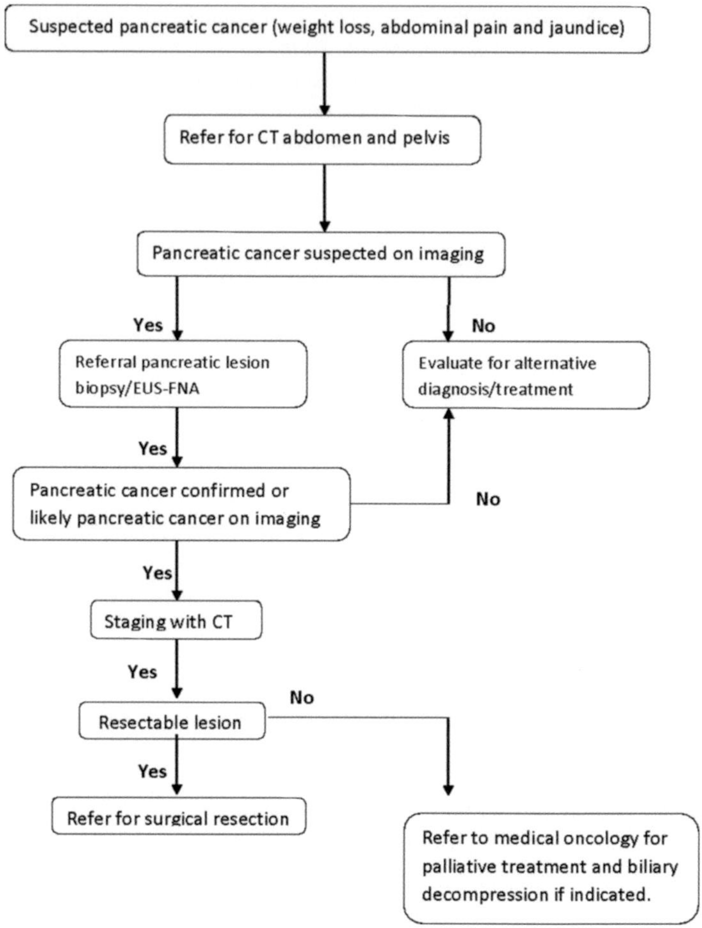

Fig. 45.2 Management of pancreatic cancer algorithm

45.7 Pancreatic Neuroendocrine Neoplasm (PNET)

Pancreatic neuroendocrine neoplasms arise from endocrine cells of the pancreas, which compromise a group of rare sporadic pancreatic tumors and are less commonly associated with genetic syndromes like multiple endocrine neoplasia type 1 and Von Hipple–Lindau syndrome. The majority of PNET are nonfunctional while few are functional, manifested by the secretion of active hormones (highly malignant tumors with distant metastasis) (Fig. 45.3).

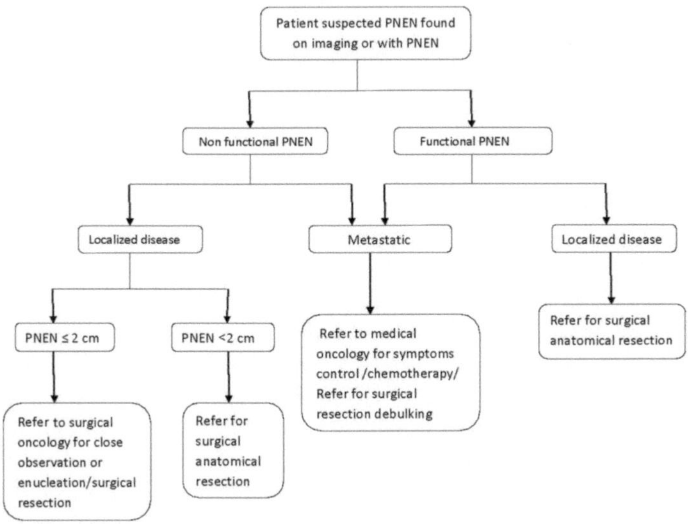

Fig. 45.3 PNET management algorithm

45.8 Insulinoma

Presentation: Patients present with the Whipple triad: fasting hypoglycemia, symptoms of hypoglycemia (tremor, weakness, diaphoresis, palpitation, irritability, blurry vision and confusion), and symptom relief with glucose administration.

Diagnosis: Decrease serum glucose, increase insulin level, C-peptide, and proinsulin during hypoglycemic episode. CT pancreas protocol, MRI abdomen, and EUS will demonstrate a hypoechoic pancreatic lesion.

Management: Referral to HBP/surgical oncology for enucleation or anatomic resection in patients with resectable symptomatic insulinoma. Referral to IR for hepatic artery embolization or RFA for metastatic liver lesions. Referral to medical oncology for chemotherapy in patients with metastatic insulinoma.

45.9 Gastrinoma

Presentation: Patients present with abdominal pain, diarrhea, heartburn, gastric and duodenal ulcers refractory to medical treatment.

Diagnosis: Fasting gastrin level >1000 pg/ml and confirmation with secretin stimulation test. CT pancreas protocol, MRI abdomen, and EUS will demonstrate a hypoechoic pancreatic lesion.

Management: Referral to HBP/surgical oncology for segmental pancreatic resection in patients with localized tumor and for palliative cytoreduction surgery for symptom control in patients with localized metastatic disease. For patients with unresectable metastatic disease, treatment should focus on symptom control with acid reduction medication and somatostatin analogs to decrease gastric release and acid secretion.

45.10 Somatostatinoma

Patients present with steatorrhea, symptoms of diabetes, and gallstones.

Diagnosis: Fasting serum somatostatin level >160 pg/ml. CT pancreas protocol, MRI abdomen will demonstrate a hypoechoic pancreatic lesion. Localization could be performed with EUS, somatostatin receptor scintigraphy, and 68Ga-DOTATATE PET scan if CT or MRI are unable to localize the tumor.

Management: Given the high potential of malignant disease, referral to HBP or surgical oncology for anatomic resection is warranted in patients with resectable disease.

45.11 VIPoma

Patients present with diarrhea, hypokalemia, metabolic acidosis, and achlorhydria.

Diagnosis: Elevated fasting vasoactive intestinal peptide (VIP) level of 223–2000 pg/ml. CT pancreas protocol, MRI abdomen, and EUS will demonstrate a hypoechoic pancreatic lesion.

Management: Given the high potential of malignant disease, referral to HBP or surgical oncology for anatomic resection is warranted in patients with resectable disease. Medical management with hydration and somatostatin analogs for unresectable disease.

45.12 Glucagonoma

Patients present with symptoms of diabetes mellitus, weight loss, skin rashes (necrolytic migratory erythema), and DVT.

Diagnosis: Fasting glucagon level >1000 pg/ml. CT pancreas protocol, MRI abdomen, and EUS will demonstrate a hypoechoic pancreatic lesion.

Management: Glucagonoma has high malignant potential; thus, referral to HBP/surgical oncology for anatomic resection in patients with resectable disease is warranted.

A summary of referral guidelines and pre-referral recommendation is presented in Tables 45.3 and 45.4.

Table 45.3 Pancreatic solid and cystic lesions on CT scan

Refer to emergency room	Urgent surgical referral	Nonurgent surgical referral	Refer to GI medicine	Management by PCP
Cholangitis Acute pancreatitis Infected pancreatic pseudocyst with sepsis Panccreaticoduodenal arteries pseudoaneurysm bleed	Symptomatic patient (abdominal pain, jaundice, and weight loss) Pancreatic lesions with worrisome and high-risk features	Asymptomatic patient with worrisome and high-risk features	Symptomatic and asymptomatic patient with high-risk features or worrisome features for EUS +FNA and surveillance	Cyst> 1 cm without high-risk or worrisome features Repeat MRI in one year then every 2 years until 5 years Stop surveillance if the lesion is stable

Table 45.4 Tests and imaging to perform prior to surgical referral

Pancreatic solid lesion	Suspected IPMN/MCN/SCN	Suspected insulinoma	Suspected gastrinoma	Suspected somatostatinoma	Suspected glucagonoma
CT pancreas protocol or MRI Refer to GI for EUS + FNA Ca 19-9	CT pancreas protocol or MRI Refer to GI for EUS + FNA + cyst fluid analysis	CT pancreas protocol or MRI Serum blood glucose Serum C peptide Serum pro insulin	CT pancreas protocol or MRI Secretin stimulation test	CT pancreas protocol or MRI Serum somatostatin level	CT pancreas protocol or MRI Fasting glucagon level

Suggested Readings

1. Sabiston Textbook of Surgery: The Biological Basis of Modern Surgical Practice, 21st ed. Ch. 56: Exocrine pancreas, Cystic neoplasms of the pancreas.
2. https://pubmed.ncbi.nlm.nih.gov/15131794/.
3. https://seer.cancer.gov/statfacts/html/pancreas.html.
4. https://www.ncbi.nlm.nih.gov/pmc/articles/PMC5890653/.
5. https://www.sciencedirect.com/science/article/pii/S1424390317305161.

Splenic Lesions

46

Sage A. Vincent and Francesco Palazzo

46.1 Introduction

The spleen, located intraperitoneally in the left upper quadrant, plays an important role in the hematologic and reticuloendothelial systems. The spleen may harbor a number of abnormal lesions that vary in their biologic behavior, appearance, and need for further workup. Splenic lesions can be quite heterogeneous, which is felt to be due, in part, to the organ's unique structural composition[1, 8, 12, 15]. Red pulp comprises the majority of the splenic parenchyma and is rich in macrophages, whose function consist in the removal of damaged erythrocytes and platelets. Red pulp envelopes tufts of white pulp, which serve primarily an immune func-

S. A. Vincent · F. Palazzo (✉)
Thomas Jefferson University Hospital, Philadelphia, PA, USA
e-mail: Sage.Vincent@jefferson.edu; Francesco.Palazzo@jefferson.edu

G. P. Kohn et al. (eds.), *The SAGES Manual of Surgical Referral for Primary and Emergency Care*,
https://doi.org/10.1007/978-3-031-92678-5_46

tion. These distinct tissues can play host to a number of different lesions, some of which require surgical referral and intervention, which will be reviewed below. While the majority of splenic lesions can be asymptomatic and are found incidentally during the workup of unrelated conditions, others are brought to a provider's attention based on vague abdominal symptoms (i.e., vague abdominal pain, distension, nausea, vomiting, early satiety) related to the close proximity of the spleen to adjacent organs. Retrospective reviews in the trauma literature have found that 1–1.5% of imaging studies will identify incidental splenic lesions; these rates are increasing in recent years, in part as a result of the broader access and utilization of cross-sectional imaging.

The ideal imaging modality for characterizing splenic lesions remains a subject of discussion. Particularly from the outpatient setting, splenic lesions may first be noted on ultrasound, regarded as a quick and noninvasive means of looking at the organ. Ultrasound can pick up on heterogeneity of the spleen, a departure from the typically uniform echogenicity, indicating some sort of lesion. Further characterization typically requires true cross-sectional imaging, preferably a contrast-enhanced computed tomography (CT) or magnetic resonance imaging (MRI). A CT helps distinguish subtle differences in the Hounsfield units (HU) between the lesion and surrounding parenchyma in order to characterize the lesion. Known for their high definition and detail, MRI can also be particularly helpful in differentiating splenic lesions, though in many circumstances may not be readily or quickly available.

Despite increasing identification of splenic lesions, there remains minimal guidelines or recommendations to guide clinicians in the care of their patients. For example, it remains unclear what surveillance is needed for splenic lesions, if any. Radiology literature seems to suggest that surveillance imaging is only indicated for patients in whom there is diagnostic uncertainty, though this has not been formally recommended or studied in clinical medicine. It is important to note that this chapter will not discuss splenic trauma, pediatric splenic lesions, or medical splenomeg-

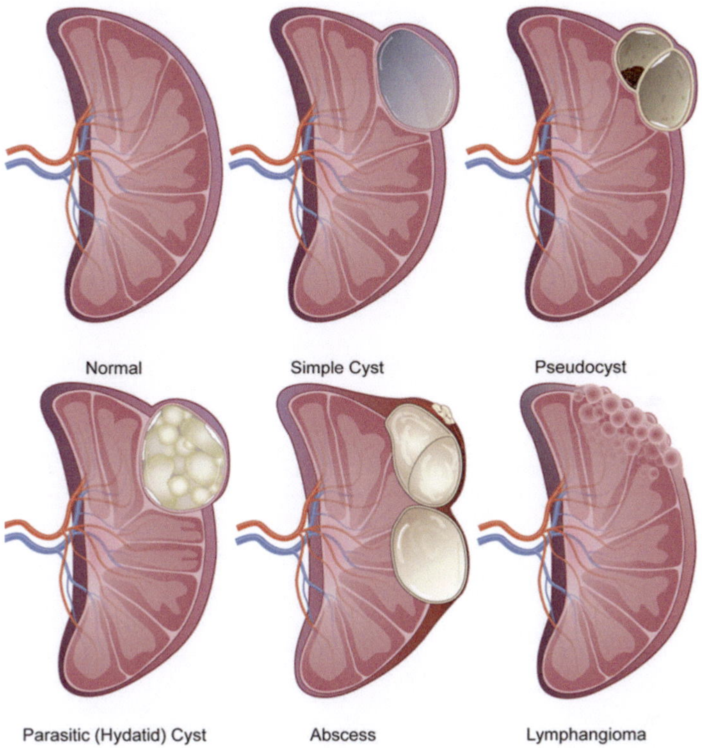

Fig. 46.1 Illustrative representations of the commonly encountered cystic lesions of the spleen. (Figure created courtesy of, and published with express permission of, medical illustrator, Jennifer Brumbaugh, MA; Thomas Jefferson University Hospital, Department of Surgery)

aly due to a variety of etiologies, including splenic vein thrombosis or infectious mononucleosis. As the majority of splenic lesions will be first noted on an imaging study, this chapter will utilize the imaging characteristic of solid versus cystic as a means of subcategorization (Figs. 46.1 and 46.2) in order to aid providers in their management and referral patterns.

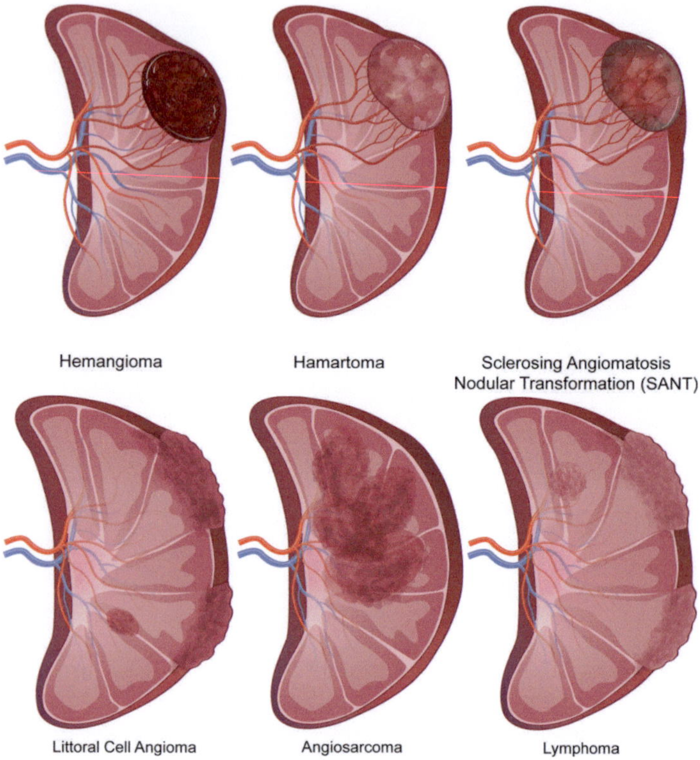

Fig. 46.2 Illustrative representations of the commonly seen solid lesions of the spleen. (Figure created courtesy of, and published with express permission of, medical illustrator, Jennifer Brumbaugh, MA; Thomas Jefferson University Hospital, Department of Surgery)

46.2 General Principles

While many splenic lesions are diagnosed incidentally via imaging studies, some patients may present with symptomatic lesions. In general, splenic lesions become symptomatic as they enlarge, with the constellation of chief complaints reflecting compression or displacement of adjacent organs. Mass effect on the stomach may result in early satiety, nausea, vomiting, or dyspepsia, while mass effect on the colon may cause constipation or obstructive symptoms. Upward pressure on the diaphragm may result in dyspnea or shortness of breath. As the spleen enlarges, patients may also develop associated hematologic abnormalities, including thrombocytopenia and anemia. Because these presenting symptoms are nonspecific and can overlap different splenic lesions, providers will often rely on imaging findings to determine the specific pathology. With a high-enough index of suspicion, patients may be referred for surgical evaluation to discuss splenectomy. When the diagnosis is uncertain, histologic confirmation via percutaneous biopsy is reasonable and demonstrates a high degree of accuracy, >90%. In the past, there was concern regarding the safety of percutaneous biopsy, with unacceptably high rates of postprocedural bleeding; however, contemporary studies have found the procedure to be quite safe with morbidity of any type limited to 5% of patients. Many splenic lesions can be safely monitored over time without the need for surgical intervention, while others warrant surgical referral at the time of diagnosis in order to expedite splenectomy. The nuances of and rationale for these differences will be discussed below and summarized in Tables 46.1 and 46.2.

Table 46.1 Summary of frequently encountered cystic splenic lesions and their associated recommendations for surgical referral

Cystic lesion	Characteristics	Surgical referral
Simple cyst	Common, benign Imaging: thin-walled, hypo-attenuating	Size >5 cm Mass effect symptoms
Pseudocyst	Most common type of splenic cyst Female to male predominance 2:1 Imaging: thick wall, calcifications	Size >5 cm Mass effect symptoms
Parasitic cyst	Typically seen in endemic regions Biopsy contraindicated due to the risk of anaphylaxis Imaging: thin-walled, hypo-attenuating	Refer at the time of diagnosis
Abscess	Common in patients with endocarditis, immunocompromised state Consider IR drainage Imaging: rim enhancing	Failure of medical, percutaneous therapy
Lymph-angioma	Usually seen in patients <30 years old Imaging: hypoattenuating, subcapsular	Size >5 cm Mass effect symptoms

Table 46.2 Summary of frequently encountered solid splenic lesions and their associated recommendations for surgical referral

Solid lesion	Characteristics	Surgical referral
Hemangioma	Most common solid splenic tumor Risk of malignant transformation Imaging: hypo-attenuating with delayed peripheral enhancement	Refer at the time of diagnosis
Hamartoma	Rare Associated with other solid organ malignancies (i.e., renal, thymus) Imaging: arterial enhancement	Size >5 cm Mass effect symptoms
SANT	Rare Requires tissue diagnosis	Mass effect symptoms Uncertain diagnosis
Littoral cell angioma	Rare Requires tissue diagnosis Risk of malignant transformation when large	Size >5 cm Mass effect symptoms
Angiosarcoma	Rare Aggressive, high metastatic potential	Refer at the time of diagnosis
Lymphoma	Most common malignant lesion of the spleen Treatment is medical primarily	Mass effect symptoms
Metastasis	Melanoma, breast, lung, and ovarian are the most common primary	Refer at the time of diagnosis

46.3 Cystic Splenic Lesions

46.3.1 Simple Cyst

Also referred to as primary cysts, simple cysts are frequently asymptomatic, solitary, and benign. Simple cysts are considered to be true cysts, containing an epithelial lining and account for about 15–20% of all splenic cysts. These may vary widely in size and complexity, ranging from small, unilocular to large and multilocular. These are often identified incidentally on imaging as thin-walled and hypo-attenuating. When simple cysts enlarge, patients may present with symptoms related to mass effect, such as early satiety, nausea, vomiting, and painless abdominal mass.

Although there are no universally accepted guidelines for the treatment of splenic cysts, it is generally acceptable to manage simple cysts nonoperatively when they are small, <5 cm, and asymptomatic. There is limited evidence to support a cutoff size of <5 cm for operative intervention and is certainly appropriate to refer symptomatic patients or those with rapidly enlarging simple splenic cysts for consideration of resection prior to meeting the 5 cm cutoff. There have been reports of splenic cyst rupture leading to peritonitis, hemoperitoneum, and sepsis, outcomes that serve as the basis for surgical excision. Percutaneous drainage of simple splenic cysts has been shown to have a high rate of recurrence, as well as inflammatory adhesion formation, and should be reserved only for patients who are not suitable operative candidates.

46.3.2 Pseudocyst

Pseudocysts are the most common of all splenic cysts, accounting for 80–90% of cysts. In contrast to simple cysts, pseudocysts do not contain an epithelial cell lining. They arise as the result of splenic insult, frequently in the setting of trauma, ischemia, or infection, such as mononucleosis, tuberculosis, or malaria. Pseudocysts are most frequently identified in young and middle-aged adults, with a female-to-male predominance of 2:1, the rationale for which is unknown but may be related to hormonal differences. Pseudocyst walls often become thickened and develop characteristic calcifications as a result. The pseudocyst itself is typically filled with a combination of serous fluid, necrotic debris, and old hematoma, depending on its etiology.

Similar to simple splenic cysts, the management of pseudocysts is dependent on their size and degree of symptoms. Symptomatic patients or those whose cysts exceed 5 cm in size are appropriate for referral for consideration of resection, which may include splenectomy or partial splenectomy depending on the location of the lesion and its depth of involvement.

46.3.3 Parasitic Cyst

Most commonly due to *Echinococcus granulosus*, parasitic cysts, or hydatid cysts, are the most common type of splenic cyst seen outside the Western world. Sometimes mistaken for simple cysts given their similar appearance on imaging studies, parasitic splenic cysts are the result of fecal-oral transmission in which a human incidental host ingests *E. granulosus* tapeworm eggs that are able to penetrate intestinal mucosa to enter the lymphatic system and travel to visceral organs, including the spleen. These cysts enlarge over time as the parasitic life cycle continues and the cyst fills with hydatid fluid.

Patients typically present with symptoms related to mass effect, including vague abdominal pain, reflux, and dyspnea, although as many as 30% of cases are identified incidentally on imaging studies. Parasitic splenic cysts are often solitary, cystic lesions. Depending on the timing of the parasitic life cycle, daughter cysts, seen as septations, may also be visible. It is important to have a high degree of suspicion for parasitic cyst in patients from endemic regions with these imaging findings. Diagnosis can be confirmed using serologic testing. Although some splenic cysts can be biopsied or aspirated percutaneously to establish a diagnosis, this is strictly contraindicated for patients in whom there is concern for parasitic infection given the risk of echinococcal spillage (seeding the peritoneal cavity) and anaphylaxis.

Antihelminth therapy, typically albendazole, is recommended at the time of diagnosis of a parasitic splenic cyst, although this does not represent definitive management. Medical management alone has a failure rate of 25–50%, and relapse is common even years after therapy is discontinued. Splenectomy is the gold standard for the eradication of parasitic splenic cysts, particularly when large; however, it is not without its risks. Parasitic cyst rupture carries a high risk of anaphylaxis and disseminated echinococcosis, as well as an operative rate as high as 4% independent of operative technique.

46.3.4 Abscess

Cysts due to infection may form complex abscesses in the splenic parenchyma. These are rarely incidentally found and are often accompanied by fevers, chills, malaise, and lab findings, including leukocytosis and positive blood cultures. Abdominal imaging findings will note rim-enhancing collections in the splenic parenchyma, and left pleural effusion may be seen in >85% of patients at presentation. Splenic abscesses are often concomitantly found with liver and renal abscesses as well as lymphadenopathy. Microbiologic speciation is typically gram-negative bacteria or fungi. Patients who are found to have splenic infections are often immunocompromised and have underlying endocarditis or a previous splenic lesion such as infarct or solid lesion, which predispose abscess formation.

Treatment of splenic abscesses varies greatly based on patient characteristics, size, degree of splenic involvement, and provider preference. In patients with multiple collections, smaller collections, or difficult anatomy, antibiotics alone may be sufficient. Solitary, unilocular collections are appropriate for management with percutaneous drainage; however, failure rates may be upward of 33%. In the spirit of splenic preservation, percutaneous drainage is preferable in young patients. Patients with complex, multilocular, multicentric collections not amenable to drainage or those who have failed drainage procedures should be considered for operative intervention. It is worth noting that there is no difference in mortality from splenic abscess in patients treated with antibiotics, percutaneous drainage, or splenectomy.

46.3.5 Lymphangioma

Lymphangiomas are small, slow-growing, and indolent splenic lesions that are often detected during childhood or young adulthood[15]. They represent a congenital abnormality of lymphatic tissue in the spleen, with disorganized tissue forming lesions. In most cases, lymphangiomas are cystic appearing on imaging, but may be more solid if they are cavernous or capillary subtypes. They are typically found adjacent to the splenic capsule, consistent with the anatomic location of lymphatic channels, and are surrounded by thin walls, making them well circumscribed.

Splenic lymphangiomas are often asymptomatic and incidentally found; however, as they enlarge, patients may present with symptoms related to mass effect. The treatment of choice for definitive management of splenic lymphangioma is splenectomy, either partial or total, in order to reduce the risk of rupture, infection, or expansion. Partial splenectomy is associated with a 9.5% risk of recurrence, but does preserve immune function. It is reasonable to monitor patients with splenic lymphangiomas <5 cm as the risk of rupture is low. Aspiration, with or without sclerosing agents, and drainage have been attempted, though with high rates of recurrence. Malignant transformation in patients with splenic lymphangiomas has been reported but is exceedingly rare.

46.4 Solid Splenic Lesions

46.4.1 Hemangioma

Splenic hemangiomas are benign tumors that arise as a result of abnormal proliferation of blood vessels, which is felt to reflect a congenital anomaly. They are the most common benign primary tumor the spleen, with an incidence of 0.03–14% of the population. These are often solitary, although occasionally may be multifocal[8]. As many as 80% of patients are asymptomatic at the time of diagnosis, with much of the remaining patients presenting with classic mass effect symptoms. In rare instances, patients may be brought to medical attention with thrombocytopenia, hemolytic anemia, and coagulopathy, the so-called Kasabach–Merritt syndrome. Imaging findings will note a characteristic hypoattenuating lesion with delayed peripheral enhancement.

The natural course of a splenic hemangioma is slow, indolent growth over many years. The risk of spontaneous hemangioma rupture has been well documented, with historic rates of around 25% over a lifetime. Malignant transformation is a known, and feared, complication of splenic hemangiomas, with increasing risk with size greater than 4 cm. Given these risks, early surgical referral is warranted in patients found to have hemangiomas.

46.4.2 Hamartoma

Lesions that are the result of malformation of the red and white pulp are referred to as hamartomas. These rare tumors are benign and quite rare, with an estimated incidence of 0.024–0.13%. Imaging studies will note characteristic homogeneous arterial enhancement. Most splenic hamartomas are sporadic but some may be the result of genetic syndromes, particularly tuberous sclerosis and Wiscott–Aldrich-like syndrome. As such, there is a strong association between splenic hamartomas and other solid tissue tumors, including thymoma, renal cell carcinomas, and squamous cell carcinomas.

There is a risk of rupture, particularly as the lesions grow in size. Symptoms, rapid growth, and size >5 cm are reasonable indications for surgical intervention, although as it is a benign pathology, the decision ultimately requires a high degree of joint discussion between provider and patient.

46.4.3 Sclerosing Angiomatosis Nodular Transformation (SANT)

Sclerosing angiomatosis nodular transformation (SANT) is a relatively rare solid, vascular lesion of the spleen. More commonly diagnosed in women, SANT has been reported across a wide age range and in some instances is only diagnosed on pathologic review of a splenic specimen resected for another indication. As a vascular lesion of the spleen, it is often radiographically and clinically indistinguishable from hemangiomas and hamartomas, requiring histologic examination for formal diagnosis. Although morphologically similar to hemangiomas and hamartomas, there is no definitive evidence or validated reports that SANT lesions carry a risk of rupture. As such, there are some who argue that patients with a confirmed diagnosis of SANT can be monitored clinically regardless of size, provided they are asymptomatic. However, given its similarity to other splenic lesions that do carry risk of rupture and malignancy, it has been argued that splenectomy is the safest means of eliminating those risks altogether. In patients with inconclusive pathology and unknown diagnoses, splenectomy can be diagnostic and therapeutic. It is also important to consider a patient's personal preference with regard to watchful waiting versus surgical resection, which can certainly be taken into consideration during joint decision-making conversations.

46.4.4 Littoral Cell Angioma

Littoral cell angioma is an exceedingly rare vascular splenic tumor that arises from abnormal overgrowth of the cells from the edge of the red pulp and affects patients of all ages and genders. This benign tumor is typically multifocal and has architecture that resembles vascularized anastomosing ducts with cystic infiltration. As the angioma grows, the spleen becomes enlarged with diffuse nodularity with resultant splenomegaly. Morphologically, littoral cell angiomas contain old blood products, which may lead to heterogeneous uptake on imaging studies. Despite this, there is no characteristic diagnostic imaging criteria for the identification of littoral cell angioma and percutaneous biopsy is frequently indicated in order to establish a diagnosis.

Littoral cell angiomas are unique in that they carry a risk of malignant growth and metastatic disease, which increases with lesion size. Given the theoretical risk of rupture, as well as the malignant potential, surgical referral and subsequent splenectomy are recommended when littoral cell angiomas enlarge to >5 cm or become symptomatic.

46.4.5 Angiosarcoma

Splenic angiosarcomas are aggressive, rapidly growing, and rare primary vascular lesions. Angiosarcomas are the result of malignant proliferation of the splenic sinusoidal epithelial cells. Affected patients are typically in their fourth or fifth decades of life with a slight female predominance. Presenting symptoms are often related to mass effect, including abdominal pain as well as constitutional symptoms such as fever, chills, fatigue, and weight loss. In part due to the vague initial symptomatology, as well as the aggressive biologic cellular behavior, splenic angiosarcomas are frequently advanced at the time of diagnosis. Metastases are common in the disease course, with 69–100% of patients developing metastatic deposits at some point, most frequently to the liver, followed by lungs, lymph nodes, and bone.

The gold standard treatment for splenic angiosarcoma is splenectomy; however, given the aggressive nature of the pathology, surgical resection is often inadequate alone. That being said, early resection is still advocated for as soon as a diagnosis is made, in part due to the increasing likelihood of rupture as the tumor grows. In fact, as many as 25% of splenic angiosarcomas are diagnosed after rupture requiring splenectomy. Angiosarcoma rupture has significant implications on overall mortality rate as well, with one study demonstrating survival time after splenectomy to be 4.4 months in patients undergoing splenectomy after rupture compared to 14.4 months in patients undergoing splenectomy on an elective basis.

46.4.6 Lymphoma

Not surprisingly, as the largest lymphoid organ of the body, the most commonly diagnosed splenic malignancy is lymphoma. However, splenic lymphoma is fairly uncommon as a manifestation of hematologic malignancies, comprising 1–2% of all cases of lymphoma. Patients may present with symptoms related to splenomegaly and mass effect on adjacent organs, as well as classic symptoms of lymphoma, including fever, chills, night sweats, weight loss, and lymphadenopathy. CT, PET, and MRI have all been studied for their utility in identifying splenic lymphoma, with PET and MRI demonstrating slightly improved accuracy. Diagnosis of primary splenic lymphoma is challenging because in many circumstances it requires tissue; however, the use of percutaneous needle biopsy is controversial given the risk of bleeding. In cases of diagnostic uncertainty, splenectomy can sometimes be performed, particularly when the level of suspicion is high.

Management of splenic lymphoma requires treatment of the underlying hematologic malignancy, which will hinge on medical oncologic input. Splenectomy is only recommended as a therapy for splenic lymphoma in cases of severely symptomatic splenomegaly or rupture. Laparoscopy has been found to have decreased postoperative pain, shorter length of stay, and similar outcomes; however, a larger extraction site is often necessary to ensure the specimen is removed intact.

46.4.7 Metastasis

There are relatively few solid tumors that metastasize to the spleen; however, it is important that these metastases are recognized early as resection can have a significant survival benefit. Melanoma, breast, lung, and ovarian cancers are the most frequent primary malignancies identified[12]. Splenic metastases can be difficult to diagnose, in part because of their rarity, but also because of their lack of distinguishable imaging findings. Radiologic reviews have noted differences in enhancement, degree of infiltration and size depending on the primary tumor and previous treatment modalities. As such, providers need a high degree of suspicion in patients with other known solid malignancies. Particularly in the case of solitary and large metastases, or those that are symptomatic, referral for splenectomy is advisable, both for oncologic benefit and to eliminate the morbidity of rupture. Not surprisingly, the management of splenic metastases varies greatly based on primary tumor, and consultation with medical and surgical oncologic teams is recommended.

46.5 Conclusion

Splenic lesions are being increasingly identified on routine imaging studies, and given the complexity of the organ, there is a large differential of pathologic diagnoses. Characterizing splenic lesions as solid or cystic can be helpful in narrowing the differential. When the diagnosis of a splenic lesion remains questionable, percutaneous biopsy can be considered, with the exception being patients with generalized splenomegaly or those with high pretest probability of splenic lymphoma. Although percutaneous biopsy was historically considered to be unsafe due to the risk of bleeding, contemporary literature has shown it to be safe and efficacious. In many instances, benign splenic lesions do not require intervention and can be watched over time, though the time interval for surveillance is highly provider dependent and may be unnecessary in patients with diagnostic certainty. In patients with symptoms related to mass effect, concern for malignancy or growth >5 cm that increases the risk of rupture, referral to surgical colleagues is warranted. Referral may often be elective; however, if there are clinical or radiographic findings that are concerning, such as rapid rate of growth, worsening abdominal pain, and suggestion of impending rupture on imaging, more urgent surgical referral is appropriate.

Acknowledgement The authors thank **Jennifer Brumbaugh, MA,** Medical Illustrator, at the Department of Surgery at Thomas Jefferson University, for her contribution in creating the illustrations for this chapter.

Suggested Readings

1. Malgras B, Najah H, Dohan A, et al. Diagnosis and treatment of focal splenic lesions. J Visc Surg. 2022;159(2):121–35.
2. Hansen MB, Moller AC. Splenic cysts. Surg Laparosc Endosc Perc Tech. 2004;14(6):316–22.
3. Corvino A, Granata V, Tafuri D, et al. Incidental focal splenic lesions: integrated imaging and pattern recognition approach to differential diagnosis. Diagnostics. 2023;13(15):2536.
4. Thut D, Smolinksi S, Morrow M, et al. A diagnostic approach to splenic lesions. Appl Radiol. 2017;46(2):7–22.

47 Adrenal Lesions

Justin D. Leavitt, Colston A. Edgerton, and William W. Hope

47.1 Anatomy and Physiology

The adrenal glands are paired organs located superior and anteromedial to the kidneys. They are triangle-shaped (right is pyramidal and left is crescent-shaped), about 5 cm long (side-to-side), and 3 cm tall. The outer cortex contains the zona glomerulosa, zona fasciculata, and zona reticularis, where mineralocorticoids, glucocorticoids, and androgens are synthesized, respectively. The medulla, which lies deep to the cortex, is composed of chromaffin cells that synthesize catecholamines. The terms adenomas and incidentalomas refer to adrenocortical adenomas, whereas pheochromocytoma refers to benign medullary tumors.

On noncontrast CT, the glands appear slightly less dense than other solid organs like the liver and spleen. The glands are supplied by several arteries and have extensive arterial networks. These characteristics are seen in CT imaging. The Hounsfield unit (HU) is the measurement of radiation attenuation that estimates tissue density. Most abdominal solid organs measure 20–50 HU,

J. D. Leavitt · C. A. Edgerton · W. W. Hope (✉)
New Hanover Regional Medical Center/Novant Health, Wilmington, NC, USA
e-mail: william.hope@novanthealth.org

G. P. Kohn et al. (eds.), *The SAGES Manual of Surgical Referral for Primary and Emergency Care*,
https://doi.org/10.1007/978-3-031-92678-5_47

water 0 HU, and fatty tissue are −50 to −100 HU. Iodinated contrast measures 100–500 HU depending on the concentration administered and timing of the image. These physical and imaging characteristics are frequently discussed in the evaluation of adrenal masses and are helpful to recall, with benign fatty-filled adenomas typically less than 10 HU, and more concerning lesions greater than 20 HU.

47.2 Indications for Surgery

The two primary reasons for adrenalectomy are hormone-producing (functional) tumors or concern for malignancy. All patients with incidentalomas should be assessed for primary hypercortisolism, hyperaldosteronism, and pheochromocytoma. Concern for malignancy is largely based on the size and imaging characteristics. Of all adrenalectomies, over 80% are performed for benign tumors.

47.3 Cortisol-Producing Tumors

Cortisol-producing tumors are the most common functional tumor and represent up to 10% of benign incidentalomas. All incidentalomas should be evaluated for excess cortisol production. Hypercortisolism may present overtly as Cushing syndrome or much more commonly as mild autonomous cortisol secretion (MACS—this term has replaced "subclinical Cushing syndrome"). Patients with MACS have an increased risk of, and should be assessed for, hypertension, diabetes, obesity, and osteopenia.

Initial laboratory evaluation should begin in the primary physician office, where such testing has become more commonplace due to the prevalence of adrenal incidentalomas (Table 47.1). If at any point a primary care physician is unsure of the next step or

Table 47.1 Testing prior to surgeon referral

Imaging	Noncontrast CT abdomen
Labs	Functional (hormone-producing) testing: **Hypercortisolism** *All patients* Dexamethasone suppression test (DST) Confirmatory test—high-dose DST or urine test (practices vary) ACTH (if DST positive) **Hyperaldosteronism** *Only if suspected due to unexplained hypokalemia and hypertension* Plasma renin/aldosterone ratio **Pheochromocytoma** *For any patients with imaging not consistent benign adenomas.* Plasma free metanephrines OR urinary fractionated metanephrines Any patients with positive or indeterminate lab findings should be referred to a surgeon, oncologist, or endocrinologist

test while pursuing a diagnosis, the patient should be referred to a surgeon or endocrinologist. Evaluation for hypercortisolism begins with a 1 mg overnight dexamethasone suppression test (DST). High-dose suppression tests are sometimes performed to confirm positive 1 mg DST results; however, the evidence for high-dose and urine tests is mixed and recommendations vary. Dehydroepiandrosterone sulfate (DHEAS) measurement is frequently recommended, and low values are sensitive and specific for MACS. An abnormal DST should be followed by ACTH. In the case of bilateral incidentalomas with evidence of MACS, adrenal vein sampling should be performed to localize the hormone-producing tumor. Adrenalectomy is recommended for unilateral cortisol-producing tumors with consideration of patient preferences and surgical risk factors. While individualizing care, be aware of the risks of increasing size over time and hormone exposure through the patient's anticipated lifespan.

47.4 Aldosterone-Producing Tumors

Patients with unexplained hypokalemia and hypertension should be evaluated for primary aldosteronism, but laboratory screening for this is not routinely performed upon discovery of adrenal incidentaloma. Evaluation includes plasma renin/aldosterone ratio, and abnormal findings should result in a surgical referral. Because primary aldosteronism can be caused by adenomas or hyperplasia (unilateral or bilateral), a consulting surgeon may recommend adrenal venous sampling to determine laterality.

Adrenalectomy is recommended in cases of aldosterone-secreting adenomas. If surgery is not appropriate (i.e., comorbid conditions, or bilateral hyperplasia), then patients should be treated with mineralocorticoid receptor antagonist therapy.

47.5 Pheochromocytoma

Unlike benign-appearing cortical adenomas (nonfunctional, cortisol, or aldosterone producing), pheochromocytomas of the medulla typically appear heterogeneous and more dense on CT. Imaging is discussed further below; however, any adrenal lesion without typical features of a benign adenoma should undergo evaluation with plasma-free metanephrines or urinary fractionated metanephrines. Elevated plasma-free metanephrines are very sensitive for pheochromocytoma. If false-positive or indeterminate results occur, the tests should be repeated after ensuring proper technique and body positioning.

The presence of symptoms should not be relied on before testing as many patients with pheochromocytoma do not have the prototypical phenotype, and some with the phenotype do not have pheochromocytoma. Pheochromocytoma has the highest heritability among adrenal lesions (approximately 40 percent are part of a familial disorder such as MEN syndrome) and genetic evaluation should be considered, especially in cases of bilateral pheochromocytoma.

Patients with pheochromocytoma should undergo adrenalectomy. In select cases, cortical-sparing adrenalectomy can be considered to preserve steroid production. Because physical manipulation of the gland during surgery can cause sudden and dangerous releases of catecholamines, patients should start a selective or nonselective alpha-blocker at least 7 days before surgery. Adequate alpha blockade is often determined clinically when a patient endorses orthostasis.

47.6 Sex Hormone-Producing Tumors

Benign adenomas do not typically produce androgens, and serum levels are not routinely measured. Sex hormones and their precursors should be evaluated for masses concerning for adrenocortical carcinoma, which tend to produce androgens rather than corticosteroids.

47.7 Malignancy and Imaging Characteristics

Diagnosis, workup, and surgical evaluation begin with and are heavily influenced by imaging. Benign adenomas are typically fatty and less dense than normal adrenal cortical tissue, and thus have lower HU measurement on noncontrast CT (<10 HU). Because iodinated contrast rapidly accumulates in the glands and thus will appear much brighter on CT, contrast-enhanced CT cannot be used to distinguish benign from malignant adrenal tumors. Noncontrast CT is the recommended first imaging modality for all incidentalomas (this includes lesions seen on contrast-enhanced CT).

Adenomas with density <10 HU, size <4 cm, that are smooth and regular-shaped (homogeneity) have a very low likelihood of malignancy. The most recent guidelines from the American Association of Endocrine Surgeons (2022) and European Society of Endocrinology (2023) recommend no further imaging or routine follow-up for nonfunctioning adenomas that meet the above criteria. Most benign adenomas do not increase in size, and evaluation should proceed to the assessment of hormone secretion outlined in the previous paragraphs.

Patients with high-risk characteristic findings should be referred to a surgeon if not done so already, and multidisciplinary care (MDC) is strongly encouraged. Further imaging, which need not be requested by the referring physician and can be ordered by the surgeon, may include FDG-PET/CT, chest CT ± contrast, and abdominal/pelvic CT or MRI with contrast, and should be performed to evaluate for regional and distant metastasis. Adrenalectomy is recommended for localized tumors with high-risk characteristics. While further imaging is not recommended for benign appearing nonfunctional adenomas, and surgery is recommended for high-risk-appearing tumors, care should be individualized for patients with indeterminate-risk tumors, such as benign-appearing tumors >4 cm, or tumors ≤4 cm but are 10–20 HU. If surgery is not performed after patient-centered discussions, interval imaging is typically recommended every 6–12 months with noncontrast CT or MRI. These intervals are guidance; however, there are no strict recommendations for these individualized cases and they should be coordinated by the consulting surgeon or MDC team. Development of high-risk characteristics should prompt re-evaluation.

Percutaneous biopsy is not routinely performed during the evaluation of benign or malignant-appearing adrenal lesions because it does not frequently provide additional information to guide management. In cases of adrenocortical carcinoma, specificity is over 95%; however, sensitivity is only 70%. The most common circumstance when biopsy is recommended is to determine whether an adrenal lesion is an extra-adrenal metastasis in cases where this information would impact decision-making.

47.8 Surgical Referral

Any adrenal tumor that is functional or has malignant characteristics should be referred to a surgeon with expertise in adrenal gland surgery and/or an endocrinologist for evaluation (Table 47.2). The surgeon will be able to continue the diagnostic evaluation and make surgical recommendations. Like any surgical evaluation, patient-centered decision-making will guide the discussion of

Table 47.2 Referral recommendations

Conditions requiring emergency department evaluation and treatment	Conditions requiring emergency surgical evaluation are very rare but may possibly include adrenal hemorrhage (very rare) or the results of mass effect from very large tumors.
Conditions requiring urgent surgical review	Any adrenal tumors associated with severe symptoms due to excess hormone secretion or mass effect.
Conditions requiring nonurgent surgical review	Any functional (hormone-producing) benign adenoma. Any tumor with high-risk imaging characteristics at risk of malignancy (>10 HU, >4 cm, heterogeneous appearing). Any tumor with indeterminant imaging or laboratory results.
Conditions appropriate for PCP management	Evaluation of low-risk benign adenomas (<10 HU, <4 cm, homogeneous appearing) that are not hormone-producing. CT surveillance of indeterminate-risk adenomas.

risks and benefits of surgery while accounting for the patient's health and goals.

For benign-appearing lesions, the minimally invasive (laparoscopic and robotic assisted) approach has increasingly become the recommended approach for adrenalectomy because of its associated shorter hospital stays and decreased surgical pain. The open surgical approach has traditionally been recommended for malignant appearing tumors; however, most contemporary guidelines state that the minimally invasive approach is appropriate within certain circumstances. For malignant-appearing tumors, the surgical approach should be determined on a case-by-case basis according to the tumor characteristics, patient's anatomy, patient's preferences, and whether negative margins (R0 resection) can be confidently achieved by the surgeon.

47.9 Summary

The adrenal incidentaloma and its subsequent diagnostic evaluation have become a very common occurrence for practitioners around the world. Most physicians have become knowledgeable about the initial evaluation and should become familiar with their local resources and when patients should be referred. Surgery represents the definitive treatment for any adrenal pathology. Whether this treatment is appropriate and will benefit the patient should be evaluated by a surgeon and a multidisciplinary team when possible. As such, referral to a surgeon to aid in diagnosis, provide surgical recommendations, and assist the patient in their decision-making should be considered at any point in the evaluation of functional tumors or adenomas with any concerning radiographic features.

Suggested Readings

1. Fassnacht M, Tsagarakis S, Terzolo M, et al. European Society of Endocrinology clinical practice guidelines on the management of adrenal incidentalomas, in collaboration with the European Network for the Study of Adrenal Tumors. Eur J Endocrinol. 2023;189(1):G1–G42. https://doi.org/10.1093/ejendo/lvad066.
2. Kebebew E. Adrenal incidentaloma. N Engl J Med. 2021;384(16):1542–51. https://doi.org/10.1056/NEJMcp2031112.
3. Lenders JW, Duh QY, Eisenhofer G, et al. Pheochromocytoma and paraganglioma: an endocrine society clinical practice guideline [published correction appears in J Clin Endocrinol Metab. 2023 Apr 13;108(5):e200]. J Clin Endocrinol Metab. 2014;99(6):1915–42. https://doi.org/10.1210/jc.2014-1498.
4. Yip L, Duh QY, Wachtel H, et al. American association of endocrine surgeons guidelines for adrenalectomy: executive summary. JAMA Surg. 2022;157(10):870–7. https://doi.org/10.1001/jamasurg.2022.3544.
5. Young WF Jr. Clinical practice. The incidentally discovered adrenal mass. N Engl J Med. 2007;356(6):601–10. https://doi.org/10.1056/NEJMcp065470.

Polyps on Colonoscopy 48

Emily Miraflor

48.1 Key Points

It is safe to endoscopically resect most complex polyps.

Polyps that harbor invasive cancer should be evaluated for the need for surgical resection.

48.2 Management of the Complex Polyp

Advances in endoscopic imaging and resection techniques in the last decade have shifted the management of large polyps away from traditional surgical resection for two reasons. First, there are advanced methods of visualizing the surface of a polyp using narrow band imaging or chromoendoscopy to better categorize a polyp as being likely benign or likely malignant. Secondly, endoscopic resection techniques have advanced such that polyps can be resected en bloc without traditional surgery using the technique of submucosal resection. As experience has grown with submucosal resection, studies have shown that most complex polyps can be

E. Miraflor (✉)
UCSF East Bay, San Francisco, CA, USA
e-mail: emiraflor@alamedahealthsystem.org

G. P. Kohn et al. (eds.), *The SAGES Manual of Surgical Referral for Primary and Emergency Care*,
https://doi.org/10.1007/978-3-031-92678-5_48

resected using this technique and any bleeding or inadvertent perforation that occurs can be safely managed with endoscopic clips. Thus, in the past when it may have been appropriate to refer a patient with a large polyp for surgical resection, now referral to an advanced endoscopist may be more appropriate. There are specific situations where surgical referral for management of polyps is appropriate and will be discussed further.

There are several different grading systems to assist in classifying polyps as complex or simple. The goal of each of these different classification schemas is to predict whether a polyp has the potential to be invasive. In other words, when assessing a polyp, a key step in the algorithm for treatment is to classify it as likely benign or likely malignant. A polyp that is likely malignant may prompt further consideration of cancer staging and surgical planning, whereas a polyp that is assuredly benign may be removed by endoscopic means.

Delineating each of the polyp classification systems is beyond the scope of this chapter; however, there are some common themes that predict both how amenable a polyp would be to endoscopic resection and how likely a polyp is to harbor a malignant focus.

The first thing to consider is polyp size. A polyp that is smaller than 20 mm is likely to be benign and is typically removed with endoscopic techniques practiced by most endoscopists. Polyps that are more than 20 mm in size are more likely to contain foci of invasive cancer (though some may still be completely benign) and for that reason should be removed by an endoscopist with advanced training in techniques that can assure complete removal of the lesion such as endoscopic mucosal resection (EMR) or endoscopic submucosal resection (ESR).

In addition to size, location needs to be considered as some polyps may not be completely reachable with endoscopy. The situations where surgical resection should be considered are polyps growing into or arising from the appendiceal orifice, polyps growing along the ileocecal valve or located behind a fold. Polyps in these locations may be considered for surgical resection rather than endoscopic resection regardless of size. Additionally, polyps that are in the distal rectum near the anal opening may be better approached with an open surgery or with a transanal minimally invasive surgery (TAMIS), which employs traditional laparoscopic instrumentation via a trans-anal access device. TAMIS procedures are typically performed by colorectal specialists rather than general surgeons.

Polyps that harbor malignant foci tend to have a particular appearance. Features that raise concern for malignancy include an irregular vascular pattern (determined with narrow band imaging or chromoendoscopy during the diagnostic colonoscopy) and a morphology with an appearance described to be excavated (Fig. 48.1). Additional concerning features include lesions that are ulcerated or have a fixed or tethered appearance on endoscopy. Polyps with these features despite small size can still be considered for surgical intervention rather than endoscopic resection. If endoscopic resection is performed, the region should be tattooed so that if a cancer is identified on pathology, surgical resection of the lymphatic-bearing tissue can be performed.

Interestingly, even if an endoscopically removed polyp is found to harbor a malignancy on final pathology, if appropriate cancer care is subsequently given, it has been shown that there is no adverse effect in terms of survival and recurrence. Thus, it is reasonable to attempt endoscopic resection in lieu of surgery without fear of negatively impacting the patient's oncologic outcome.

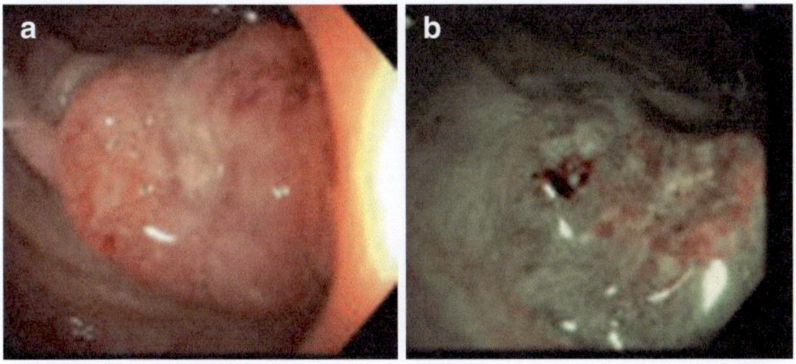

Fig. 48.1 Colon polyp showing excavated appearance on white light endoscopy (**a**) and heterogeneous vascularity with missing vessels on narrow band imaging (**b**). While the polyp is small, the excavated appearance and heterogeneous vascularity led to suspicion for cancer. Surgical resection confirmed invasive cancer with lymph node involvement

The finding of a cancer in a resected polyp does not necessarily mean the patient needs to go on to have a surgical resection. Polyps that have been completely removed endoscopically that are found to harbor cancer need to be evaluated for depth of invasion and factors that would predict lymph node involvement to determine the need for additional surgical resection. Histologic findings that predict lymph node spread and necessitate surgical resection for staging include undifferentiated or mucinous tumors, lymphovascular invasion, tumor budding, cancerous cells extending to the base of a pedunculated polyp, or submucosal invasion depth of greater than 1000 micrometers. If none of these findings are present, endoscopic resection is sufficient (Fig. 48.2).

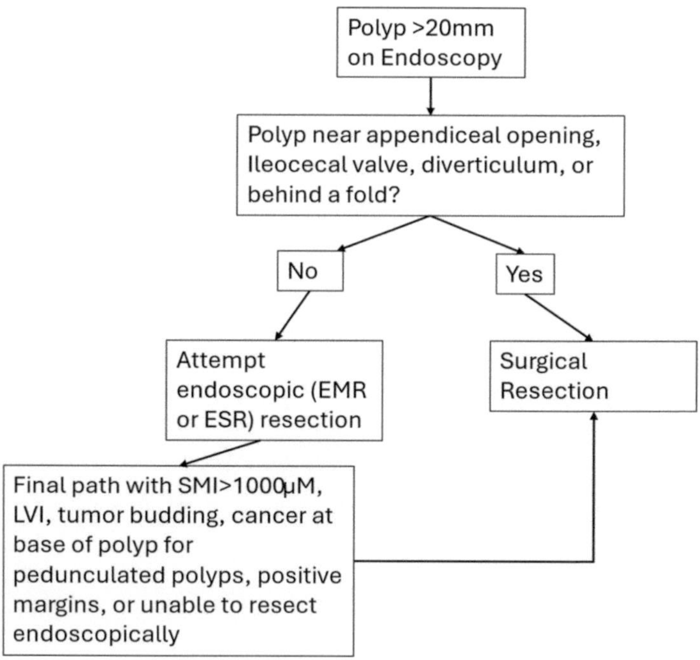

Fig. 48.2 Algorithm to determine the need for surgical resection when a complex polyp is found on endoscopy. *EMR* endoscopic mucosal resection, *ESR* endoscopic submucosal resection, *SMI* submucosal invasion, *LVI* lymphovascular invasion

48.3 Management of Simple Polyps

Surveillance protocols for patients found to have simple adenomatous polyps without villous components and are not otherwise at elevated risk for the development of colon cancer have been developed by the United States Multi Society-Task Force. These protocols assume that the patient has no personal or family history of colon cancer, and that they do not have inflammatory bowel disease. Patients with inflammatory bowel disease are typically surveyed on a schedule determined by their gastroenterologist. Surveillance colonoscopies are performed at varying intervals based on the number of polyps removed and the completeness of their resection as shown in Table 48.1.

Table 48.1 Surveillance interval recommendations based on initial colonoscopy findings

Initial colonoscopy finding	Recommended surveillance interval
1–2 tubular adenoma <10 mm	7–10 years
3–4 tubular adenoma <10 mm	3–5 years
5–10 tubular adenoma <10 mm	3 years
Adenoma >10 mm, or with villous histology or dysplasia	3 years
>10 adenomas	1 year
Piecemeal resection of a polyp >20 mm	6 months

48.4 Polyp Syndromes

Although rare, there are several polyp syndromes that may come to the attention of the primary care physician, including familial adenomatous polyposis (FAP), juvenile polyposis syndrome (JPS), and Peutz–Jeghers syndrome.

FAP is often thought of as a disease that comes to attention in adolescence; however, there are attenuated forms of FAP that may go undetected until adulthood. This type of attenuated FAP arises through a different genetic mutation than traditional FAP; however, the finding of hundreds of polyps is common to both. In the situation where hundreds of polyps are identified on colonoscopy, the patient should be referred to a colorectal surgeon or general surgeon familiar with complex gastrointestinal surgery. The surgical treatment options are a total abdominal colectomy with an ileorectal anastomosis if there are few polyps in the rectum or a total proctocolectomy with either a permanent end ileostomy or ileo pouch anal anastomosis (J-pouch). The indication for surgery is an inability to adequately survey the polyps and the high likelihood of cancerous transformation during the patient's lifetime. There is no need for a staging CT scan or CEA levels prior to surgical referral unless there is already strong suspicion that one of the polyps harbors cancer.

Juvenile polyposis syndrome, despite its name, is not a disease of juveniles but rather refers to the immature histology of the polyps seen on tissue biopsy. The disease features numerous polyps throughout the GI tract. Endoscopic resection is performed for symptomatic polyps or polyps more than 5 mm in size. Surgical referral is only necessary in the case of invasive cancer, intussusception, refractory anemia, or hypoproteinemia due to protein loss from a large number of polyps.

Peutz–Jeghers syndrome can result in polyps throughout the gastrointestinal tract, including the small and large bowel. The polyps can be large and result in bowel obstructions caused by intussusception with the polyp acting as a lead point. Surgical referral is necessary for large polyps or intussusception; otherwise, the polyps can be surveyed with endoscopy every 2–3 years.

Table 48.2 Pre-referral evaluation

Referral indication	Labs	Imaging
Polyp not amenable to endoscopic resection without concern for malignancy	CBC and chemistry	No specific imaging
Polyp concerning for malignancy	CBC, chemistry, CEA	CT of chest, abdomen, and pelvis
Polyposis syndrome without identified malignancy	CBC, chemistry	No specific imaging
Polyposis syndrome with concern for malignancy	CBC, chemistry, CEA	CT of the chest, abdomen, and pelvis

Once it has been determined that the patient will require referral to either an advanced endoscopist or a surgical specialist, it is prudent to consider additional laboratory or imaging studies that may be desired by the specialist. While individual specialists may have specific presurgical evaluations, commonly a complete blood count, electrolyte panel, and in older patients an electrocardiogram are needed prior to surgical interventions. When there is high suspicion for cancer, a carcinoembryonic antigen (CEA) level and a CT scan of the chest, abdomen, and pelvis to assess for metastatic disease are done (Table 48.2).

48.5 Summary Table

When should the patient seek emergency care?	Post-polypectomy bleeding or perforation	Signs and symptoms: Blood per rectum, severe abdominal pain, rapid heart rate.
	Obstruction from size of polyp or intussusception of polyp	Signs and symptoms: abdominal pain, inability to pass flatus or stool, vomiting, and abdominal distention.
When is urgent surgical review necessary?	Concern for malignant polyp	Signs of possible malignancy: Size >20 mm sessile or ulcerated polyps with heterogenous vascularity.

(continued)

When is nonurgent surgical review necessary?	Large polyps with benign appearance, polyposis syndromes	Examples: polyps in locations not amenable to advanced endoscopic techniques (Fig. 48.2) or patient with newly diagnosed polyposis syndromes such as FAP.
Which polyps can be managed by the PCP?	Adenomatous polyps	Examples: completely removed adenomatous polyps can be surveyed following the guidelines shown in Table 48.1. Complex polyps that do not require surgery may be referred for removal with advanced endoscopic techniques using the algorithm in Fig. 48.2.

Suggested Readings

1. Copland AP, et al. AGA clinical practice update on appropriate and tailored polypectomy: expert review. Clin Gastroenterol Hepatol. 2023;22(3):470–9.
2. Gupta S, et al. Recommendations for follow up after colonoscopy and polypectomy: a consensus update by the US multi-society task force on colorectal cancer. Am J Gastroenterol. 2023;115(3):415–34.
3. Kyriakidid F, et al. Updated perspectives on the diagnosis and management of familial adenomatous polyposis. Appl Clin Genet. 2023;16:139–53.
4. Matsumoto T. Clinical guidelines for diagnosis and management of Juvenile polyposis syndrome in children and adults. J Anus Rectum Colon. 2023;7(2):115–25.
5. Moreira P, et al. Endoscopic submucosal dissection, endoscopic mucosal resection, and transanal minimally invasive surgery for the management of rectal and anorectal lesions: a narrative review. J Clin Med. 2023;12(14):4777.
6. NCCN Guidelines Version 4.2023 Colon Cancer.
7. Yamamoto H, et al. Clinical guidelines for diagnosis and management of Peutz-Jeghers syndrome in children and adults. Digestion. 2023;104(5):335–47.

Part IV

Miscellaneous

49 Feeding Tube Placement

Neil Patel

49.1 Introduction

Enteral nutrition is commonly provisioned in both pediatric and adult populations. The use of home enteral nutrition has increased significantly in the United States over the previous 20 years. The indications for feeding tube placement are wide. Careful patient selection is important to achieve the desired therapeutic outcomes and avoid iatrogenic harm. Enteral access can be accomplished through a number of different techniques ranging from temporary nasoenteric (e.g., nasogastric, nasojejunal) tube placement, endoscopic or radiographic-guided percutaneous placement, and surgical placement. Many devices exist to facilitate short- and long-term enteral access. This chapter aims to review common indications for feeding tube access and provide general guidelines on the most appropriate referral pathway depending on the indication and patient situation.

N. Patel (✉)
Creighton University Medical Center, Omaha, NE, USA
e-mail: NeilPatel@creighton.edu

G. P. Kohn et al. (eds.), *The SAGES Manual of Surgical Referral for Primary and Emergency Care*,
https://doi.org/10.1007/978-3-031-92678-5_49

49.2 Indications

Percutaneous endoscopic gastrostomy (PEG) tubes are the most commonly placed type of durable enteral access. The most common indication for enteral tube placement is dysphagia, most commonly following stroke. Friginal-Ruiz and Lucendo provide a scheme to classify indications for PEG tube placement based on the acuity of the underlying disease and prognosis for recovery (Table 49.1). More broadly, patients appropriate for enteral access include those unable to meet their nutritional requirements through ordinary dietary intake who possess a functional GI tract. A list of common indications for enteral access is summarized in Table 49.1. For many conditions, permanent enteral access may not be required (e.g., head and neck cancer expected to regress following treatment). Whereas in other conditions, the need for access is expected to be permanent, for example, amyotrophic lateral sclerosis (ALS). Durable enteral access is generally not indicated in situations where the duration of treatment is anticipated to be less than 4–6 weeks. For potentially reversible conditions such as dysphagia following stroke, aggressive treatment should be undertaken, including evaluation by speech and language pathology to prevent avoidable feeding tube placement. Discharge disposition may also factor into the decision to place a transabdominal feeding tube. Many rehabilitation and long-term care facilities do not accept patients with nasoenteric tubes. Similarly, in pediatric patients, some neonatal units may not discharge patients who are geographically remote from care without durable enteral access. Thus, in a patient otherwise medically appropriate for transition of care, a transabdominal feeding tube may be indicated to facilitate discharge to the next level of care.

Altered gastric function such as gastroparesis or post-surgical/post-traumatic anatomic alteration (e.g., gastrectomy) may require creation of post-pyloric, that is, jejunal, durable enteral access. A multidisciplinary approach involving the treating clinicians and specialist services such as dieticians and speech and language pathologists is ideal to determine the need for enteral access.

Table 49.1 Common indications for enteral access

Neurologic diseases
Stroke
Motor neuron disease, e.g., amyotrophic lateral sclerosis (ALS), Guillain–Barré syndrome
Muscular dystrophies
Congenital myopathies
Cerebral palsy
Parkinson disease
Traumatic brain injury
Dementia
Anorexia nervosa
Anatomic obstructive disease
Head and neck cancer
Esophageal cancer
Esophageal stricture
Gastric outlet obstruction
Malignant bowel obstruction (venting gastrostomy)
GI tract alteration due to trauma or other surgery
Catabolic conditions
Critical illness, e.g., severe burns, pancreatitis
Cystic fibrosis
Short gut syndrome
Inflammatory bowel disease
Pediatric indications
Premature infant with oral aversion
Congenital malformations resulting in dysphagia
Catabolic surgical or medical disease
Special dietary needs or metabolic diseases
Short gut syndrome
Maintenance of nutrition during chemotherapy

49.3 Contraindications and Specific Considerations

49.3.1 Dementia

The decision to place a feeding tube must be individualized. Patients with dementia may develop oral aversion and malnutrition as their disease severity progresses. Unfortunately, feeding tube placement does not confer any survival benefit and generally does not reverse malnutrition. Feeding tube placement in patients with advanced dementia is not recommended.

49.3.2 Life Expectancy

Enteral access is not recommended when the patient's life expectancy is estimated to be less than 30 days. Venting gastrostomy tube placement may be considered for palliation in situations where life expectancy is less than 30 days.

49.3.3 Contraindications

Contraindications for feeding tube placement are generally related to the specific technique chosen for enteral access. Ascites, uncorrectable coagulopathy, and inability to endoscopically access the gastric lumen are all contraindications to PEG tube placement. Ascites and uncorrectable coagulopathy may also preclude radiographic enteral access. Surgically placed feeding tubes generally require general anesthesia; therefore, inability to tolerate anesthesia presents an additional contraindication. Absence of a full-thickness abdominal wall at the planned access site is a common contraindication regardless of technique chosen. Cirrhosis and portal hypertension may be considered relative contraindications for enteral access but should be evaluated on an individual basis.

49.4 Referral

Once an appropriate indication has been identified, referral for enteral access is appropriate. The majority of indications for enteral access can be satisfied by a percutaneous endoscopic gastrostomy (PEG) tube placement, which is the most commonly placed type of durable enteral access. This procedure can be performed by appropriately trained gastroenterologists or surgeons. The specific choice of referral is dependent on local expertise and referral patterns.

There are several situations that may preclude PEG tube placement in which referral to a surgeon or interventional radiologist may be appropriate. Inability to endoscopically access the gastric lumen due to stricture or obstruction precludes safe PEG tube placement and referral for surgical feeding tube placement is advisable. Altered gastrointestinal anatomy is another relative indication for surgical referral. Patients who have undergone bariatric surgery and Roux-en-Y gastric bypass may benefit from surgical referral as the remnant stomach is the preferred gastrostomy site and is typically not endoscopically accessible with a single-stage endoscopic procedure. Laparoscopic gastrostomy tube placement as opposed to endoscopic placement is common in pediatric patients to facilitate placement of a low-profile "button" device with detachable tubing at the onset. This is more commonly performed by a pediatric surgeon.

When feeding distal to the stomach is indicated such as in the case of gastroparesis or pyloric obstruction, then referral for surgical jejunostomy tube placement may be appropriate. An alternative is placement of a gastrojejunostomy tube where the tube enters the stomach through the overlying skin but has an internal extension that is directed from the stomach through the pylorus to feed directly into the jejunum. These can be placed by gastroenterologists, surgeons, or radiologists depending on local norms. In the case of esophageal cancer where esophagectomy and gastric pull-up is being considered, a gastrostomy tube does not seem to be inferior to jejunostomy in terms of oncologic outcomes. There is a small risk of tumor seeding in the setting of head and neck cancer when an endoscopic technique is utilized; therefore, a radiographic or surgical technique may be preferred in this scenario. Radiographically guided feeding tube placement may be considered in situations where endoscopic placement is contraindicated or has failed or for situations where a patient is not able to tolerate general anesthetic for surgical feeding tube placement.

Preoperative information that may be helpful to obtain prior to referral includes clinical tolerance of tube feedings and imaging in some instances (Table 49.2). In patients in whom gastric tube feedings have not been tolerated, preoperative imaging such as an upper GI series may be helpful and identify a need for a more distally placed feeding tube. Similarly, in a patient with suspected congenitally or surgically altered anatomy, upper GI, or cross-sectional imaging such as a CT with enteric contrast may be helpful for planning purposes. However, in general, for a patient who is clinically tolerating tube feeding by a nasogastric route no routine preoperative imaging is necessary.

Table 49.2 Preoperative management and workup

Study or test	Recommendation
Clinical information	Tolerance of gastric feedings should generally be established clinically prior to placement of a transabdominal feeding tube. A trial of post-pyloric feeding may be helpful prior to jejunostomy placement in patients who do not tolerate gastric feeds. Surgical history is also pertinent to establish which technique of feeding tube placement is most likely to succeed.
Coagulation studies	For most patients without a history of clotting disorder these studies can be omitted. Local protocol may require pre-op coagulation studies for surgically placed feeding tubes.
Upper GI series	Consider for patients with a history of intolerance to gastric tube feeds or surgically altered anatomy.
CT abdomen	Generally not needed but may be performed at the request of proceduralist to assess for anatomy when there is a history of congenital abnormality or prior surgery. May be helpful for the proceduralist to assess the feasibility of feeding tube placement and likelihood of success.

49.5 Postplacement Management and Follow-Up

Establishing a plan of care prior to placement is helpful to optimize the utility of a feeding tube. The timing of tube feed initiation is typically determined by the proceduralist and may depend on the method of feeding tube placement. In general, after uncomplicated placement, a PEG tube may be used immediately following placement, but there is likely significant practitioner variation in this regard. The tube feeding formulation should be determined by the treating practitioner. Consultation with a dietician or nutritional specialist may be beneficial for patients with specific nutritional needs such as altered absorption requiring elemental tube feed formulations.

When tube feeding placement is performed, it is important to work with local resources such as social workers and case managers to ensure that the necessary tube feeding equipment, home healthcare resources, teaching, and tube feeds are available for patients at discharge. Ideally these arrangements are made prior to tube placement and include determination of the caregivers to manage feeding regimens, supplies, and tube replacements in the future. Guidance should be provided to monitor for tolerance of tube feeds, and patients should be educated on indications to return to the clinic or Emergency Department (Table 49.3). For most endoscopically placed or radiographically guided feeding tube placements, routine follow-up with the proceduralist is not necessary. The need for follow-up for surgically placed feeding tube should be addressed with the surgeon.

There is no standard timing for exchange or replacement of a feeding tube. Feeding tubes may be left in place until there is a specific indication for exchange or replacement if the tube remains functional. Some patients may benefit from replacement of a PEG tube with a long external component with a low-profile tube. This can generally be performed in the clinic setting after 4–6 weeks to allow for maturation of the gastrostomy tract. Referral to the placing practitioner is appropriate depending on the comfort and experience of the managing provider. Other indications for

Table 49.3 Postprocedure management

Referral to the Emergency Department
Dislodgement of the gastrostomy tube less than 2–4 weeks after placement.
Nausea/vomiting and obstructive symptoms particularly in the early postplacement period or when the feeding tube is a jejunostomy.
Bleeding from the stoma not controlled with pressure or blood in the tube suggestive of an intraluminal source.
Urgent surgical review
Dislodgement of the gastrostomy tube more than 4 weeks after placement. When surgical consultation is not available within 8 h, consider referral to the Emergency Department for replacement.
Minor bleeding from the peristomal site.
Nonurgent surgical review
Failure of the fistula tract to close more than 72 h after gastrostomy tube removal.
Endoscopic or surgical removal of a feeding tube.
Persistent peristomal leakage or skin irritation.
Replacement of a deteriorating or clogged tube if no experienced nonsurgical practitioner available.

replacement of the feeding tube include tube deterioration, which may be evident from discoloration of the tube, loss of pliability, and malodor. The objective is to maintain a functional tube and avoid interruptions in enteral access.

Dislodgement of the tube can be an indication for urgent referral to the Emergency Department. PEG tubes are held in position by an internal bumper or balloon and an external bolster that apposes the stomach against the abdominal wall. The gastrostomy tract is typically mature by 4 weeks at which point the stomach will remain apposed to the abdominal wall while the tube serves to maintain the patency of the tract. Inadvertent dislodgement of the PEG tube prior to maturation of the tract can result in peritonitis from a free gastric perforation; therefore, referral to the emergency care setting is appropriate. Attempts at replacement of a dislodged tube in this setting are recommended only in consultation with the appropriate proceduralist. Surgically placed and some radiographically guided feeding tube placements are done with gastropexy of the stomach that reduces the risk of peritonitis and leak in the event of early tube dislodgement. Consultation with the proceduralist is recommended when there is any doubt.

After 4 weeks, replacement of the tube can be safely attempted in the clinic setting. The tract will generally begin to close within 8 h of tube dislodgement and will completely close within 24–72 h. To avoid the need to place a new feeding tube, attempts should be made to replace the tube as soon as possible after dislodgement. The practitioner replacing the tube should be comfortable confirming placement by either aspiration of gastric contents or with a radiographic study utilizing contrast through the feeding tube. Unrecognized creation of a false passage can necessitate the need for additional procedures.

Routine postplacement management of a feeding tube requires attention to wound healing in the early postoperative feeding and monitoring for complications throughout the duration of placement. Excess granulation tissue can also form at the stoma site. This is typically benign and can be managed with local application of silver nitrate and/or topical treatments in the ambulatory setting. Late development of granulation tissue can occur after either trauma to the site or in response to a tube becoming too tight. Children with gastrostomy tubes commonly require longer low-profile tubes with weight gain and increased thickness of the abdominal wall to prevent granulation tissue formation.

Peristomal leakage of gastric contents can occur early or late after feeding tube placement. Early leakage will generally resolve after maturation of the tract. Attention should be directed to ensuring the external bolster does not result in excessive compression of the abdominal wall. The feeding tube should spin freely and be able to slide in and out a short distance. Excessive tension on the tube or an overly tight bolster can cause erosion at the gastrostomy site resulting in troublesome leakage. Local wound care to protect the surrounding skin is crucial, and consultation with a wound care specialist should be considered. Additionally, referral to the placing proceduralist is recommended for persistent leakage or skin breakdown. Cellulitis and fungal infections are additional complications to monitor for. Localized infections can be managed with oral antibiotics while ensuring satisfactory position of the tube.

A clogged feeding tube is a common complication. Patients and caregivers should be provided liquid drug formulations whenever possible. Pills should be crushed into fine powders and feeding tubes should be flushed with 15–30 mL of water after each use to ensure continued patency. Initial attempts at relieving a blocked feeding tube can be performed prior to referral to the proceduralist. Flushing a tube with warm water is the recommended first step and can be attempted by the patient or caregiver. A solution of pancreatic enzymes and bicarbonate may be used to attempt to dissolve the obstruction. A cytology brush may be used to attempt to mechanically clear an obstruction, failing simpler techniques. Should these maneuvers fail, replacement of the tube can be performed in the ambulatory setting by an appropriately trained practitioner.

Clinically significant bleeding is an uncommon complication but can be observed after feeding tube placement. Minor bleeding typically occurs around the stoma site itself and can be the result of irritation of the local tissue. This bleeding can be managed with direct pressure. Bleeding that does not stop or bleeding that appears to be coming through the tube from the gastric lumen should prompt referral to the Emergency Department for further evaluation and management.

Gastrostomy tubes rarely result in intestinal obstruction due to the volume of the gastric lumen. The much smaller diameter of the proximal bowel can result in intestinal obstruction by the balloon or bumper of a jejunostomy tube. In a patient with obstructive symptoms, checking the balloon for overinflation is prudent. To avoid this complication, many surgically placed jejunostomy tubes do not utilize a balloon; therefore, consultation with a surgeon is appropriate when in doubt.

Once a feeding tube is no longer necessary, removal can typically be performed in the ambulatory setting. Many PEG tubes are designed to be removed by a traction method and can be removed by constant steady pulling on the tube until it dislodges. Not all feeding tubes are designed to be removed using a traction method; therefore, it is important to identify the type of tube prior to attempts at removal. Some PEG tubes require endoscopic removal. Feeding tubes with inflatable balloons can typically be removed in a similar fashion as PEG tubes after deflation of the balloon. A dressing should be applied to control any gastric effluent. The fistula tract will begin to close within 8 h, and most are completely closed within 24–72 h. Failure of the tract to close after 72 h with significant leakage should prompt surgical referral for further evaluation.

49.6 Conclusions

There is a wide array of indications to establish durable enteral access. Careful patient selection is critical to achieving the desired outcomes. Gastric feeding by PEG tube is generally the first-choice option, and referral to a gastroenterologist or surgeon is appropriate depending on local practice patterns and resources. Situations precluding PEG tube placement or the need for feeding distal to the stomach where a gastrojejunostomy tube is not feasible should be considered for surgical referral.

Suggested Reading

1. Arvanitakis M, Gkolfakis P, Despott EJ, et al. Endoscopic management of enteral tubes in adult patients – Part 1: definitions and indications. European Society of Gastrointestinal Endoscopy (ESGE) guideline. Endoscopy. 2021;53:81–92. https://doi.org/10.1055/a-1303-7449.
2. Bischoff SC, Austin P, Boeykens K, et al. ESPEN guideline on home enteral nutrition. Clin Nutr. 2020;39:5–22. https://doi.org/10.1016/j.clnu.2019.04.022.
3. Friginal-Ruiz AB, Lucendo AJ. Percutaneous endoscopic gastrostomy: a practical overview on its indications, placement conditions, management, and nursing care. Gastroenterol Nurs. 2015;38:354–66. https://doi.org/10.1097/SGA.0000000000000150.
4. Kwon RS, Banerjee S, Desilets D, et al. Enteral nutrition access devices. Gastrointest Endosc. 2010;72:236–48. https://doi.org/10.1016/j.gie.2010.02.008.
5. Ley D, Austin K, Wilson KA, Saha S. Tutorial on adult enteral tube feeding: indications, placement, removal, complications, and ethics. J Parenter Enteral Nutr. 2023;47:677–85. https://doi.org/10.1002/jpen.2510.

50 Vascular Access Considerations

Travis Hughes

50.1 Introduction

Arterial and venous vascular access are critical for modern medical care. Access sites provide the ability to both remove blood for study, filtration, or oxygenation and for infusion of a wide range of medications and treatments. The purpose for which the line will be used often determines if it will be peripheral or central and arterial or venous. While a variety of practitioners can provide vascular access, surgeons are among those commonly consulted for the placement of devices. Since the timeframe in which access is needed often guides referral patterns (Table 50.1), it is uncommon for extensive pre-referral studies to be performed. However, when feasible, a duplex ultrasound of the vessels to be targeted for line placement can be of assistance (Table 50.2) . In this chapter, we will discuss the different types of vascular access, their indications, and complications that may arise.

T. Hughes (✉)
University of Kentucky, Lexington, KY, USA
e-mail: travis.hughes@uky.edu

G. P. Kohn et al. (eds.), *The SAGES Manual of Surgical Referral for Primary and Emergency Care*,
https://doi.org/10.1007/978-3-031-92678-5_50

Table 50.1 When to refer to a surgeon

Emergent, refer to the emergency room	Suppurative thrombophlebitis with abscess formation or with soft tissue necrosis Infection of tunneled catheter or subcutaneous port Pneumothorax Phlegmasia cerulea dolens Ischemia (from atheroembolism, dissection, or thrombosis)
Urgent	Arteriovenous fistula Pseudoaneursym
Nonurgent	Superficial venous thrombosis >5 cm length or <3 cm from deep vein
Referral not required	Uncomplicated thrombophlebitis

Table 50.2 Investigations to order so as to be available for surgeon's review

No investigations required before emergent referral to the emergency room
Duplex ultrasound before urgent referral if this will not delay the process of referral
Ultrasound before nonurgent referrals

50.2 Peripheral Venous Access

The least invasive and most common vascular access is the butterfly needle, which range from 18 to 27 gauge; however, most needles used are 21–23 gauge. These are frequently used for blood draws in both the inpatient and outpatient settings. There is no catheter associated with the needle, and they cannot be used for intravenous infusion.

The most common peripheral venous access for infusion is the peripheral intravenous catheter. The placement of these catheters involves intraluminal placement of a needle and then advancement of a catheter over the needle. Long term these patients may require midlines, peripherally inserted central lines, or central lines for better intravenous access.

Care should be taken not to access near hemodialysis fistula, areas of previous injury, or previous operative fields; additionally, there will be patients who have contraindications to peripheral access in an extremity. When placing ultrasound-guided peripheral venous catheters, the most common sites for successful cannulation are the basilic and cephalic veins; occasionally, the deep brachial veins are suitable for cannulation; however, accidental arterial cannulation, nerve injury, and brachial sheath hematoma are possible complications.

50.3 Complications of Peripheral Venous Access

The primary complications of peripheral venous access are pain, bleeding, bruising, superficial venous thrombosis, and thrombophlebitis. Pain and bruising should be treated with non-opiate pain medications, and nearly all peripheral venous bleeding resolves with manual pressure. Superficial thrombophlebitis is inflammation or infection of the superficial vein. This frequently presents with pain, erythema along the vein, and a palpable cord. Thrombophlebitis may or may not be associated with a superficial venous thrombosis. Superficial thrombophlebitis is uncomplicated if there are no signs of infection, whereas suppurative thrombophlebitis is inflammation of the superficial vein with infection. Uncomplicated thrombophlebitis should be treated with warm compress, nonsteroidal anti-inflammatory drugs, and elevation. Suppurative thrombophlebitis should be treated with systemic antibiotics, drainage of associated abscess, and debridement of necrotic tissue. The mainstay of catheter-associated superficial venous thrombosis of the upper extremity is warm compression, elevation, and nonsteroidal anti-inflammatory drugs. There is compelling data to support anticoagulation for spontaneous superficial venous thrombosis of the lower extremity that is within 3 cm of the deep venous system or greater than 5 cm of thrombosis. There is no similar data to support anticoagulation of catheter-associated upper extremity superficial venous thrombosis; however, it is reasonable to consider in particular if the patient does not improve with standard therapy.

50.4 Intraosseous Access

Intraosseous access is a reasonable access when emergent intravascular access is required; however, no peripheral vein is available, and central venous access cannot be readily obtained. This is an excellent bailout access for first responders; however, it is periodically the optimal initial access in the emergent setting. This access is most frequently used in the pediatric population; however, it may be used in adults. The intraosseous needle may be placed into the proximal or distal tibial, proximal humerus, anterior superior iliac crest, or sternum. Intraosseous access can be used for fluid infusions, and infusion of medications including medications required for cardiopulmonary resuscitation. Contraindications to placement include fracture or previous orthopedic procedure to target bone, local infection, and nearby vascular injury. The intraosseous access should be removed as soon as alternative access is obtained, and ideally within 24 h of placement. Complications of intraosseous access include cellulitis, abscess, osteomyelitis, fracture, and compartment syndrome secondary to extravasation.

50.5 Peripheral Arterial Access

The least invasive peripheral arterial access is an arterial stick performed for an arterial blood gas measurement. Most frequently this is drawn from the radial artery. After the needle is removed, it is important to hold at least 5 min of pressure on the artery to avoid the formation of a pseudoaneurysm.

Peripheral arterial access may be required for hemodynamic monitoring, assess volume status, titrate vasoactive medications, frequent arterial blood gases, or intra-arterial intervention. Most commonly these are placed in the radial artery; however, it is recommended that an Allen's test should be performed on all patients prior to radial arterial cannulation. To perform an Allen's test, both the radial and ulnar arteries should be compressed, and the patient is instructed to clench their fist repeatedly until the hand blanches. The ulnar artery is released, and the hand should return to its previous color. If the patient is unable to follow commands, then pressure can be held until the hand blanches, or a transcutaneous pulse oximeter can be placed on the index finger. Once the pulse oximeter decreases below 90% and the waveform becomes dampened, the ulnar artery can be released; if the waveform returns to normal and the oxygen saturation returns to baseline, then this is sufficient.

50.6 Complications of Peripheral Arterial Access

Arterial access complications require rapid identification as many require intervention. The general categories of arterial access complication are arterial injury, arteriovenous fistula creation, and ischemia. Arterial injury most commonly presents as pseudoaneurysm, arteriovenous fistula, or dissection.

Pseudoaneurysm most frequently presents as an expanding pulsatile mass at the site of arterial access and may be associated with bleeding and distal neurologic deficit. A pseudoaneurysm is an injury to the arterial wall in which blood enters the surrounding tissue with persistent communication with the injured artery. Rapid expansions, hemorrhage, distal ischemia, and distal neurologic deficit are indications for urgent vascular surgical consultation; however, stable pseudoaneurysm and asymptomatic pseudoaneurysm are not a surgical emergency.

Arteriovenous fistula creation rarely requires emergent intervention; however, it should prompt vascular surgical evaluation. Indications for emergent intervention are ischemia and high-output cardiac failure. If a patient develops ischemia after placement, attempted placement, or removal of peripheral arterial access, the patient should undergo a thorough neurovascular evaluation of the limb, ultrasound or angiography to identify the location of the ischemia, and urgent vascular surgical evaluation. Patients with ischemia of an extremity after arterial access should be placed on a heparin drip unless there is strong contraindication such as gastrointestinal or intracranial hemorrhage. If there is a postprocedural concern or complication after peripheral arterial access for intervention, it is important to perform a neurovascular exam of the affected extremity. Additionally, it is important to determine the procedure performed, the largest sheath size placed, and the closure device used.

50.7 Central Venous Access

Central venous access can be achieved by direct access of a central vein or by placing a peripherally inserted central catheter (PICC). The catheter used will be dependent on the length of time the catheter is to be used and what the catheter will be used for. PICCs can be used for short- to mid-term infusions. They are ideal for IV antibiotic infusions; however, they would not have the infusion rate for large volume infusions and would not have the long-term patency and reliability required for chemotherapy. There are no specific medications that cannot be placed in a PICC line; however, it is important to review medication compatibility when infusing multiple drugs through the line.

Short-term central venous access can be obtained via internal jugular, subclavian, and femoral veins. Long-term central venous access is most commonly placed via the internal jugular or subclavian veins using a tunneled catheter or port. These lines are placed by interventional radiologists, interventional radiologists, and surgeons. Tunneled catheters have a polymer cuff that creates a barrier along the catheter track to prevent infections from skin flora. The specific indications for long-term central venous access are myriad; however, the general indications are long-term infusions, poor peripheral venous access with chronic disease, and hemodialysis. Central to the care of these catheters is meticulous sterile technique during access and cleanliness of the catheter and access site between use.

50.8 Complications of Central Venous Access

Central venous complications can arise from the placement or result from long-term catheter use.

Placement complications include misplacement into the nearby artery or pneumothorax. In the age of ultrasound-guided placement of central venous catheters, there has been a reduction in misplacement; however, this still occurs. The catheter may enter the artery directly or enter the artery through the intended venous structure. Internal jugular vein catheters may be misplaced into the common carotid artery, subclavian vein catheters may be misplaced into the subclavian artery, and femoral venous catheters may be misplaced into the superficial femoral, common femoral, or external iliac arteries. The primary concern for arterial placement is thrombus formation and distal embolization. Distal embolization carries the greatest risk for misplaced internal jugular vein catheter, which can cause stroke; however, misplaced subclavian vein catheters into the subclavian artery can cause stroke due to thrombus formation with embolization and from disrupting plaque in the aortic arch causing atheroembolization. Additionally, misplaced subclavian vein catheters can cause upper extremity ischemic complications. Misplaced femoral vein catheters carry a risk for lower extremity ischemic complications. All catheters placed through the target vein into a nearby artery risk the formation of arteriovenous fistula. Once a catheter is recognized as arterial, the catheter should be removed by a vascular surgeon as expeditiously as possible. The role of anticoagulation once catheter misplacement is recognized is unclear; however, this is generally recommended. Repair of the arteriotomy may be performed through an incision, covered with a percutaneous stent, or closed with a percutaneous closure device. Of note, catheters of the upper extremity may be misplaced through the posterior wall of the target artery and into the mediastinum; this is frequently recognized by the inability to aspirate from the ports or on postprocedure X-ray. These catheters should be removed and pressure held on the venotomy; no medications should be infused through these catheters.

Another procedural complication with central venous catheter placement with internal jugular or subclavian vein is pneumothorax. This typically occurs when the access needle is placed too far, violates the pleura causing, and causes an injury to the lung. Postprocedural chest X-ray typically identifies these pneumothoraces. Most pneumothoraces after central line placement are small and resolve spontaneously; however, all should be monitored with serial chest X-ray until resolution. Patients who have symptomatic or enlarging pneumothoraces should undergo small-bore thoracostomy tube placement. The thoracostomy tube should be placed to suction for the first 24 h; initial chest X-ray after thoracostomy tube placement should show resolution of pneumothorax. If the pneumothorax is no longer visible on chest X-ray at 24 h, then the chest tube should be placed to water seal. If serial chest X-ray while water sealed shows no re-accumulation of the pneumothorax, then the thoracostomy tube may be removed.

Long-term complications of central venous catheter include deep venous thrombosis, central venous stenosis, and infection. Deep venous thrombosis associated with a central venous catheter should be treated with anticoagulation. The catheter should be removed if it is not necessary for the care of the patient or nonfunctional. Thrombosed catheters may be salvaged by allowing tissue plasminogen activator or urokinase to dwell in the lumen of the central line. Central venous catheter infections are a dangerous result of long-term catheter use and carry an approximately 10% mortality. Central venous catheter infections include redness or drainage from the insertion site, bacteremia, and systemic infectious symptoms. It is important to establish if the patient has implants that could be infected as this will factor into the treatment course of IV antibiotics. While there is literature describing catheter salvage in low-risk patients, the author's recommendation is to remove infected central catheters as soon as possible and establish alternative intravenous access for IV antibiotic delivery. Bacteremia should be cleared for at least 48 h prior to replacement. Bacteremia should be treated with IV antibiotics for 7–14 days depending on patient risk factors and bacteria species. Central venous stenosis occurs caused by fibrotic changes of the vein in response to long-term central venous catheter placement.

This can result in facial and upper extremity swelling, and typically does not require intervention unless the patient develops respiratory symptoms. Central venous stenosis can also decrease future hemodialysis options in patients requiring long-term hemodialysis.

50.9 Venous Complications

Complication	Treatment	Surgical/procedural intervention
Uncomplicated thrombophlebitis or superficial vein thrombosis	Warm compression, elevation, NSAIDS Therapeutic AC if <3 cm from deep vein or ≥ 5 cm of thrombosis	No surgical intervention
Suppurative thrombophlebitis	Systemic antibiotics + treatment for uncomplicated thrombophlebitis	Drainage—abscess Excision—soft tissue necrosis
Catheter infection	Blood cultures, catheter removal, IV antibiotics	Tunneled lines and ports require removal with local anesthetic
Pneumothorax	Serial chest X-ray and monitoring	Thoracostomy tube placement if enlarging or symptomatic
Misplacement (arterial)	Heparin drip and vascular surgery consult	Surgical removal of line and repair of artery
Deep venous thrombosis	Anticoagulation (minimum of 3 months), removal of unnecessary or nonfunctional catheters	Vascular surgical consult for phlegmasia (rare)

50.10 Arterial Complications

Complication	Treatment	Surgical/ procedural intervention
Pseudoaneurysm	Thrombin injection, stent placement, or open repair	Vascular surgical consult
Arteriovenous fistula	Stent placement or open repair	Vascular surgical consult
Ischemia (atheroembolism, dissection, thrombosis)	Heparin drip, treatment varies depending on degree, site of stenosis or occlusion, and patient status	Vascular surgical consult

Reference

1. Rosenberg H, Cheung WJ. Intraosseous access. Canad Med Assoc J. 2013;185(5):E238.

Dialysis Access

51

Tanvi Subramanian
and Stephen P. Haggerty

Abbreviations

CKD	Chronic kidney disease
ESRD	End-stage kidney disease
RRT	renal replacement therapy
HD	hemodialysis
PD	peritoneal dialysis
GFR	glomerular filtration rate
KDOQI	Kidney Disease Outcomes Quality Initiative
KDIGO	Kidney Disease Improving Global Outcomes
AER	albumin excretion rate
ACR	albumin creatinine ratio
AVF	arteriovenous fistula
CMS	Centers for Medicare and Medicaid Services
AVG	arteriovenous graft

T. Subramanian
Department of Surgery, University of Chicago, Chicago, IL, USA
e-mail: tanvi.subramanian@uchicagomedicine.org

S. P. Haggerty (✉)
Department of Surgery, Division of Gastrointestinal and General Surgery, Endeavor Health, Evanston, IL, USA
e-mail: shaggerty@northshore.org

G. P. Kohn et al. (eds.), *The SAGES Manual of Surgical Referral for Primary and Emergency Care*,
https://doi.org/10.1007/978-3-031-92678-5_51

BL	basic laparoscopic
AL	advanced laparoscopic
ISPD	International Society for Peritoneal Dialysis
SAGES	Society of American Gastrointestinal and Endoscopic Surgeons

51.1 Introduction

Chronic kidney disease (CKD) is a common health problem in the United States, affecting more than 37 million people. In 2002, clinical practice guidelines were developed by the Kidney Disease Outcomes Quality Initiative (KDOQI) from the National Kidney Foundation, and this group defined CKD as abnormalities of kidney structure or function present for >3 months with implications for health. Specific abnormalities included albuminuria, urine sediment abnormalities, electrolyte/other abnormalities due to tubular dysfunction, abnormalities detected by histology on biopsy, structural abnormalities identified by imaging, and abnormal glomerular filtration rate (GFR) (<60 ml/min per 1.73 m^2). They also proposed a system to stage CKD based on GFR (Fig. 51.1). The Kidney Disease Improving Global Outcomes (KDIGO) group published guidelines in 2012 and added that the severity of CKD should be staged by GFR and degree of albuminuria, and separated stage 3 into two levels, a and b (Fig. 51.1). Category G1 indicates normal renal function of GFR >90, G2 indicates mild renal disease (GFR between 60 and 89), G3a indicates mildly to moderately decreased renal function (GFR 45–59), G3b signifies moderately to severely decreased renal function (GFR 30–44), G4 indicates severely decreased renal function (GFR 15–29), and G5 signifies kidney failure or end-stage renal disease (ESRD) with GFR <15. Three albuminuria categories are used for prognostication based on albumin–creatinine ratio (ACR, mg/d) and albumin excretion rate (AER, mg/g). Normal to mildly increased albuminuria, A1, is indicated by ACR and AER <30, while A2 is given to patients with ACR and AER between 30 and 300, indicating moderate albuminuria. Finally, patients with

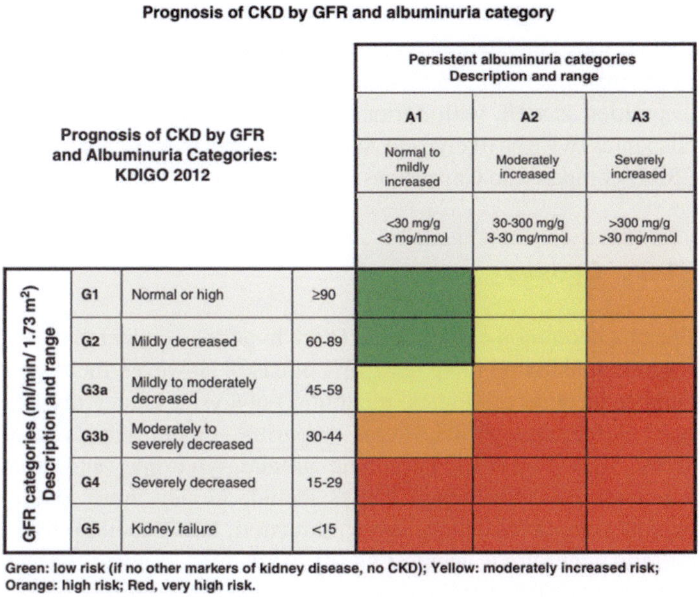

Fig. 51.1 CKD prognosis by GFR and albuminuria. (Taken from the KDIGO work group [6])

severely increased urine albumin are categorized as A3, with both ACR and AER >300. Taking both GFR and albuminuria together allows more accurate prognostication of the development of ESRD.

51.2 Epidemiology of Renal Failure

Chronic kidney disease affects more than 800 million people globally and has emerged as a leading cause of worldwide mortality. In the United States, 15% of adults are estimated to have CKD. Of this, almost 808,000 people have stage V CKD, defined as end-stage renal disease (ESRD), with 69% on dialysis and 31% post-kidney transplantation. Prevalence has increased over the last several years in association with increases in hypertension and diabetes. Age is closely correlated with low GFR (<60), and CKD is most prevalent in patients >60 years old. Women are more likely than men to have this disease. There are associated racial disparities as well, with African Americans 4 times more likely, Hispanics twice as likely, and Asians 1.4 times more likely to have ESRD compared to Caucasians.

51.3 Causes

The most common causes of CKD are hypertension and diabetes, together making up more than 50% of cases. However, there are a number of other etiologies, including polycystic kidney disease, IgA glomerulonephritis, lupus nephritis, Goodpasture's syndrome, IgA vasculitis, hemolytic uremic syndrome, and renal artery stenosis. Secondary causes include kidney injury due to hypotension, dehydration, shock, infection, heavy metal poisoning, and nephrotoxic agents. Obesity, heart disease, advanced age, and family history are the largest associated risk factors.

51.4 Approach to the Renal Failure Patient from the Primary Care Perspective

Unfortunately, chronic kidney disease is associated with progressive loss of function, ultimately leading to renal failure. CKD remains underdiagnosed as early-stage kidney disease is often asymptomatic. Therefore, it is important for primary care physicians to have a high index of suspicion and perform routine laboratory evaluation of patients to assess creatinine, blood urea nitrogen, and, most importantly, glomerular filtration rate. Obtaining these labs can allow early diagnosis and intervention to slow the progression of the disease. When CKD is identified, urine studies should be obtained. The GFR, calculated by using a prediction equation, detects chronic kidney disease more accurately than does the serum creatinine level alone; GFR also is used for disease staging, as mentioned above. Finally, in most clinical situations, analysis of random urine samples to determine the

Table 51.1 Primary care management prior to surgical referral

Tests to obtain prior to referral	Basic labs—basic metabolic panel, complete blood count, prothrombin time/international normalized ratio Glomerular filtration rate Microalbumin/creatinine ratio, urine Protein/creatinine ratio, urine
Management prior to referral	Referral to a nephrologist if not already done Referral to transplant surgeon if indicated Medical control of other comorbidities including hypertension, diabetes, sleep apnea, chronic obstructive pulmonary disorder Encourage lifestyle changes including diet, exercise, smoking/alcohol cessation Ensure patient is risk-stratified to undergo a surgical procedure Obtain further cardiac or pulmonary testing as indicated

albumin–creatinine or protein–creatinine ratio has replaced analysis of timed urine collections in staging of CKD. A summary of management strategies for the primary care physician is shown in Table 51.1.

The KDIGO guidelines suggest that primary care physicians should consider referral to a specialist when patients develop acute kidney injury or show an abrupt sustained fall in GFR, if they reach a GFR <30 ml/min/1.73 m^2 (GFR categories G4–G5), if there is a consistent finding of significant albuminuria (ACR >300 mg/g [>30 mg/mmol] or AER >300 mg/24 h, approximately equivalent to PCR >500 mg/g [>50 mg/mmol] or PER >500 mg/24 h), and if there is rapid progression of CKD. They also suggest referral if they detect urinary red cell casts, 420 per high-power field, sustained, and not readily explained. Finally, if a patient has CKD and hypertension refractory to treatment with four or more antihypertensive agents, persistent abnormalities of serum potassium, recurrent or extensive nephrolithiasis, and hereditary kidney disease referral to a nephrologist are indicated. As kidney disease reaches stage III, patients often benefit from aggressive treatment of hypertension and diabetes that can help prevent progression of the disease. Furthermore, lifestyle changes such as diet modification, increasing activity, limiting alcohol, and smoking cessation are also very beneficial. Patients who have severely impaired kidney function (stage IV, GFR 15–29) may develop symptoms of muscle cramps, fatigue, ankle edema, dyspnea on exertion, polyuria, or oliguria; diuretics are usually necessary. As the disease progresses, patients also experience anemia, undernutrition, renal bone disease, metabolic acidosis, and increased risk of cardiovascular disease. As patients develop ESRD (stage V, GFR <15), they need to strongly consider modes of renal replacement therapy. Symptoms associated with ESRD include fatigue, ankle edema, trouble concentrating, itchy or dry skin, and shortness of breath.

Once a patient has entered stage IV–V CKD, they should be under the care of a nephrologist and planning for renal replacement therapy. Surveillance becomes more frequent, with recurrent office visits and monthly laboratory testing. Options for next steps in management include renal transplant, in-center hemodialysis, home hemodialysis, or peritoneal dialysis. Despite higher satisfaction after transplant or initiation of home dialysis, patients may not be advised about all these options. This is due to several factors, including cost and nephrologist training and bias.

Early patient education and planning are critical for the best outcomes and patient satisfaction. Kidney transplant remains the best option in appropriate ESRD patients, with significant survival, cost, and quality-of-life benefits over dialysis. The first step for renal transplantation is referral to and evaluation by a transplant center. Options include either living-related or deceased donor. However, per the United Network of Organ Sharing, there are upward of 100,000 patients currently on the transplant list, with an average wait time of 3–5 years to receive a kidney. Therefore, bridging therapy must be contemplated to avoid the development of congestive heart failure and hyperkalemia, requiring emergent hospitalization and hemodialysis via a temporary venous access catheter. Early referral for either vascular or peritoneal access is paramount to avoiding this scenario.

51.5 Hemodialysis Access

Hemodialysis (HD) remains the most common approach to renal replacement therapy. Given the increased risk of complications surrounding the use of indwelling catheters, including infection and venous stenosis, the surgical creation of an arteriovenous fistula (AVF) remains the preferred method to approaching dialysis access. In comparison to other methods, these have been demonstrated to last the longest and provide an increased amount of blood flow for efficient dialysis. Creation of an AVF has been cemented as the gold-standard approach through the Fistula First Breakthrough Initiative, coined in 2003 by the Centers for Medicare and Medicaid Services (CMS), with the goal of doubling the number of ESRD patients receiving an AVF as their means of dialysis access. This requires a multidisciplinary collaboration between primary care physicians, nephrologists, vascular surgeons, and dialysis staff in order to promote early referral, optimal operative approach, and appropriate maintenance once created.

51.5.1 Preoperative Workup

Preoperative evaluation should include a thorough history to assess for any history of upper extremity trauma, previous indwelling catheter, previous dialysis access attempts, pacemaker or ICD placement, and dominant handedness. It is also important to delineate any comorbidities apart from ESRD, including hypertension, diabetes mellitus, peripheral vascular disease, or history of hypercoagulable disorder. Along with a standard physical examination, a focused examination of the upper extremities, including pulse examination, should be performed. Performance of an Allen test, which involves occluding the radial artery and observing for collateral flow from the ulnar artery, and vice versa, allows for assessment of patency of the palmar arch. Preoperative imaging is usually obtained in the form of duplex ultrasound, as well as vein mapping. To proceed with an AVF, arterial diameter must be at least 1.5–2 mm and vein diameter at least 2–3 mm.

51.5.2 Surgical Considerations

Autogenous AVF remains the best option, but this depends on the availability of a suitable vein. If able to proceed with AVF, ideal planning would involve creation of the fistula as distal as possible in the nondominant hand in order to preserve future access options. Radiocephalic fistulas are thus preferred, followed by brachiocephalic, then brachiobasilic configurations (see Fig. 51.2).

If the patient does not have appropriately sized veins for the creation of AVF, the next step is the use of prosthetic graft material. Arteriovenous grafts (AVGs) are less ideal due to the placement of non-autogenous material in a field that will be frequently accessed, leading to higher infectious complications; however, these are still preferred over indwelling catheters.

In patients who have known central vein stenosis, hemodialysis reliable outflow grafts can be used. These involve a combined open and endovascular approach with a tunneled venous outflow catheter on one end and an arterial anastomosis created with ePTFE on the other.

51.5.3 Postoperative Management

Once created, AVFs must be allowed to mature prior to use. Maturation time for an AVF is 4–6 weeks versus 2–3 weeks for a graft. Mature access requires an adequate diameter for safe access,

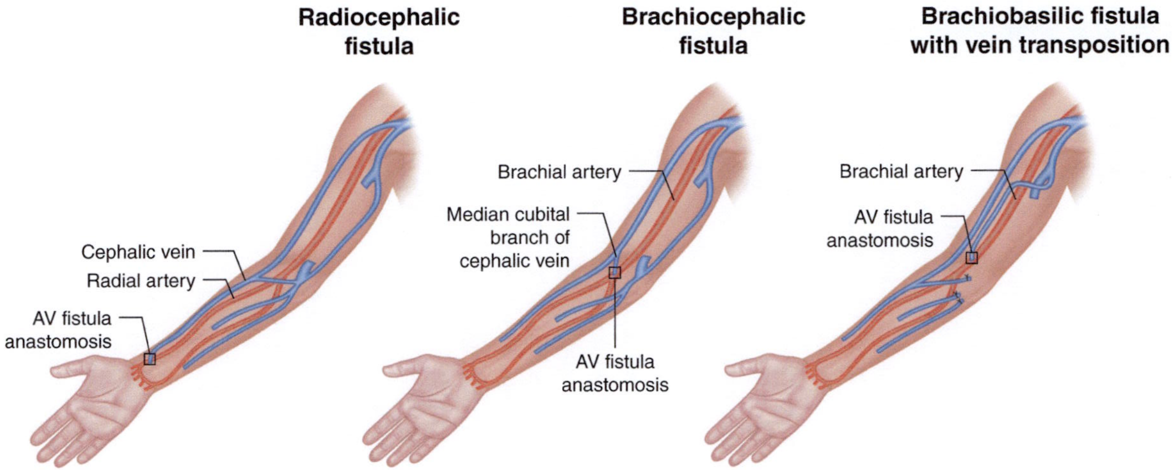

Fig. 51.2 Arteriovenous fistula configurations. (Taken from Lawson et al. [7])

adequate flow rate (≥500 mL/min), and superficial enough for safe cannulation. Following this, hemodialysis can be initiated as long as they have an audible bruit and palpable thrill, postoperative edema is resolved, and there are no signs or symptoms of infection. Postoperative monitoring includes duplex ultrasound to assess flow; if any concerns arise, formal fistulogram should be obtained.

It is crucial to monitor patients for postoperative complications. Infection and bleeding can occur secondary to frequent access. Bleeding can often be controlled with manual pressure, but may require placement of a stitch or revision in cases of uncontrollable bleeding. Infection in patients with AVG requires excision of the infected prosthetic material. Aneurysms and pseudoaneurysms can occur, especially if the same local site is accessed often; these must be addressed surgically due to rupture risk.

Steal syndrome occurs due to hand ischemia secondary to preferential blood flow through the low-resistance venous system. This can be associated with pain, numbness, coldness, weakness, and in severe cases, tissue necrosis. There are several different surgical revision options that go beyond the scope of this review.

Graft thrombosis and/or failure can also occur in the setting of low-flow states, hypercoagulability, or inadequate vein length. Weak bruit/thrill is indicative of an inflow issue. Pulsatility in the fistula is indicative of an outflow issue. Once diagnosed on either duplex ultrasound or fistulogram, first-line treatment often involves thrombectomy, angioplasty, and/or stenting. If these fail, surgical revision becomes necessary. Takeaways regarding hemodialysis access for the primary care physician are shown in Table 51.2.

Table 51.2 Takeaways regarding hemodialysis access for the primary care physician

Emergencies requiring ER presentation	Medical issues such as fluid overload and hyperkalemia Access problems such as bleeding, skin infection, suspected bacteremia, sensorimotor deficits, graft thrombosis
Requiring urgent surgical review	Acute access complications as above
Requiring nonurgent surgical review	Referral for evaluation and planning of access surgery
To be managed by PCP	Coordination of care, management of associated comorbid conditions, pain control, referral to specialty services as indicated, routine preoperative evaluation and clearance
To be managed by specialist	Dialysis management (nephrology), transplantation medications (nephrology/transplant team), fistula access institution and maintenance (vascular surgery and interventional radiology)

51.6 Peritoneal Dialysis Access

Peritoneal dialysis (PD) has been a proven mode of renal replacement therapy for over 40 years. While its usage has risen globally, it has waxed and waned in the United States. PD offers clinical and quality-of-life advantages over hemodialysis (HD), including improved patient autonomy, preservation of residual renal function, and survival benefit for the first two years. In addition, there are major cost benefits to home dialysis. In 2021, CMS passed the End-Stage Renal Disease (ESRD) Treatment Choices Model, which promoted PD and kidney transplantation as a way to improve the quality of care and reduce Medicare expenditures for patients with CKD. Therefore, PD is once again growing in the United States as a primary form of renal replacement therapy, but unfortunately only makes up about 12% of patients with renal failure. Patient selection in the United States relies heavily on nephrologist recommendations, which may be based on their fellowship training, group practice patterns, and personal bias and strength of their existing PD program.

Absolute contraindications to PD include documented ultrafiltration failure of the peritoneal membrane, severe protein malnutrition and/or proteinuria >10 g/day, and active intra-abdominal infection such as Crohn's disease, acute diverticulitis, or ischemic bowel. Relative contraindications to PD include loss of domain/unrepairable abdominal wall hernia and loss of peritoneal volume due to dense abdominal adhesions. In both these instances, surgical correction is possible if expertise is available and should be considered since it is difficult to tell preoperatively if the operation will allow successful PD. There are also "barriers to PD," such as old age, obesity, polycystic kidney disease, presence of an ostomy, prior liver transplant, congestive heart failure, portal hypertension, ascites, impaired vision, dementia or poor memory, home conditions, and employment circumstances. However, these can be overcome with correct patient selection, nephrology team education, having a surgeon with expertise in the field, and obtaining help from family and caregivers.

51.6.1 Preoperative Workup

Typically, patients decide to pursue PD based on discussion with their nephrologist and are referred to a surgeon for preoperative evaluation. Important aspects of that visit include assessing the potential risk factors for catheter dysfunction such as prior abdominal surgery, hernias, and obesity. Patients are also counseled to get preoperative education at their outpatient dialysis center such as Davita™ or Fresinius ™, and the optimal time to begin "training" is 10 days prior to the catheter insertion procedure. Finally, since these patients are at high medical risk to undergo anesthesia and surgery, thorough preoperative workup and risk stratification by the primary care physician, and cardiologist, when indicated, are paramount.

51.6.2 Surgical Considerations

Surgical techniques for the insertion of peritoneal dialysis catheters have evolved over the years, as have the configuration of the catheters. Based on current literature regarding infection and catheter dysfunction, the most commonly used catheters have either a straight or coiled tail that will ultimately rest in the deep pelvis. They also have two "cuffs," which are adhered to the mid portion catheter; the "deep cuff" and the "superficial cuff" in the subcutaneous layer about 2 cm from the skin exit site. These facilitate rapid tissue ingrowth after insertion to prevent accidental removal and retrograde bacterial migration from the skin along the catheter. Currently, three shapes are commonly available to allow the exit site to come out above or below the belt line, and away from the pannus or an ostomy. These are the straight catheter, swan neck, and extended two-piece catheter configurations (see Fig. 51.3). The surgical technique used for insertion includes open, laparoscopic, and percutaneous methods. Now both the International Society for Peritoneal Dialysis (ISPD) and Society of American Gastrointestinal and Endoscopic Surgeons (SAGES) guidelines support the use of advanced laparoscopic (AL) techniques as offering lower risk of PD catheter dysfunction over open and basic laparoscopic techniques. Over the last two decades, there has been an increasing number of PD catheters inserted by interventional radiologists and nephrologists using an image-guided percutaneous approach, usually under ultrasound and fluoroscopic guidance. Comparing image-guided percutaneous insertion to advanced laparoscopic insertion was the focus of a key question on the recent SAGES Updated Guidelines for Peritoneal Dialysis Access Surgery. The panel concluded that either AL insertion or ultrasound-guided percutaneous insertion should be used for patients needing PD catheter insertion (conditional recommendation, very low certainty evidence). The other advantages of the percutaneous technique found in this analysis included lower risk of dialysate leakage, hernia, exit-site infection, and late catheter dysfunction. However, there was a higher

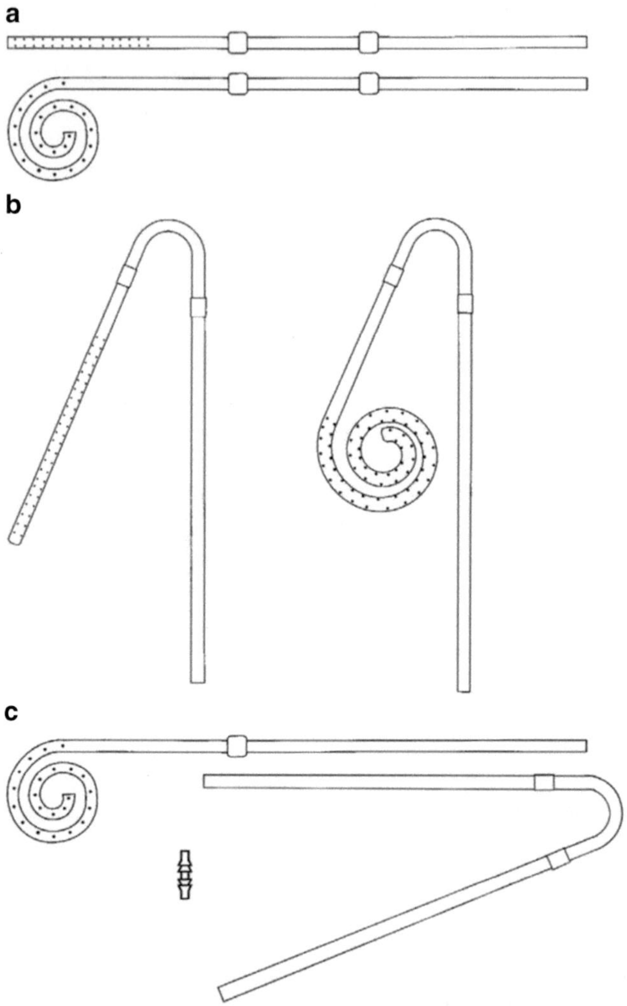

Fig. 51.3 Peritoneal dialysis catheter configurations. (Taken from Crabtree et al. [8]). (**a**) depicts a straight catheter with straight tip, and straight catheter with coiled tip. (**b**) depicts a swan neck (angled) catheter with straight tip and a swan neck (angled) catheter with coiled tip. (**c**) depicts a two piece extended catheter with coiled tip, swan neck and titanium connector piece

risk of bleeding and bowel injury, and this may be magnified in patients with prior abdominal operations.

No matter what technique is used, certain principles should be followed after the catheter is inserted. The catheter should be flushed and capped with a transfer set and secured with sterile dressing and should not be touched for one week, when the first flushing should occur. International Society of Peritoneal Dialysis guidelines recommend a "break-in" period of 2 weeks to allow healing before PD is initiated.

51.6.3 Urgent Start

Despite recommendations that patients enroll in specialist care early in the stages of CKD, many end up needing urgent or emergent dialysis due to fluid overload or hyperkalemia. In the past, these patients were given a venous catheter for inpatient HD and then discharged on scheduled outpatient HD. Once the patient developed this routine, they rarely switched to PD. However, there has been a recent movement toward "urgent start" PD as an attempt to avoid temporary HD and increase the penetration of PD. Initiating PD prior to the traditional two weeks has additional benefits of avoiding bridging HD, including preservation of vascular access, better outcome after renal transplantation, and lower risk of hepatitis B and C infection. Urgent start requires stabilization of the patient by the medical team and availability of the surgical or interventional radiology team to place a catheter before the patient is discharged. In the SAGES guideline, the panel found that urgent start of PD prior to the traditional two-week break-in period is likely associated with a higher risk of dialysate leakage, early catheter dysfunction, and bleeding. However, this question specifically addressed urgent versus traditional start when the patient has the ability to delay initiation of PD. The panel did recognize that for certain patients the benefits of avoiding HD-access procedures and interval HD may outweigh the risks associated with an urgent start of PD. They concluded that this decision should be made between the patient and physicians taking into account the aforementioned factors, and further research is indicated on this subject.

51.6.4 Complications

Complications related to PD access are fortunately rare, but present major dissatisfaction to both patient and the care team. Both infectious and mechanical complications can occur and threaten the ability to dialyze. Therefore, they must be dealt with swiftly to avoid the need to switch to hemodialysis. Peritonitis occurs in about 5% of patients and can range in severity from mild abdominal pain to life-threatening infection and sepsis. The most common complaint is the observation of cloudy PD fluid effluent, often accompanied by severe abdominal pain and tenderness. The diagnosis is confirmed by PD fluid cell count and culture. Treatment includes empiric broad-spectrum intravenous antibiotics until culture results are finalized; antibiotic choice should cover both gram-positive and -negative organisms. ISPD guidelines state that intraperitoneal antibiotics are the preferred route of administration unless the patient has features of systemic sepsis. Symptoms usually improve in 72 h, but if the effluent does not clear in five days, the chances are high that the catheter will need to be removed and the patient maintained on temporary HD. However, a PD catheter may be reinserted at a later date once the infection has been completely cleared.

Catheter dysfunction is the next most significant complication. This problem can be classified as either one-way (outflow) or two-way (inflow and outflow) and requires urgent attention. Two-way obstruction is usually due to fibrin plug or a mechanical kink in the tubing if it occurs immediately after surgery. Outflow obstruction presents as poor or slow drainage of dialysate out of the abdomen and is commonly caused by distended colon due to constipation. Other more difficult to treat causes include omental wrapping, catheter migration, and entrapment in bowel or inflammatory adhesions. The initial approach includes vigorous flushing at the center, aggressive treatment of constipation with laxatives, and X-rays to assess the position. The next step could include tissue plasminogen activator instillation as an attempt to dissolve fibrin film and plugs or interventional radiology evaluation with contrast injection and possible wire manipulation to attempt repositioning. However, operative intervention with exploratory laparoscopy and catheter revision has better long-term results and should be undertaken in a timely manner so that temporary HD may be avoided.

Exit-site infection is another vexing problem that can be encountered while a patient is on PD. The primary care physician should be on the lookout for superficial cuff extrusion, redness, or drainage from the exit site. Fluctuance and tenderness over the catheter and purulent drainage indicate tunnel infection. When these signs are present, evaluation by the nephrologist and referral to a surgeon is indicated, as well as infectious diseases when necessary. Evaluation usually involves ultrasound of the tract to assess for fluid, and a trial of antibiotics if peritonitis is not present. Incision and drainage may also be needed to drain pus. If these fail, catheter removal and replacement are definitive treatment. Takeaways regarding peritoneal dialysis access for the primary care physician are shown in Table 51.3.

Table 51.3 Takeaways regarding peritoneal dialysis access for the primary care physician

Emergencies requiring ER presentation	Acute abdominal pain and signs of peritonitis, signs of inadequate dialysis, fluid overload, hyperkalemia
Requiring urgent surgical review	Catheter-related peritonitis
Requiring nonurgent surgical review	Decreased inflow and/or outflow through peritoneal dialysis catheter, exit-site infection and granulation tissue, abdominal wall hernias, scrotal edema
To be managed by PCP	Coordination of care, management of associated comorbid conditions, pain control, referral to specialty services as indicated, routine preoperative evaluation and clearance
To be managed by specialist	Dialysis management (nephrology), transplantation medications (nephrology/transplant team), peritoneal catheter institution and maintenance (general, minimally invasive or vascular surgery, and interventional radiology)

51.7 Conclusion

CKD and ESRD remain prevalent in the United States. It is crucial for the primary care physician to diagnose this condition early and initiate appropriate specialist treatment. Next steps include renal transplantation, hemodialysis, or peritoneal dialysis, and referral to the appropriate surgical team is needed for transplant evaluation and/or creation of dialysis access. Care of these patients involves close multidisciplinary collaboration between patients, primary care physicians, nephrologists, and surgeons.

Suggested Readings

1. Kidney Disease: Improving Global Outcomes (KDIGO) CKD Work Group. KDIGO 2012 Clinical practice guideline for the evaluation and management of chronic kidney disease. Kidney Int Suppl. 2013;3:1–150.
2. Hart A, Smith JM, Skeans MA, Gustafson SK, Stewart DE, Cherikh WS, Wainright JL, Boyle G, Snyder JJ, Kasiske BL, Israni AK. Kidney. Am J Transplant. 2016;16(Suppl 2):11–46. https://doi.org/10.1111/ajt.13666. PMID: 26755262; PMCID: PMC5541687
3. Sidawy AN, Spergel LM, Besarab A, Allon M, Jennings WC, Padberg FT Jr, Murad MH, Montori VM, O'Hare AM, Calligaro KD, Macsata RA, Lumsden AB, Ascher E. Society for Vascular Surgery. The Society for Vascular Surgery: clinical practice guidelines for the surgical placement and maintenance of arteriovenous hemodialysis access. J Vasc Surg. 2008;48(5 Suppl):2S–25S. https://doi.org/10.1016/j.jvs.2008.08.042. PMID: 19000589.
4. Teitelbaum I. Peritoneal dialysis. N Engl J Med. 2021;385(19):1786–95. https://doi.org/10.1056/NEJMra2100152. PMID: 34731538.
5. Haggerty SP, Kumar SS, Collings AT, Alli VV, Miraflor E, Hanna NM, Athanasiadis DI, Morrell DJ, Ansari MT, Abou-Setta A, Walsh D, Stefanidis D, Slater BJ. SAGES peritoneal dialysis access guideline update 2023. Surg Endosc. 2024;38(1):1–23. https://doi.org/10.1007/s00464-023-10550-8. Epub 2023 Nov 21. PMID: 37989887.
6. National Kidney Foundation. K/DOQI, clinical practice guidelines for chronic kidney disease: evaluation, classification, and stratification. Am J Kidney Dis. 2002;39(2 suppl 1):S1–266.

7. Lawson JH, Niklason LE, Roy-Chaudhury P. Challenges and novel therapies for vascular access in haemodialysis. Nat Rev Nephrol. 2020;16(10):586–602. https://doi.org/10.1038/s41581-020-0333-2. Epub 2020 Aug 24. PMID: 32839580; PMCID: PMC8108319.
8. Crabtree JH, Shrestha BM, Chow KM, Figueiredo AE, Povlsen JV, Wilkie M, Abdel-Aal A, Cullis B, Goh BL, Briggs VR, Brown EA, Dor FJMF. Creating and maintaining optimal peritoneal dialysis access in the adult patient: 2019 update. Perit Dial Int. 2019;39(5):414–36.

Correction to: Impactions of the Esophagus and Upper Gastrointestinal Tract

Bright Huo, Nader Hanna,
and John Agzarian

Correction to:
Chapter 2 in: G. P. Kohn et al. (eds.),
The SAGES Manual of Surgical Referral for Primary and Emergency Care,
https://doi.org/10.1007/978-3-031-92678-5_2

The surname of the author "Bright Huo" was incorrectly spelled as "Ho" in Chapter 2. This typo has now been corrected.

The updated version of this chapter can be found at
https://doi.org/10.1007/978-3-031-92678-5_2

G. P. Kohn et al. (eds.), *The SAGES Manual of Surgical Referral for Primary and Emergency Care*,
https://doi.org/10.1007/978-3-031-92678-5_52

Appendix: SAGES Guidelines (Since 2017)

1. Kumar SS, Collings AT, Wunker C, Athanasiadis DI, DeLong CG, Hong JS, et al. SAGES guidelines for the use of laparoscopy during pregnancy. Surg Endosc. 2024;38(6):2947–63.
2. Kumar SS, Collings AT, Lamm R, Haskins IN, Scholz S, Nepal P, et al. SAGES guideline for the diagnosis and treatment of appendicitis. Surg Endosc. 2024;38(6):2974–94.
3. Kumar SS, Collings AT, Collins C, Colvin J, Sylla P, Slater BJ. Society of American Gastrointestinal and Endoscopic Surgeons guidelines development: health equity update to standard operating procedure. Surg Endosc. 2024;38(5):2315–9.
4. Haggerty SP, Kumar SS, Collings AT, Alli VV, Miraflor E, Hanna NM, et al. SAGES peritoneal dialysis access guideline update 2023. Surg Endosc. 2024;38(1):1–23.
5. Daly S, Kumar SS, Collings AT, Hanna NM, Pandya YK, Kurtz J, et al. SAGES guidelines for the surgical treatment of hiatal hernias. Surg Endosc. 2024;38(9):4765–75.
6. Vreeland TJ, Collings AT, Ozair A, Adams AM, Dirks R, Kushner BS, et al. SAGES/AHPBA guidelines for the use of minimally invasive surgery for the surgical treatment of colorectal liver metastases (CRLM). Surg Endosc. 2023;37(4):2508–16.
7. Slater BJ, Collings A, Dirks R, Gould JC, Qureshi AP, Juza R, et al. Multi-society consensus conference and guideline on the treatment of gastroesophageal reflux disease (GERD). Surg Endosc. 2023;37(2):781–806.

G. P. Kohn et al. (eds.), *The SAGES Manual of Surgical Referral for Primary and Emergency Care*,
https://doi.org/10.1007/978-3-031-92678-5

8. Kohn GP, Awad ZT, Al-Mansour MR, Salluzzo J, Miraflor E, Oliphant U, Slater BJ. Process for quality assessment review of societal guidelines-an editorial to accompany "multi-society consensus conference and guideline on the treatment of gastroesophageal reflux disease (GERD)". Surg Endosc. 2023;37(2):1611–3.
9. Irani JL, Hedrick TL, Miller TE, Lee L, Steinhagen E, Shogan BD, et al. Clinical practice guidelines for enhanced recovery after colon and rectal surgery from the American Society of Colon and Rectal Surgeons and the Society of American Gastrointestinal and Endoscopic Surgeons. Surg Endosc. 2023;37(1):5–30.
10. Ceppa EP, Collings AT, Abdalla M, Onkendi E, Nelson DW, Ozair A, et al. SAGES/AHPBA guidelines for the use of microwave and radiofrequency liver ablation for the surgical treatment of hepatocellular carcinoma or colorectal liver metastases less than 5 cm. Surg Endosc. 2023;37(12):8991–9000.
11. Antoniou SA, Huo B, Tzanis AA, Koutsiouroumpa O, Mavridis D, Balla A, et al. EAES, SAGES, and ESCP rapid guideline: bowel preparation for minimally invasive colorectal resection. Surg Endosc. 2023;37(12):9001–12.
12. Collings AT, Jeyarajah DR, Hanna NM, Dort J, Tsuda S, Nepal P, et al. SAGES 2022 guidelines regarding the use of laparoscopy in the era of COVID-19. Surg Endosc. 2022;36(5):2723–33.
13. Slater BJ, Dirks RC, McKinley SK, Ansari MT, Kohn GP, Thosani N, et al. SAGES guidelines for the surgical treatment of gastroesophageal reflux (GERD). Surg Endosc. 2021;35(9):4903–17.
14. Rogers AT, Dirks R, Burt HA, Haggerty S, Kohn GP, Slater BJ, et al. Society of American Gastrointestinal and Endoscopic Surgeons (SAGES) guidelines development: standard operating procedure. Surg Endosc. 2021;35(6):2417–27.
15. Kohn GP, Dirks RC, Ansari MT, Clay J, Dunst CM, Lundell L, et al. SAGES guidelines for the use of peroral endoscopic myotomy (POEM) for the treatment of achalasia. Surg Endosc. 2021;35(5):1931–48.

16. Kindel TL, Dirks RC, Collings AT, Scholz S, Abou-Setta AM, Alli VV, et al. Guidelines for the performance of minimally invasive splenectomy. Surg Endosc. 2021;35(11):5877–88.
17. Brunt LM, Deziel DJ, Telem DA, Strasberg SM, Aggarwal R, Asbun H, et al. Safe cholecystectomy multi-society practice guideline and state-of-the-art consensus conference on prevention of bile duct injury during cholecystectomy. Surg Endosc. 2020;34(7):2827–55.
18. Francis NK, Sylla P, Abou-Khalil M, Arolfo S, Berler D, Curtis NJ, et al. EAES and SAGES 2018 consensus conference on acute diverticulitis management: evidence-based recommendations for clinical practice. Surg Endosc. 2019;33(9):2726–41.
19. Carmichael JC, Keller DS, Baldini G, Bordeianou L, Weiss E, Lee L, et al. Clinical practice guideline for enhanced recovery after colon and rectal surgery from the American Society of Colon and Rectal Surgeons (ASCRS) and Society of American Gastrointestinal and Endoscopic Surgeons (SAGES). Surg Endosc. 2017;31(9):3412–36.

Index

G. P. Kohn et al. (eds.), *The SAGES Manual of Surgical Referral for Primary and Emergency Care*,
https://doi.org/10.1007/978-3-031-92678-5

K

L

M

MIX
Papier aus verantwortungsvollen Quellen
Paper from responsible sources
FSC® C105338

FSC
www.fsc.org

If you have any concerns about our products,
you can contact us on
ProductSafety@springernature.com

In case Publisher is established outside the EU,
the EU authorized representative is:
Springer Nature Customer Service Center GmbH
Europaplatz 3, 69115 Heidelberg, Germany

Printed by Libri Plureos GmbH
in Hamburg, Germany